Using Information and Communication Technologies (ICT) for Mental Health Prevention and Treatment

Using Information and Communication Technologies (ICT) for Mental Health Prevention and Treatment

Editors

Ana Fonseca
Jorge Osma

MDPI • Basel • Beijing • Wuhan • Barcelona • Belgrade • Manchester • Tokyo • Cluj • Tianjin

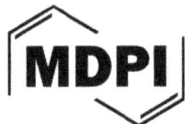

Editors
Ana Fonseca
Center for Research in
Neuropsychology and
Cognitive-Behavior Intervention,
Faculty of Psychology and
Educational Sciences,
University of Coimbra
Portugal

Jorge Osma
Universidad de Zaragoza and
Instituto de Investigación
Sanitaria de Aragón
Spain

Editorial Office
MDPI
St. Alban-Anlage 66
4052 Basel, Switzerland

This is a reprint of articles from the Special Issue published online in the open access journal *International Journal of Environmental Research and Public Health* (ISSN 1660-4601) (available at: https://www.mdpi.com/journal/ijerph/special_issues/UIACTFMHPAT).

For citation purposes, cite each article independently as indicated on the article page online and as indicated below:

LastName, A.A.; LastName, B.B.; LastName, C.C. Article Title. *Journal Name* **Year**, *Volume Number*, Page Range.

ISBN 978-3-0365-0458-2 (Hbk)
ISBN 978-3-0365-0459-9 (PDF)

© 2021 by the authors. Articles in this book are Open Access and distributed under the Creative Commons Attribution (CC BY) license, which allows users to download, copy and build upon published articles, as long as the author and publisher are properly credited, which ensures maximum dissemination and a wider impact of our publications.

The book as a whole is distributed by MDPI under the terms and conditions of the Creative Commons license CC BY-NC-ND.

Contents

About the Editors vii

Ana Fonseca and Jorge Osma
Using Information and Communication Technologies (ICT) for Mental Health Prevention and Treatment
Reprinted from: *Int. J. Environ. Res. Public Health* **2021**, *18*, 461, doi:10.3390/ijerph18020461 . . . 1

Tracy Gladstone, Katherine R. Buchholz, Marian Fitzgibbon, Linda Schiffer, Miae Lee and Benjamin W. Van Voorhees
Randomized Clinical Trial of an Internet-Based Adolescent Depression Prevention Intervention in Primary Care: Internalizing Symptom Outcomes
Reprinted from: *Int. J. Environ. Res. Public Health* **2020**, *17*, 7736, doi:10.3390/ijerph17217736 . . . 7

Bonifacio Sandín, Julia García-Escalera, Rosa M. Valiente, Victoria Espinosa and Paloma Chorot
Clinical Utility of an Internet-Delivered Version of the Unified Protocol for Transdiagnostic Treatment of Emotional Disorders in Adolescents (iUP-A): A Pilot Open Trial
Reprinted from: *Int. J. Environ. Res. Public Health* **2020**, *17*, 8306, doi:10.3390/ijerph17228306 . . . 25

Patricia Otero, Isabel Hita, Ángela J. Torres and Fernando L. Vázquez
Brief Psychological Intervention Through Mobile App and Conference Calls for the Prevention of Depression in Non-Professional Caregivers: A Pilot Study
Reprinted from: *Int. J. Environ. Res. Public Health* **2020**, *17*, 4578, doi:10.3390/ijerph17124578 . . . 43

Mª Dolores Vara, Adriana Mira, Marta Miragall, Azucena García-Palacios, Cristina Botella, Margalida Gili, Pau Riera-Serra, Javier García-Campayo, Fermín Mayoral-Cleries and Rosa Mª Baños
A Low-Intensity Internet-Based Intervention Focused on the Promotion of Positive Affect for the Treatment of Depression in Spanish Primary Care: Secondary Analysis of a Randomized Controlled Trial
Reprinted from: *Int. J. Environ. Res. Public Health* **2020**, *17*, 8094, doi:10.3390/ijerph17218094 . . . 59

Fabiana Monteiro, Marco Pereira, Maria Cristina Canavarro and Ana Fonseca
Be a Mom's Efficacy in Enhancing Positive Mental Health among Postpartum Women Presenting Low Risk for Postpartum Depression: Results from a Pilot Randomized Trial
Reprinted from: *Int. J. Environ. Res. Public Health* **2020**, *17*, 4679, doi:10.3390/ijerph17134679 . . . 81

Shu Da, Yue He and Xichao Zhang
Effectiveness of Psychological Capital Intervention and Its Influence on Work-Related Attitudes: Daily Online Self-Learning Method and Randomized Controlled Trial Design
Reprinted from: *Int. J. Environ. Res. Public Health* **2020**, *17*, 8754, doi:10.3390/ijerph17238754 . . . 99

Mariana Branquinho, Maria Cristina Canavarro and Ana Fonseca
A Blended Cognitive–Behavioral Intervention for the Treatment of Postpartum Depression: Study Protocol for a Randomized Controlled Trial
Reprinted from: *Int. J. Environ. Res. Public Health* **2020**, *17*, 8631, doi:10.3390/ijerph17228631 . . . 119

Alba Quilez-Orden, Vanesa Ferreres-Galán and Jorge Osma
Feasibility and Clinical Usefulness of the Unified Protocol in Online Group Format for Bariatric Surgery Candidates: Study Protocol for a Multiple Baseline Experimental Design
Reprinted from: *Int. J. Environ. Res. Public Health* **2020**, *17*, 6155, doi:10.3390/ijerph17176155 . . . 133

Carlos Suso-Ribera, Diana Castilla, Irene Zaragozá, Ángela Mesas, Anna Server, Javier Medel and Azucena García-Palacios
Telemonitoring in Chronic Pain Management Using Smartphone Apps: A Randomized Controlled Trial Comparing Usual Assessment Against App-Based Monitoring with and without Clinical Alarms
Reprinted from: *Int. J. Environ. Res. Public Health* **2020**, *17*, 6568, doi:10.3390/ijerph17186568 . . . 151

Laura Andreu-Pejó, Verónica Martínez-Borba, Carlos Suso-Ribera and Jorge Osma
Can We Predict the Evolution of Depressive Symptoms, Adjustment, and Perceived Social Support of Pregnant Women from Their Personality Characteristics? a Technology-Supported Longitudinal Study
Reprinted from: *Int. J. Environ. Res. Public Health* **2020**, *17*, 3439, doi:10.3390/ijerph17103439 . . . 175

Patricia Gual-Montolio, Verónica Martínez-Borba, Juana María Bretón-López, Jorge Osma and Carlos Suso-Ribera
How Are Information and Communication Technologies Supporting Routine Outcome Monitoring and Measurement-Based Care in Psychotherapy? A Systematic Review
Reprinted from: *Int. J. Environ. Res. Public Health* **2020**, *17*, 3170, doi:10.3390/ijerph17093170 . . . 191

Rocío Herrero, Mª Dolores Vara, Marta Miragall, Cristina Botella, Azucena García-Palacios, Heleen Riper, Annet Kleiboer and Rosa Mª Baños
Working Alliance Inventory for Online Interventions-Short Form (WAI-TECH-SF): The Role of the Therapeutic Alliance between Patient and Online Program in Therapeutic Outcomes
Reprinted from: *Int. J. Environ. Res. Public Health* **2020**, *17*, 6169, doi:10.3390/ijerph17176169 . . . 213

Diana Castilla, Carlos Suso-Ribera, Irene Zaragoza, Azucena Garcia-Palacios and Cristina Botella
Designing ICTs for Users with Mild Cognitive Impairment: A Usability Study
Reprinted from: *Int. J. Environ. Res. Public Health* **2020**, *17*, 5153, doi:10.3390/ijerph17145153 . . . 229

Ángel Castro, Juan Ramón Barrada, Pedro J. Ramos-Villagrasa and Elena Fernández-del-Río
Profiling Dating Apps Users: Sociodemographic and Personality Characteristics
Reprinted from: *Int. J. Environ. Res. Public Health* **2020**, *17*, 3653, doi:10.3390/ijerph17103653 . . . 251

Kathleen M. Baggett, Betsy Davis, Lisa B. Sheeber, Robert T. Ammerman, Elizabeth A. Mosley, Katy Miller and Edward G. Feil
Minding the Gatekeepers: Referral and Recruitment of Postpartum Mothers with Depression into a Randomized Controlled Trial of a Mobile Internet Parenting Intervention to Improve Mood and Optimize Infant Social Communication Outcomes
Reprinted from: *Int. J. Environ. Res. Public Health* **2020**, *17*, 8978, doi:10.3390/ijerph17238978 . . . 265

Artemisa R. Dores, Andreia Geraldo, Irene P. Carvalho and Fernando Barbosa
The Use of New Digital Information and Communication Technologies in Psychological Counseling during the COVID-19 Pandemic
Reprinted from: *Int. J. Environ. Res. Public Health* **2020**, *17*, 7663, doi:10.3390/ijerph17207663 . . . 279

About the Editors

Ana Fonseca is a PhD researcher at UC/CINEICC. She is a Clinical Psychologist and certified expert in Clinical and Health Psychology by the Portuguese College of Psychology. She is currently the principal investigator of the I&D project "BeAMom Trial, a web-based psychological intervention to promote maternal mental health", funded by the Portuguese Foundation for Science and Technology and by the Centro2020 program. She leads the Workgroup 'Prevention and Treatment Strategies in PPD' of the Riseup-PPD COST Action (COST Action 18138), which includes about 80 researchers and health professionals in the field, from different European countries and with different backgrounds and expertise. She is also a member of the Global Consortium for Depression Prevention and of the Psychology and eHealth Taskforce of the Portuguese College of Psychology. This taskforce was responsible for the development of the Portuguese Guidelines for delivering psychological services using Information and Communication Technologies. She is also an Associate Editor of the Clinical Psychology section of Frontiers in Psychology and Clinica y Salud. Ana also has a strong track record in disseminating her research, with more than 45 papers published in peer-reviewed international journals.

Jorge Osma is an Associate Professor and Coordinator of the General Health Psychology Master at the University of Zaragoza. He is the principal investigator of the "Research on Personality, Emotion & Health" research group of the Research Health Institute of Aragon (https://ipes-group.com/) and a research member of the "Research on Behavior, Health and Technologies" (S31_20D) of the Aragon Government. His research is focused on the prevention and treatment of emotional disorders using the Unified Protocol for transdiagnostic treatment of emotional disorders and also on the implementation of cost-effective intervention formats such as group therapy and Information and Communication Technologies. He is the President of the Spanish Marcé Society of Perinatal Mental Health. Dr. Osma is also the principal investigator of two national research projects, author of 3 books, 16 book chapters, and 32 papers published in peer-reviewed international journals. He is a member of the panel of expert reviewers of the Spanish Ministry of Science, Innovation and Universities and a substitute member of the e-COST Spanish Commission (Riseup-PPD). He is also a member of the Association for Behavioral and Cognitive Therapies, the Oficial College of Psychology of the Valencian Comunity, the Spanish Society of Clinical Psychology and Psychopathology, the International Marcé Society and Spanish Marcé Society of Perinatal Mental Health, and the Spanish Society for the Advancement of Clinical Psychology. He is an Associate Editor of *Frontiers in Psychology*: Health Psychology and of *Psicosomática y Psiquiatría*.

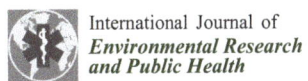

International Journal of
Environmental Research and Public Health

Editorial

Using Information and Communication Technologies (ICT) for Mental Health Prevention and Treatment

Ana Fonseca [1,*] and Jorge Osma [2,3,*]

1 Center for Research in Neuropsychology and Cognitive-Behavioral Intervention (CINEICC), Faculty of Psychology and Educational Sciences, University of Coimbra, 3000-115 Coimbra, Portugal
2 Health Research Institute of Aragon, C/San Juan Bosco, 13, 50009 Zaragoza, Spain
3 Department of Psychology and Sociology, Universidad de Zaragoza, C/Atarazanas, 4, 44003 Teruel, Spain
* Correspondence: anadfonseca@fpce.uc.pt (A.F.); osma@unizar.es (J.O.)

Received: 11 December 2020; Accepted: 29 December 2020; Published: 8 January 2021

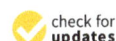

Mental disorders are a recognized population health issue, with recent estimates placing mental illness as the first in global burden of disease in terms of years lived with disability, and comparable to cardiovascular and circulatory diseases in terms of disability-adjusted life years. Common mental disorders refer to a range of anxiety and depressive disorders, which are prevalent disorders around the world (4.4% and 3.6% of the global population suffer from depression and anxiety disorders, respectively), with variations across different regions and populations [1]. Despite the human, social, and economic costs of mental disorders, mental health has been often neglected. Recently, the Lancet Commission on Global Mental Health and Sustainable Development launched a report recommending that mental health should be reframed as a fundamental human right, and that the definition of mental health should be expanded to promote mental wellbeing, prevent mental health problems, and enable recovery from mental disorders.

Despite this, we still face great inequalities in access to mental health promotion, prevention, and treatment programs worldwide (e.g., limited resources to accommodate the existent needs) and/or treatment uptake barriers, such as attitudinal barriers (e.g., stigma towards mental health) or structural barriers (e.g., geographical or financial restrictions, work constraints, or patient's physical conditions). The delivery of psychological services—including assessment/monitoring, mental health promotion, prevention, and treatment—through information and communication technologies (ICT) may be an effective way of improving individual access and use of mental healthcare services [2]. ICT-delivered psychological services include (but are not restricted to) web-based interventions, mobile apps, videoconferencing systems (telepsychology), or virtual reality systems, and may be used complementary to face-to-face services or as the sole means of access to psychological interventions. The use of ICT-delivered psychological services has several advantages, related with increased accessibility and flexibility, self-monitoring integrated into treatment, and empowerment promotion, as well as increased novelty and appeal. However, we cannot exclude that they also have challenges and limitations, related with low digital literacy or with safety and privacy issues, among others [2].

The present Special Issue focuses on acceptability, cost-effectiveness, potentialities, and limitations of ICT-based psychological services for mental health promotion, prevention, and treatment. Sixteen articles are included in this special issue from different international research teams working in China, Portugal, Spain, and the United States.

Five of the studies included in this Special Issue focused on the assessment of ICT tools for the prevention [3,4] and treatment [5,6] of mental disorders, or the promotion of mental health [7], in different populations. Specifically, these studies examined the interventions' effectiveness, clinical utility, acceptability, or feasibility through pilot trials or randomized controlled trials.

Two of the studies focused on the adolescent population. Gladstone et al. [3] examined the effects of an online preventive intervention for depression disseminated through primary care settings targeting adolescents at moderate-to-high risk for depression (Competent Adulthood Transition with Cognitive-behavioral, Humanistic, and Interpersonal—CATCH-IT), compared with a health education online program. Although long-term reductions of depressive symptoms were found in both groups, participants in the CATCH-IT group also showed a cross-over effect for anxiety symptoms, suggesting the potential for transdiagnostic interventions targeting underlying mechanisms shared by both disorders. Moreover, the study showed that the presence of some pre-conditions (e.g., supportive environmental factors such as a supportive relationship with a physician and adequate paternal monitoring) may favor the benefits of the CATCH-IT intervention among adolescents. On the other hand, Sandín et al. [5] performed a pilot trial where they examined the feasibility, acceptability, and clinical utility of the internet-delivered version of the Unified Protocol for Transdiagnostic Treatment of Emotional disorders in Adolescents (UP-A). The internet-delivered version of the UP-A showed high feasibility and acceptability, with all participants and responsible parents reporting an improvement in the adolescents' ability to cope with emotions. Moreover, the results of the pilot trial were also promising, showing preliminary evidence of the program's efficacy in improving outcomes (anxiety and depression) and vulnerability of transdiagnostic mechanisms.

An additional study focused on the prevention of depression among non-professional caregivers at risk for depression, which are an often-neglected group, despite the high burden and negative consequences of the caregiving responsibilities. Otero et al. [4] conducted a pilot study to examine the efficacy and feasibility of a brief cognitive-behavioral intervention for depression prevention delivered through a smartphone app combined with positive and corrective feedback provided by a psychologist through conference calls. The results provided preliminary evidence of the efficacy of the intervention in reducing depressive symptoms and the risk of developing depression, both at postintervention and in the follow-up assessments, and show good indicators of adherence and satisfaction with the intervention, encouraging further research on the topic.

Finally, two other studies targeting different populations investigated the effectiveness of interventions by considering, as primary outcomes, not mental illness indicators (e.g., depression and anxiety symptoms), but positive mental health indicators (positive affect and positive mental health). Vara et al. [6] provided us with a secondary analysis of a randomized controlled trial that assessed the efficacy of a low-intensity internet intervention aimed to promote positive affect in depressive patients in primary care, as an adjunct therapy to improved treatment as usual. The results of this study supported not only that the promotion of positive affect might have an impact on the decline in clinical symptomatology and improve positive functioning, but that both the improvements in depression and in positive affect can be responsible for the long-term changes in wellbeing. Moreover, the profile of patients who can benefit most from the intervention was analyzed. Monteiro et al. [7] conducted one of the first trials examining the effectiveness, acceptability, and feasibility of a self-guided web-based intervention that was originally developed for preventing postpartum depression among high-risk women, in promoting positive mental health among women presenting low risk for postpartum depression, as even those women face significant challenges to their adjustment and may benefit from mental health promotion interventions. The results showed that women in the intervention group presented a larger increase in positive mental health compared to women in the waiting-list control group, with a large proportion of women showing good acceptability of the intervention.

Moreover, focusing on a different context (organizational context), Da et al. [8] explored, through a randomized controlled trial design, the effectiveness and feasibility of a brief online intervention (20 min during 5 days) to enhance psychological capital in workplaces (PsyCap intervention). Participants randomized to the experimental condition received daily online links with some lectures to read and activities to practice regarding how to develop efficacy, hope, resilience, and optimism. Those in the placebo condition were asked to write down self-reflections during the same timeline. Nothing was sent to the control group. The preliminary results have shown increases in psychological capital, job satisfaction and reductions in turnover intention after the intervention and at one-week follow-up.

In addition to effectiveness studies, this Special Issue includes the description of two study protocols using internet. The first one, by Branquinho et al. [9], is a two-arm, non-inferiority randomized controlled trial comparing a cognitive behavioral blended intervention to usual treatment for postpartum depression provided in healthcare centers. The blended condition will integrate face-to-face sessions with a web-based program called Be a Mom. This approach has the advantage of being dynamic and flexible, given that it allows using technology for motivating, monitoring, giving support, and treating patients, but without losing treatment sessions face-to-face. The study will explore the efficacy and cost-effectiveness of both conditions, and will offer greater support to evidence-based psychological treatments for postpartum depression. The second one, presented by Quilez et al. [10], is a pilot study with a repeated single-case experimental design (multiple baseline design) in a public mental health unit in Spain. The main focus is to further explore the clinical utility and feasibility of an online transdiagnostic emotion regulation-based intervention (the Unified Protocol) delivered in group format to people waiting for bariatric surgery with emotional symptoms or disorders. Expected outcomes will be reductions in anxiety and depression symptoms and weight maintenance over the two years follow-up period after the intervention.

Two of the studies included in this Special Issue focus on how ICT tools can be helpful in the screening and monitoring of different symptoms. Suso-Ribera et al. [11] examined if the Monitor de Dolor app—which allows daily assessment of pain through ecological momentary assessments—would be an effective option for patient monitoring, in terms of improvement of chronic musculoskeletal pain management. The authors performed a randomized controlled trial in which they compared three conditions: the usual monitoring method (onsite retrospectively), usual monitoring plus app without alarms, and usual monitoring plus app with predefined alarms sent to clinicians to make treatment adjustments. In addition to allowing the collection of patients' pain-related data in an automated way, the results of this study were suggestive of the effectiveness of telemonitoring in pain and other mental health outcomes (e.g., depressive symptoms), particularly if an alarm system that allow changes in pain management can be implemented. Andreu-Pejó et al. [12] examined a sample of 85 pregnant women who participated in a web-based platform HappyMom (Mamáfeliz), which longitudinally assessed a set of risk factors for the development of perinatal emotional disorders. The results showed that certain personality characteristics (e.g., high neuroticism) may be a risk factor to pregnant women's wellbeing deterioration and therefore should be assessed early during pregnancy mental health screening, which might be facilitated through the use of ICT tools. In a related topic, Gual-Montolio et al. [13] presented a systematic review about the use of ICTs for routine outcome monitoring (ROM) and measurement-based care (MBC) in face-to-face psychological interventions for mental health problems. The eighteen articles revised showed that handheld technologies such as smartphone apps, tablets, or laptops were used for assessment and feedback during psychological interventions (including ROM and MBC), providing evidence about their feasibility and acceptability.

The remaining five studies cover different aspects related to ICTs. Considering the association between therapeutic alliance to treatment outcomes in psychotherapy and the increased use of internet-based interventions, Herrero et al. [14] adapted The Working Alliance Inventory for online interventions (WAI-TECH-SF), based on the WAI Short Form [15]. Authors found good psychometric properties of the WAI-TECH-SF and its association with positive therapeutic outcomes (changes in depressive symptoms) and satisfaction with the treatment in a sample of 193 participants with depressed diagnosis.

Castilla et al. [16] studied the needs of 28 participants (58–95 years old) with a diagnosis of mild cognitive impairment, regarding an ICT-based intervention tool design for elderly care. Interesting results were found about the need to place main interaction elements in the center of the screen instead of in the peripheral areas, and also that speed of audio help had a significant impact on performance. Other usability recommendations for this specific sample are described in the article.

ICTs have changed different aspects of our daily life; one of them is the way we interact with other people searching for a romantic and/or sexual partner. In this sense, Castro et al. [17] explored, in a sample of 1705 university students, the association between present and past use of dating apps, sociodemographic data, and bright and dark personality traits. Results indicated that being men, older youth, and members of sexual minorities were more likely to be current and previous dating app users. It was not expected that dark personality showed no predictive ability. These studies are needed in order to personalize both prevention and promotion interventions of healthy romantic and sexual relationships in different target groups.

In the context of enhancing the access to a mobile-based intervention for improving maternal mood and increasing parent practices in a sample of postpartum women, Bagget et al. [18] explored the differential efficacy of three referral approaches (i.e., community agency staff referral, research staff referral, and maternal self-referral). Among the results obtained, we highlight that women who self-referred and those who were referred by community gatekeepers were as likely to eventually consent to study participation and initiate the intervention in comparison with those referred by research staff.

Finally, during the COVID-19 outbreak, mental healthcare delivery was imposed with sudden challenges. Dores et al. [19] explored changes in the delivery of psychological services through ICT during the COVID-19 pandemic. The results showed that psychologists have adopted ICTs to continue to provide mental healthcare during the COVID-19 outbreak. Despite the challenges identified, they globally assessed the experience of delivering psychological services through ICT tools as positive and with similar results, suggesting a change in attitudes towards the use of such tools.

This Special Issue bring us the ability to acknowledge some of the possibilities that ICTs in mental health offer to researchers and mental health professionals. From a clinical point of view (prevention, promotion, and treatment), as we previously explained in brief, some of the manuscripts have described different ways to solve one of the main gaps in mental health fields nowadays, that is to reach as many people in need as possible. Through ICTs, people can benefit from evidence-based prevention and treatment psychological interventions without losing their privacy, and integrating the intervention in their normal daily routine (e.g., perinatal women). As we can see, ICTs can also provide important benefits over the psychotherapy process, maintaining the therapeutic alliance and allowing clinicians to assess and get feedback of certain health or clinical variables over the interventions. Additionally, from a technology point of view (usability, feasibility, acceptability, etc.), we have seen also some examples highlighting the importance of studying the psychometric properties of measures administered through the internet, the improvements on the usability aspects of devices, especially if we want to work with special populations (e.g., elderly people), and the necessary study of users' profiles to personalize ICTs and future interventions. Despite the limitations of the studies included in this Special Issue, in general, we can say that ICT-based interventions applied for mental health prevention or treatment have proved to be effective, feasible, and well-accepted by users. We hope that the studies, outcomes, and limitations described in this Special Issue would encourage clinicians and researchers around the world to continue working to increase the scientific evidence about the cost-effectiveness and implementation of the ICTs in mental health prevention, promotion, and treatment interventions.

Author Contributions: A.F. and J.O. were both responsible for the conceptualization of the paper and for the original draft preparation, as well as for reviewing and editing the final version of the manuscript. All authors have read and agreed to the published version of the manuscript.

Funding: Jorge Osma was funded by Gobierno de Aragón (Departamento de Innovación, Investigación y Universidad) and Feder 2014–2020 "Construyendo Europa Desde Aragón", research group grant S31_20D.

Acknowledgments: As Guest Editors of this Special Issue, we would like to acknowledge the contribution of all the authors that participated in this Special Issue, for sharing their expertise and research within this topic.

Conflicts of Interest: The authors declare no conflict of interest.

References

1. World Health Organization. *Depression and Other Common Mental Disorders: Global Health Estimates*; World Health Organization: Geneva, Switzerland, 2017.
2. Lal, S.; Adair, C. E-mental health: A rapid review of the literature. *Psychiatr. Serv.* **2014**, *65*, 24–32. [CrossRef] [PubMed]
3. Gladstone, T.; Buchholz, K.R.; Fitzgibbon, M.; Schiffer, L.; Lee, M.; Voorhees, B.W.V. Randomized Clinical Trial of an Internet-Based Adolescent Depression Prevention Intervention in Primary Care: Internalizing Symptom Outcomes. *Int. J. Environ. Res. Public Health* **2020**, *17*, 7736. [CrossRef] [PubMed]
4. Otero, P.; Hita, I.; Torres, Á.J.; Vázquez, F.L. Brief Psychological Intervention Through Mobile App and Conference Calls for the Prevention of Depression in Non-Professional Caregivers: A Pilot Study. *Int. J. Environ. Res. Public Health* **2020**, *17*, 4578. [CrossRef]
5. Sandín, B.; García-Escalera, J.; Valiente, R.M.; Espinosa, V.; Chorot, P. Clinical Utility of an Internet-Delivered Version of the Unified Protocol for Transdiagnostic Treatment of Emotional Disorders in Adolescents (iUP-A): A Pilot Open Trial. *Int. J. Environ. Res. Public Health* **2020**, *17*, 8306. [CrossRef] [PubMed]
6. Vara, M.D.; Mira, A.; Miragall, M.; García-Palacios, A.; Botella, C.; Gili, M.; Riera-Serra, P.; García-Campayo, J.; Mayoral-Cleries, F.; Baños, R.M. A Low-Intensity Internet-Based Intervention Focused on the Promotion of Positive Affect for the Treatment of Depression in Spanish Primary Care: Secondary Analysis of a Randomized Controlled Trial. *Int. J. Environ. Res. Public Health* **2020**, *17*, 8094. [CrossRef]
7. Monteiro, F.; Pereira, M.; Canavarro, M.C.; Fonseca, A. Be a Mom's Efficacy in Enhancing Positive Mental Health among Postpartum Women Presenting Low Risk for Postpartum Depression: Results from a Pilot Randomized Trial. *Int. J. Environ. Res. Public Health* **2020**, *17*, 4679. [CrossRef]
8. Da, S.; He, Y.; Zhang, X. Effectiveness of Psychological Capital Intervention and Its Influence on Work-Related Attitudes: Daily Online Self-Learning Method and Randomized Controlled Trial Design. *Int. J. Environ. Res. Public Health* **2020**, *17*, 8754. [CrossRef] [PubMed]
9. Branquinho, M.; Canavarro, M.C.; Fonseca, A. A Blended Cognitive–Behavioral Intervention for the Treatment of Postpartum Depression: Study Protocol for a Randomized Controlled Trial. *Int. J. Environ. Res. Public Health* **2020**, *17*, 8631. [CrossRef]
10. Quilez-Orden, A.; Ferreres-Galán, V.; Osma, J. Feasibility and Clinical Usefulness of the Unified Protocol in Online Group Format for Bariatric Surgery Candidates: Study Protocol for a Multiple Baseline Experimental Design. *Int. J. Environ. Res. Public Health* **2020**, *17*, 6155. [CrossRef] [PubMed]
11. Suso-Ribera, C.; Castilla, D.; Zaragozá, I.; Mesas, Á.; Server, A.; Medel, J.; García-Palacios, A. Telemonitoring in Chronic Pain Management Using Smartphone Apps: A Randomized Controlled Trial Comparing Usual Assessment against App-Based Monitoring with and without Clinical Alarms. *Int. J. Environ. Res. Public Health* **2020**, *17*, 6568. [CrossRef]
12. Andreu-Pejó, L.; Martínez-Borba, V.; Suso-Ribera, C.; Osma, J. Can We Predict the Evolution of Depressive Symptoms, Adjustment, and Perceived Social Support of Pregnant Women from Their Personality Characteristics? A Technology-Supported Longitudinal Study. *Int. J. Environ. Res. Public Health* **2020**, *17*, 3439. [CrossRef] [PubMed]
13. Gual-Montolio, P.; Martínez-Borba, V.; Bretón-López, J.M.; Osma, J.; Suso-Ribera, C. How Are Information and Communication Technologies Supporting Routine Outcome Monitoring and Measurement-Based Care in Psychotherapy? A Systematic Review. *Int. J. Environ. Res. Public Health* **2020**, *17*, 3170. [CrossRef]
14. Herrero, R.; Vara, M.D.; Miragall, M.; Botella, C.; García-Palacios, A.; Riper, H.; Kleiboer, A.; Baños, R.M. Working Alliance Inventory for Online Interventions-Short Form (WAI-TECH-SF): The Role of the Therapeutic Alliance between Patient and Online Program in Therapeutic Outcomes. *Int. J. Environ. Res. Public Health* **2020**, *17*, 6169. [CrossRef]
15. Hatcher, R.L.; Gillaspy, J.A. Development and validation of a revised short version of the working alliance inventory. *Psychother. Res.* **2007**, *16*, 12–25. [CrossRef]
16. Castilla, D.; Suso-Ribera, C.; Zaragoza, I.; Garcia-Palacios, A.; Botella, C. Designing ICTs for Users with Mild Cognitive Impairment: A Usability Study. *Int. J. Environ. Res. Public Health* **2020**, *17*, 5153. [CrossRef] [PubMed]

17. Castro, Á.; Barrada, J.R.; Ramos-Villagrasa, P.J.; Fernández-del-Río, E. Profiling Dating Apps Users: Sociodemographic and Personality Characteristics. *Int. J. Environ. Res. Public Health* **2020**, *17*, 3653. [CrossRef]
18. Baggett, K.M.; Davis, B.; Sheeber, L.B.; Ammerman, R.T.; Mosley, E.A.; Miller, K.; Feil, E.G. Minding the Gatekeepers: Referral and Recruitment of Postpartum Mothers with Depression into a Randomized Controlled Trial of a Mobile Internet Parenting Intervention to Improve Mood and Optimize Infant Social Communication Outcomes. *Int. J. Environ. Res. Public Health* **2020**, *17*, 8978. [CrossRef] [PubMed]
19. Dores, A.R.; Geraldo, A.; Carvalho, I.P.; Barbosa, F. The Use of New Digital Information and Communication Technologies in Psychological Counseling during the COVID-19 Pandemic. *Int. J. Environ. Res. Public Health* **2020**, *17*, 7663. [CrossRef] [PubMed]

Publisher's Note: MDPI stays neutral with regard to jurisdictional claims in published maps and institutional affiliations.

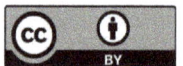

© 2021 by the authors. Licensee MDPI, Basel, Switzerland. This article is an open access article distributed under the terms and conditions of the Creative Commons Attribution (CC BY) license (http://creativecommons.org/licenses/by/4.0/).

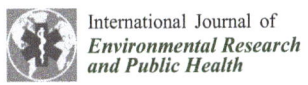

Article

Randomized Clinical Trial of an Internet-Based Adolescent Depression Prevention Intervention in Primary Care: Internalizing Symptom Outcomes

Tracy Gladstone [1,*], Katherine R. Buchholz [1], Marian Fitzgibbon [2,3,4], Linda Schiffer [3], Miae Lee [2] and Benjamin W. Van Voorhees [2]

[1] The Robert S. and Grace W. Stone Primary Prevention Initiatives, Wellesley Centers for Women, Wellesley College, Wellesley, MA 02481, USA; katherine.buchholz@wellesley.edu
[2] Department of General Pediatrics, College of Medicine, University of Illinois at Chicago, Chicago, IL 60612, USA; mlf@uic.edu (M.F.); mlee9@uic.edu (M.L.); bvanvoor@uic.edu (B.W.V.V.)
[3] Institute for Health Research and Policy, School of Public Health, University of Illinois at Chicago, Chicago, IL 60608, USA; lschiff@uic.edu
[4] University of Illinois Cancer Center, University of Illinois at Chicago, Chicago, IL 60612, USA
* Correspondence: tgladsto@wellesley.edu; Tel.: +1-781-283-2558

Received: 30 September 2020; Accepted: 20 October 2020; Published: 22 October 2020

Abstract: Approximately 20% of people will experience a depressive episode by adulthood, making adolescence an important developmental target for prevention. CATCH-IT (Competent Adulthood Transition with Cognitive-behavioral, Humanistic, and Interpersonal Training), an online depression prevention intervention, has demonstrated efficacy in preventing depressive episodes among adolescents reporting elevated symptoms. Our study examines the effects of CATCH-IT compared to online health education (HE) on internalizing symptoms in adolescents at risk for depression. Participants, ages 13–18, were recruited across eight US health systems and were randomly assigned to CATCH-IT or HE. Assessments were completed at baseline, 2, 6, 12, 18, and 24 months. There were no significant differences between groups in change in depressive symptoms (b = −0.31 for CATCH-IT, b = −0.27 for HE, $p = 0.80$) or anxiety (b = −0.13 for CATCH-IT, b = −0.11 for HE, $p = 0.79$). Improvement in depressive symptoms was statistically significant ($p < 0.05$) for both groups ($p = 0.004$ for CATCH-IT, $p = 0.009$ for HE); improvement in anxiety was significant for CATCH-IT ($p = 0.04$) but not HE ($p = 0.07$). Parental depression and positive relationships with primary care physicians (PRPC) moderated the anxiety findings, and adolescents' externalizing symptoms and PRPC moderated the depression findings. This study demonstrates the long-term positive effects of both online programs on depressive symptoms and suggests that CATCH-IT demonstrates cross-over effects for anxiety as well.

Keywords: web-based interventions; internalizing symptoms; depressive symptoms; adolescents; prevention; primary care

1. Introduction

Depression is a significant public health concern for adolescents. It is estimated that as many as 20% of people will experience a depressive episode before adulthood [1]. Depression is associated with significant impairments in day-to-day functioning, and it can affect developmental trajectories in adolescence and early adulthood [2–4]. Episodic in its course, a single depressive episode increases the risk of future episodes that are often more severe [2,3]. Depressive symptoms, including subthreshold symptoms, are associated with an increased risk of depressive episodes, physical health problems, comorbid mental health concerns, and suicide [4–7]. The personal and societal cost of depression can be eased through depression prevention interventions [8,9].

A recent Cochrane review revealed that depression prevention programs for adolescents are associated with a moderate reduction in depressive episodes (risk difference = −0.03) across one-year follow-up [10], and a meta-analysis of 19 randomized preventive trials revealed that, for adolescents with elevated symptoms of depression, preventive interventions are associated with benefits across a two-year follow-up [11]. Several trials of specific depression prevention approaches for adolescents at risk for depression also have been found to be effective for certain subsets of teens [12–17]. The majority of these interventions involve in-person groups that rely on training therapists and recruiting participants who can attend regular sessions; these approaches are limited by lack of access due to barriers related to seeking in-person interventions [14–17]. Therefore, it can be difficult to provide these interventions cost-effectively to the large number of adolescents who may benefit from them. Given the high rate of depression among adolescents and the long-term consequences of depression, public health interventions that can reach a broad population of adolescents are needed.

Similar to depression, anxiety is a significant public health problem among adolescents. In fact, anxiety, frequently grouped with depression as an internalizing disorder, is the most common mental health concern among adolescents [18,19]. The lifetime prevalence of anxiety disorders in adolescents is just over 30% [18]. Developmentally, anxiety has an earlier age of onset than depression [18,20,21]. Some studies have found that anxiety starting in childhood precedes depression that begins in adolescence [22,23], while other studies report that there is a bidirectional relationship between anxiety and depression in children and adolescents [24,25]. Comorbid presentations result in poorer overall prognosis [26]. With both disorders, onset during childhood or adolescence is associated with chronic symptoms or functional impairment in adulthood [27,28]. Anxiety often co-occurs with depression [29–32], and adolescents with depression have been found to be at greater risk for also having an anxiety disorder compared to adolescents without depression [32,33]. Epidemiological studies suggest that 30–75% of children or adolescents with depression have comorbid anxiety [33]. Therefore, prevention and treatment of depression in adolescents must consider anxiety.

Given the high rates of co-occurring depression and anxiety, research has focused on identifying transdiagnostic factors that may represent shared etiological mechanisms or latent factors that underlie both disorders [34]. These transdiagnostic factors include negative affectivity or emotionality [35], cognitive or information processing biases [36], emotional awareness [37], and emotional regulation skills [38]. Given that comorbidity is more common than just anxiety or depression in clinical settings [26], researchers have recently developed transdiagnostic treatments to address the underlying factors associated with both depression and anxiety [39,40]. However, it has been suggested that treatments developed for depression or anxiety alone may also have cross-over effects on comorbid symptoms. In fact, clinical research confirms that many treatments developed for depression also result in decreased symptoms of anxiety. One meta-analysis [41] reviewing randomized clinical treatment or prevention trials found that crossover effects were present in both depression treatments and anxiety treatments, although the effects were stronger for the targeted symptoms. That is, depression treatments had a greater effect on depressive symptoms than anxiety symptoms, and anxiety treatments had a greater effect on anxiety symptoms than depressive symptoms. However, there were no significant cross-over effects of depression or anxiety prevention interventions.

To address the need for preventive interventions that may reduce a range of symptoms in adolescents, CATCH-IT (Competent Adulthood Transition with Cognitive-behavioral, Humanistic, and Interpersonal Training), an online prevention intervention, was developed as a low cost, universally available intervention. Disseminated through primary care settings, CATCH-IT uses a population-health based model (screening and outreach in settings where youth and their families usually receive care) [42]. CATCH-IT contains elements of CBT and interpersonal psychotherapy in a highly interactive interface, which is described in more detail in previous publications [42,43]. Early pilot studies demonstrated that participants who used CATCH-IT reported decreases in symptoms of depression at 6, 12, and 30 months, relative to baseline [13,44,45]. A more recent randomized clinical trial found CATCH-IT to be efficacious in preventing depressive episodes at six months, relative to an attention-control condition that combined usual care with monitoring and an online general health education program (HE) in adolescents who were experiencing elevated symptoms of depression, though not in the full intention to treat analysis [12]. These initial findings suggest that CATCH-IT may have great potential as a public health intervention for adolescents at risk of developing Major Depressive Disorder (MDD). As an online intervention, CATCH-IT is easy to access, cost-effective, decreases stigmatization through anonymity, and does not require highly trained professionals [46].

Even though no cross-over effects on anxiety were reported for depression prevention interventions, there is some indication that CATCH-IT may affect symptoms of anxiety as well as depression. A study of CATCH-IT adapted for Chinese adolescents found that participants in the CATCH-IT condition demonstrated a decrease in symptoms of both depression and anxiety at eight-months [47]. While CATCH-IT is specifically designed for depression prevention, many of the skills it teaches may affect transdiagnostic factors, and therefore, decrease symptoms of anxiety as well. For example, cognitive behaviorally-based A-B-C exercises presented in CATCH-IT may increase emotional awareness, and the cognitive restructuring taught in CATCH-IT may decrease negative cognitive biases as well as negative affectivity. These effects could positively impact symptoms of anxiety in addition to depression. Given the accessibility, reach, and potential public health impact of the CATCH-IT intervention, it is important to investigate and understand the potential cross-over effects that CATCH-IT may offer.

The current study uses data from the randomized clinical trial comparing CATCH-IT to HE, an online program providing general health education, in a sample that was composed of adolescents with an intermediate to high risk of depression recruited from primary care settings [43]. As mentioned above, at six months, CATCH-IT, compared to HE, prevented depressive episodes in high-risk adolescents with significant subthreshold depressive symptoms at baseline [12], and additionally, depressive symptoms significantly decreased in both conditions. Moreover, preventive effects for CATCH-IT were found for up to 24 months for those with low levels of hopelessness or adequate levels of paternal monitoring [48]. The current study expands these initial findings to examine the possibility that the CATCH-IT intervention has long-term preventive effects on symptoms of anxiety as well as on symptoms of depression, and also to examine moderators of intervention effects on symptoms of both disorders. We hypothesize that participants in the CATCH-IT condition will have experienced greater decreases in self-reported symptoms of anxiety and depression, relative to participants in the HE group. Secondary analyses will examine potential moderators that may affect findings across both groups.

2. Materials and Methods

2.1. Study Design and Setting

This study utilized a hybrid type I efficacy-implementation design to evaluate the effectiveness of CATCH-IT in a scalable setting [49]. The efficacy of CATCH-IT was evaluated while simultaneously gathering information on CATCH-IT's implementation to prepare for scaling up [12]. This trial was implemented in eight major US Health Systems ($N = 31$ primary care sites, 42,310 adolescents) in a population health approach (screen all youth, offer intervention, assessment, refer those in need of treatment) with over 1200 primary care staff consented and trained. This process has been previously described in further detail [43,50]. Data were collected from urban and suburban clinics located in Chicago, Illinois, and surrounding areas including northern Indiana, and Boston, Massachusetts and surrounding areas. The protocol, CONSORT statement, and a description of the implementation process have been described previously [43,50]. Institutional review board (IRB) approval was received from the University of Chicago IRB (protocol # 2011-0505), the IRB of record, on 15 December 2011, and also by local review boards. A data safety and monitoring board (DSMB) reviewed the trial and results twice per year.

2.2. Participants

The final sample included 369 adolescents, ages 13 to 18 years old, who were at risk for depression as indicated by elevated symptoms of depression (score of 8–17 on the 10-item or score of ≥16 on the 20-item Center for Epidemiologic Studies Depression scale (CES-D)) and/or a history of a major depressive episode or dysthymia. Exclusion criteria included a DSM-IV diagnosis of major depressive disorder (MDD), bipolar disorder, schizophrenia, psychosis, or current drug/alcohol abuse. Additionally, adolescents were excluded if they were in current treatment for MDD, had a significant developmental disability or reading impairment, were assessed to be at imminent risk of suicide, or were being treated for serious medical conditions [13,44].

2.3. Study Procedures

Participants were recruited from February 2012 to July 2016 through posted flyers, recruitment letters sent by primary care offices (sent to all families of adolescents in the targeted age range), and information given directly by the primary care physician (PCP) during clinic visits. Following verbal consent from a parent, the study staff administered a phone screen to assess adolescents for eligibility (Figure 1). Eligible adolescents and their parents attended an enrollment appointment at the office of their PCP. Informed consent was obtained before the completion of the baseline assessment. Depression risk was assessed by the KSADS, a clinician-administered, semi-structured interview. All baseline assessments were completed before informing the participants, their parents, or their PCPs of the intervention assignment. Follow-up assessments were conducted at 2, 6, 12, 18, and 24 months following baseline.

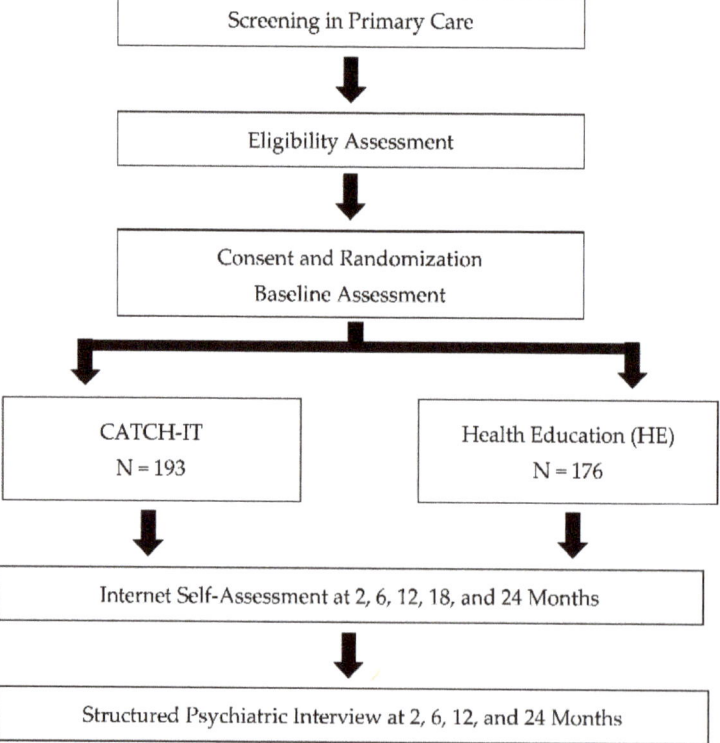

Figure 1. Study design.

2.4. Randomization and Blinding

A computer-generated sequence blocked by site and time of entry was used to randomly assign participants to CATCH-IT or HE. Participants were also stratified by age (13–14 years vs. 15–18 years), gender, and severity of their risk of a depressive episode (high risk: elevated score on the Center for Epidemiological Studies-Depression Scale (CES-D$_{10}$) and prior depressive episode; low risk: elevated CESD or prior depressive episode). The assignment of participants to HE versus CATCH-IT was 1:1. Assessors were blinded for the duration of the study, while investigators were blinded until all 12-month data were collected. PCPs were not blinded, since they provided motivational interviews to the adolescent participants in the CATCH-IT intervention.

2.5. Treatment Arms

2.5.1. The CATCH-IT Intervention

CATCH-IT consists of 14 online modules designed to help adolescents develop coping strategies to decrease symptoms related to depression and prevent depressive episodes, plus an additional, optional module to address symptoms of anxiety. CATCH-IT was adapted from the Coping with Depression Adolescent Course, a group cognitive-behavioral intervention. It also includes elements of behavioral activation strategies as well as Interpersonal Psychotherapy techniques [51–53]. The program was designed using the Instructional Design Theory to maximize learning and maintain the learner's attention [53]. In addition to the online modules, phone coaching by research staff (one to three calls) and a series of three motivational interviews conducted by the PCP (baseline, 2 months, and 12 months) were provided to support participants' use of CATCH-IT. Parents were also invited to complete four online modules to support their child's skills development, as well as an optional module for parents who worry they may themselves be depressed. Parent modules have been described in detail in previous publications [12,43,54].

2.5.2. The Health Education Intervention

The HE intervention consists of 14 online modules providing general health information, and it was used as the control intervention. The first 13 modules of the HE program provide general health information, while the final module focuses on identifying mood symptoms, the importance of treating mental health issues, and how mental health stigma may interfere with seeking treatment. In addition to the online modules, up to three check-in calls were provided to each HE participant to ensure that they had access to the website within three weeks of the study enrollment. Parents were also invited to complete four modules consisting of similar information to the adolescent modules.

2.6. Measures

Measures were chosen to capture the range of ways that internalizing symptoms are expressed by adolescents and possible mediators and moderators of intervention response. All measures were descriptive and were appropriate for adolescents ages 13–18.

Demographics. Demographic information including sex, race, ethnicity, and maternal education was collected from adolescents and their parents at baseline.

Kiddie Schedule for Affective Disorders and Schizophrenia (KSADS). The KSADS is a semi-structured, clinician-administered, clinical interview that was used to determine if participants met the criteria for depression and/or were experiencing suicidal thinking [55]. Additionally, the KSADS was used to assess global functioning (GAS score) at baseline. The GAS score can range from 1–100, with higher scores indicating higher functioning.

Center for Epidemiological Studies-Depression Scale (CES-D$_{10}$). The CES-D$_{10}$ is a 10-item self-report or clinician-administered measure that assesses symptoms of depression over the past week. Scores can range from 0–30, with higher scores indicating higher levels of depressive symptoms. Adolescents and parents completed the CES-D$_{10}$ at all time points [56]. Internal consistency of the CES-D in this sample was $\alpha = 0.71$ for youth report, and $\alpha = 0.84$ for parent report.

Screen for Child Anxiety Related Emotional Disorders (SCARED). The SCARED is a 41-item self-report measure that assesses symptoms of anxiety. Scores can range from 0–82, with higher scores indicating higher levels of anxiety symptoms [57]. The internal consistency of the SCARED in this sample was $\alpha = 0.91$ for youth report.

Disruptive Behaviors Disorder Scale (DBD). The DBD is a 41-item self-report measure that assesses behavioral concerns in adolescents. The Attention Deficit Disorder (ADHD) subscale, which includes both the Inattentive and Hyperactivity/Impulsivity domains, and the Oppositional Defiant Disorder/Conduct Disorder (ODD/CD) subscale of the DBD can range from 0–3, with a higher score indicating more externalizing behavior [58]. Internal consistency for youth report in this sample was $\alpha = 0.84$ for the ADHD subscale, and $\alpha = 0.87$ for the ODD/CD subscale.

Social Adjustment Scale (SAS-SR). The SAS-SR is a 36-item self-report measure that assesses social functioning over the past two weeks. Scores can range from 0–4 with a higher score indicating a lower level of functioning [59]. The internal consistency of the SAS-SR in this sample was $\alpha = 0.79$ for youth report.

Beck Hopelessness Scale (BHS). The BHS is a 21-item self-report measure that assesses pessimism about the future. Scores can range from 0–20, with a higher score indicating greater hopelessness [60]. The internal consistency of the BHS in this sample was $\alpha = 0.82$ for youth report.

Child Report of Parental Behavior Inventory (CRPBI). The CRPBI is a 15-item measure that assesses a child's relationship with their parents. Six subscales were used in this study: maternal and paternal acceptance (range = 10–30), psychological control (range = 8–24), and monitoring (range = 5–15). Higher scores indicate higher acceptance, control, and monitoring [61]. Internal consistency for youth report in this sample was $\alpha = 0.91$ for maternal acceptance, $\alpha = 0.78$ for maternal control, $\alpha = 0.80$ for maternal monitoring, $\alpha = 0.92$ for paternal acceptance, $\alpha = 0.82$ for paternal control, and $\alpha = 0.87$ for paternal monitoring.

Theory of Planned Behavior (TPB). The TPB Scale is a 19-item self-report measure that assesses attitude toward participating in a depression prevention intervention. Scores range from 1–5, with a higher score indicating a more positive attitude [62]. The internal consistency of the TPB in this sample was $\alpha = 0.87$ for youth report.

Trans-Theoretical Model. The Trans-Theoretical Model Scale is a 10-item self-report measure that asks the adolescent to rate the importance of preventing an episode of clinical depression, plus their ability and readiness to reduce their depression risk. Scores can range from 1–10, with a higher score indicating a higher overall intention to prevent future episodes [63]. The internal consistency of the Trans-Theoretical Model Scale in this sample was $\alpha = 0.86$ for youth report.

The Adolescent Life Events Questionnaire (ALEQ). The ALEQ is a retrospective self-report measure that asks about life events in the past 6 months. Scores can range from 0–51, with a higher score indicating more life events [64].

Engagement. Engagement in each of the interventions was assessed by the number of modules completed by parents and the number of modules completed by adolescents. A third variable was created to assess overall family engagement by summing the number of modules completed by an adolescent with the number of modules completed by the parent.

Positive Relationships in Primary Care (PRPC). The PRPC was administered at two months and asked the adolescent about their most recent interview with their primary care provider. For CATCH-IT participants, this may have been a motivational interview; for HE participants, it was their last PCP visit. The measure included both general questions ("I feel the primary care provider listened to me") and questions specific to the intervention ("It was helpful to focus on behaviors I would like to change.") Scores can range from 1–5, with higher scores indicating a more positive rating [44,65].

2.7. Statistical Analysis

Linear mixed-effect growth models with random intercept and slope were used to examine differences between groups in change over time in CES-D_{10} and SCARED scores. The CES-D_{10} analysis was conducted with and without a square root transformation of the time scale to improve linearity. All models were adjusted for sex, ethnicity (Hispanic, non-Hispanic), race (white, non-white), baseline age, and site, and the SCARED analysis was also adjusted for baseline teen CES-D_{10}. The p-value for the group*time interaction was used to test for a significant difference in slopes between CATCH-IT and HE. Within-group changes over time were estimated using simple slopes, and adjusted mean change over 24 months was calculated by multiplying the estimated slope by 24 (or the square root of 24 in the time-transformed model).

We also examined the moderating effects of theory-based covariates by including interaction terms in the models. The p-value of the group * time * moderator interaction was used to test for potential moderation of the effect of the intervention. For both the CES-D_{10} and SCARED outcomes, we examined the following potential moderators: demographics (sex, race, ethnicity, maternal education), site (Chicago or Boston), engagement (modules completed by teens, parents, teens + parents), PRPC scores at two months, and baseline scores for GAS, CRAFFT, DBD (ADHD, ODCD), SAS-SR, Theory of Planned Behavior, ALEQ, BHS, Trans-Theoretical Model, Parent CES-D_{10}, and the CRPBI (3 maternal and 3 paternal scales). We also tested SCARED as a potential moderator of the CES-D_{10} outcome and vice versa. In the moderator models with CES-D_{10} as the outcome variable, time was square-root transformed to improve linearity.

Completion or use of the supplementary CATCH-IT anxiety module was not included as a potential moderator in the analyses since only 18 (9.3%) teens completed the module, simply not a large enough percentage of the sample to allow us to test the effects of the module on anxiety and depressive symptoms. Additionally, our models included both CATCH-IT and HE participants to allow us to look for between-group differences. Therefore, we were unable to include variables that only applied to CATCH-IT as either covariates in the model or potential moderators.

Multivariable logistic regression models were used to test for differences between participants with and without CES-D_{10} or SCARED data at 12 and 24 months, including the following covariates: site, intervention group, age at baseline, gender, ethnicity, race, maternal education, parents' marital status, birth order (firstborn, other), past depressive episode at study entry, and high CES-D score at study entry. All analyses were conducted using SAS, version 9.4 (SAS Institute, Cary, NC, USA).

3. Results

3.1. Participants

One hundred ninety-three participants were randomized to CATCH-IT and 176 to HE. The mean age of the participants was 15.4 years (SD = 1.5), and 21% of the participants identified as Hispanic, 26% non-Hispanic black, 43% non-Hispanic white, 4% Asian, and 6% multiracial or other. Over half of the adolescents' parents reported having no more eduction than a high school diploma (60% of mothers and 53% of fathers), and 39.4% reported not being married. Clinically, 62% of participants reported a past sub-threshold or full depressive episode that had ended at least two months before study enrollment. Participants reported a mean score of 25.3 (SD = 12.3) on the SCARED, and a mean score of 9.4 (SD = 4.6) on the CES-D_{10} at baseline.

Site differences were found between the Chicago and Boston participants. Participants from Boston reported higher levels of parent education and a greater likelihood that parents were married. Additionally, the Boston sample was comprised of a lower percentage of ethnic minority participants, and a greater percentage of adolescents in Boston qualified for the study based on only a prior depressive episode. A complete description of the cohort data at baseline is provided in a prior publication [12].

Regarding attrition over the study period, at 24 months CESD scores were available for 182 participants (49.3%), and SCARED scores were available for 93 participants (25.2%). For the CES-D_{10}, missing scores at 24 months were associated with CATCH-IT assignment, the Chicago site, higher age at baseline, lower parent education, and elevated depressed mood at baseline (see Table S1); for the SCARED, missing scores at 24 months were associated with CATCH-IT assignment, the Chicago site, and lower maternal education (see Table S2).

3.2. Symptoms of Anxiety and Depression

There was not a significant difference between groups in change over time for either the SCARED ($p = 0.79$) or the CES-D_{10} ($p = 0.80$), see Table 1. Anxiety appeared to improve in both groups, though the change was only statistically significant in CATCH-IT. The estimated slope for SCARED scores was -0.13, SE = 0.06, $p = 0.04$ for CATCH-IT and -0.11, SE = 0.06, $p = 0.07$ for HE. The estimated mean change from baseline to 24 months was -3.1 (SE = 1.5) points in the CATCH-IT group and -2.6 (1.4) points in the HE group. Depressive symptoms improved significantly in both groups. The estimated slope for the CES-D_{10} scores with time square-root transformed was -0.31, $p = 0.004$ for CATCH-IT and -0.27, $p = 0.009$ for HE. The estimated mean change from baseline to 24 months was -1.5 (SE = 0.5) points for CATCH-IT and -1.3 (0.5) points for HE.

Table 1. Internalizing symptoms, baseline to 24 months.

Outcome Variables	Unadjusted Means						Within-Group Slopes [1]							Btw Grp Diff
	CATCH-IT (N = 193)			HE (N = 176)				CATCH-IT			HE			
	N	Mean	SD	N	Mean	SD	Time Variable	b	SE	p	b	SE	p	p
SCARED [2] total score (0–82)							Months	−0.13	(0.06)	0.04	−0.11	(0.06)	0.07	0.79
Baseline	171	25.5	(12.7)	141	25.2	(11.9)								
2 months	94	26.2	(13.1)	90	25.7	(14.3)								
6 months	74	25.1	(15.0)	92	24.0	(13.9)								
12 months	83	22.4	(13.0)	73	23.2	(13.6)								
18 months	64	25.6	(13.3)	81	23.2	(13.4)								
24 months	39	19.6	(12.2)	54	20.9	(13.7)								
CES-D$_{10}$ (0–30)							Months	−0.06	(0.02)	0.01	−0.04	(0.02)	0.10	0.44
Baseline	190	9.5	(4.5)	172	9.4	(4.6)	Sqrt (months)	−0.31	(0.11)	0.004	−0.27	(0.10)	0.009	0.80
2 months	123	9.2	(4.2)	140	7.9	(5.2)								
6 months	116	8.2	(4.9)	133	7.9	(4.7)								
12 months	115	7.9	(5.3)	126	7.1	(4.7)								
18 months	67	7.9	(5.9)	81	7.5	(5.6)								
24 months	79	7.7	(5.8)	103	8.1	(5.6)								

[1] From linear mixed effect growth models with random intercept and slope, adjusted for sex, ethnicity (Hispanic, non-Hispanic), race (white, non-white), baseline age, site, and baseline teen CES-D$_{10}$. Within-group estimated slopes and p-values are from estimates of simple slopes. The p-value for the visit*time interaction is used to test for a significant difference between slopes. [2] Higher scores indicate greater anxiety.

3.3. Analyses of Potential Moderators

Symptoms of Anxiety. Two significant moderators of the effect of CATCH-IT and HE on change in SCARED scores across the 24-month study period were identified: parental CES-D10 scores at baseline (b = −0.05, p = 0.004) and positive relationships in primary care scores at 2 months (b = −0.41, p = 0.009) (Table 2). Anxiety appeared to decrease more in the HE group than in the CATCH-IT group when parental depressive symptoms at baseline were very low. When parental CES-D10 was set to 0 in the model, the estimated slope for HE was −0.25 (SE = 0.09), and the estimated slope for CATCH-IT was 0.04 (0.09), p = 0.03 (see Table S3). However, anxiety decreased more in the CATCH-IT group than the HE group when parental depressive symptoms at baseline were very high. When parental CES-D10 was set to 27, the maximum score in our sample, the estimated CATCH-IT slope was −0.62 (0.23), while the estimated HE slope was 0.36 (0.26), p = 0.005. At intermediate parental CES-D10 scores (25th percentile, median, 75th percentile), the model did not show significant differences between groups in anxiety change.

Table 2. Summary of moderator analyses for Screen for Child Anxiety Related Emotional Disorders (SCARED): Group*Visit*Moderator Interaction Term.

Moderator	N [1]	Beta	Standard Error	p [2]
Sex = male (reference = female)	362	0.16	0.19	0.41
Race = not white (reference = white) [3]	362	0.14	0.18	0.43
Ethnicity = Hispanic (reference = not Hispanic)	362	−0.17	0.25	0.50
Site = Boston (reference = Chicago)	362	0.29	0.17	0.09
Maternal education= college degree (reference = no college degree)	352	0.15	0.19	0.43
Teen GAS, baseline	360	0.00	0.01	0.66
Teen CES-D_{10}, baseline	362	0.02	0.02	0.17
Parent CES-D_{10}, baseline	332	−0.05	0.02	0.004
ADHD (DBD-A), baseline	196	0.12	0.26	0.64
ODCD (DBD-A), baseline	193	0.28	0.52	0.59
Social adjustment (SAS-SR), baseline	212	0.15	0.23	0.51
Hopelessness (BHS), baseline	270	−0.01	0.03	0.74
Maternal acceptance (CRPBI), baseline	196	−0.04	0.02	0.06
Maternal control (CRPBI), baseline	197	0.04	0.03	0.18
Maternal monitoring (CRPBI), baseline	187	−0.10	0.06	0.12
Paternal acceptance (CRPBI), baseline	176	−0.04	0.02	0.07
Paternal control (CRPBI), baseline	176	0.00	0.03	0.88
Paternal monitoring (CRPBI), baseline	170	−0.04	0.04	0.25
Positive relationships in primary care, 2 months	133	−0.41	0.16	0.009
Theory of planned behavior, baseline	164	−0.47	0.25	0.06
Stressful life events (LEQ), baseline	300	−0.02	0.02	0.24
Trans-theoretical model, baseline	191	−0.07	0.05	0.12
Teen modules completed	362	0.00	0.01	0.83
Parent modules completed	340	−0.03	0.04	0.45

[1] Number of participants included in the analysis. Participants with missing data for the moderator variable or baseline CESD (covariate) were excluded. [2] From linear mixed effect growth models with random intercept and slope and a group*visit*moderator interaction term, adjusted for sex, ethnicity (Hispanic, non-Hispanic), race (white, non-white), baseline age, site, and baseline teen CES-D_{10}. [3] No significant effects of race were detected when the race categorization was changed to Black or multi-racial vs. all others.

Similarly, anxiety appeared to show greater improvement in the HE group than the CATCH-IT group when adolescents gave a very low score to their most recent interaction with their primary care provider (see Table S4). When PRPC was set to 1.0 in the model, the estimated slope for HE was −1.05 (SE = 0.31), while the estimated slope for CATCH-IT was 0.20 (0.37), p = 0.01. However, when PRPC was set to the maximum score of 5.0, the estimated slope was 0.18 (0.14) for HE but −0.22 (0.14) for CATCH-IT, p = 0.050. The model did not predict significant differences in anxiety change between groups at intermediate PRPC scores.

Symptoms of Depression. Three significant moderators of the effect of CATCH-IT and HE on change in adolescent CES-D10 scores across the 24-month study period were identified: baseline DBD-ADHD subscale score (b = 1.42, p = 0.004), baseline DBD-ODD/CD subscale score (b = 2.37,

$p = 0.01$), and PRPC score at two months (b = −0.60, $p = 0.046$) (Table 3). In the ADHD moderator model, CATCH-IT appeared superior to HE in reducing CES-D10 scores when ADHD scores were low, but HE appeared superior when ADHD scores were high (see Table S5). When the ADHD score was set to 0 in the model, the estimated slope for CATCH-IT was −0.31 (SE = 0.28), while the estimated slope for HE was 0.89 (0.32), $p = 0.006$. CATCH-IT still appeared superior when ADHD was set to the approximate 25th percentile in our sample (0.5), though the difference between slopes was smaller: −0.25 (0.16) for CATCH-IT vs 0.24 (0.18) for HE, $p = 0.04$. However, when ADHD was set to the maximum value for our sample (2.0), the estimated CES-D10 slope was only −0.06 (0.43) for CATCH-IT but −1.70 (0.44) for HE, $p = 0.008$. For ADHD scores at the median and 75th percentiles for our sample, the model did not predict a significant difference between groups.

Table 3. Summary of moderator analyses for CESD: Group*Visit*Moderator Interaction Term.

Moderator	N [1]	Estimate	SE	p [2]
Sex = male (reference = female)	369	0.06	0.33	0.86
Race = not white (reference = white)	369	0.54	0.30	0.07
Ethnicity = Hispanic (reference = not Hispanic)	369	−0.09	0.38	0.81
Site = Boston (reference = Chicago)	369	0.01	0.31	0.98
Maternal education = college degree (reference = no college degree)	359	0.03	0.31	0.91
Teen GAS, baseline	367	0.00	0.02	0.93
Anxiety (SCARED), baseline	312	0.00	0.01	0.99
Parent CES-D_{10}, baseline	338	0.01	0.03	0.84
ADHD (DBD-A), baseline	196	1.42	0.48	0.004
ODCD (DBD-A), baseline	193	2.37	0.93	0.01
Social adjustment (SAS-SR), baseline	212	−0.22	0.45	0.64
Hopelessness (BHS), baseline	270	0.03	0.05	0.55
Maternal acceptance (CRPBI), baseline	196	−0.04	0.05	0.40
Maternal control (CRPBI), baseline	197	0.07	0.06	0.23
Maternal monitoring (CRPBI), baseline	187	0.02	0.10	0.86
Paternal acceptance (CRPBI), baseline	176	−0.05	0.04	0.21
Paternal control (CRPBI), baseline	176	0.06	0.06	0.35
Paternal monitoring (CRPBI), baseline	170	−0.07	0.07	0.29
Positive relationships in primary care, 2 months	134	−0.60	0.30	0.046
Theory of planned behavior, baseline	164	−0.91	0.50	0.07
Stressful life events (LEQ), baseline	302	0.05	0.03	0.10
Trans-theoretical model, baseline	191	0.08	0.10	0.42
Teen modules completed	369	0.00	0.03	0.88
Parent modules completed	346	−0.05	0.08	0.52

[1] Number of participants included in the analysis. Participants with missing data for the moderator variable were excluded. [2] From linear mixed effect growth models with random intercept and slope and a group*visit*moderator interaction term, adjusted for sex, ethnicity (Hispanic, non-Hispanic), race (white, non-white), baseline age, and site. Time square-root transformed to improve linearity.

Results were similar for the DBD-ODCD subscale (see Table S6). When ODCD was set to 0 in the model, the estimated improvement in depressive symptoms was greater in the CATCH-IT group: slope = −0.29 (0.19) for CATCH-IT and 0.38 (0.23) for HE, $p = 0.03$. When ODCD was set to the maximum score in our sample (still quite low at 1.25), the estimated slopes were 0.18 (0.71) for CATCH-IT and −2.11 (0.65) for HE, $p = 0.02$. The model did not predict significant differences between slopes at intermediate values of ODCD.

As was noted for anxiety, the HE group showed a greater estimated reduction in depressive symptoms than the CATCH-IT group when the PRPC rating was very low (see Table S7). With PRPC set to 1 (minimum score) in the model, the estimated CATCH-IT slope was 0.76 (0.70), but the HE slope was −1.22 (0.58), $p = 0.03$. However, the model did not show significant differences between groups at any other PRPC value tested, including the maximum score of 5.

4. Discussion

In a long-term follow-up investigation, the current study examined symptoms of anxiety and depression in at-risk adolescents who were recruited through primary care and were assigned randomly to the CATCH-IT prevention intervention or HE. Consistent with data from a 6-month follow-up of this sample [12], adolescents assigned to both the CATCH-IT intervention and the HE intervention experienced decreasing depressive symptoms over the course of 24 months. Moreover, differences in score trajectories were not found between the conditions, suggesting that both interventions had a positive effect on depressive symptoms. The multiple study contacts (i.e., screenings, assessments, safety calls) that accompanied both intervention approaches may have obscured group differences. In addition, while the content of the HE program focused on health behaviors and not on mental health, participants and parents may have received some sense of mastery and self-efficacy from completing the program, which may account for lower depression scores for HE participants.

The current study also provided evidence for cross-over effects in the CATCH-IT group. Although there was not an overall group difference in anxiety symptoms, teens at risk for depression who were assigned to CATCH-IT experienced a significant decrease in symptoms of anxiety across the 24 months, while there was no significant change in anxiety symptoms for teens assigned to HE. This finding is consistent with results from Ip et al. [47], who found that adolescents who used a Chinese adaptation of the CATCH-IT prevention intervention, Grasp the Opportunity, reported fewer symptoms of anxiety at 8 months, relative to adolescents assigned to a control (attention) intervention. Evidence of cross-over effects from CATCH-IT suggests that this prevention intervention, which was developed to address risk for depression only, may in fact target shared underlying mechanisms for both depression and anxiety. These results are counter to Garber et al. [41], who, in a meta-analysis exploring cross-over effects for depression and anxiety treatment and prevention interventions, reported no evidence of cross-over effects for depression prevention programs. It is possible that the recruitment process, intervention engagement, and motivational interviews that accompany the CATCH-IT intervention, all of which emphasize building resilience, managing stressors, and working toward goals in addition to preventing low mood and depression, may help teens to generalize depression prevention skills to other distressing symptoms such as anxiety. It is also true that the CATCH-IT intervention includes an optional anxiety module (Module #15), which addresses symptoms of anxiety more directly and provides instructions for exercises such as progressive muscle relaxation. Because so few adolescents ($N = 18$) in our sample completed the anxiety module, however, it is more likely that the observed improvement in anxiety symptoms is explained by participants' use of other skills taught in CATCH-IT, such as cognitive restructuring and behavioral activation, both of which are commonly used to treat symptoms of anxiety in adolescents [66–68].

Secondary analyses revealed that parental depression moderates the trajectory of anxiety symptoms in teens assigned to CATCH-IT compared to HE. Specifically, when parents had no or low-level symptoms of depression at baseline, their adolescents reported a greater improvement in anxiety when assigned to HE; when parents had high-level symptoms of depression at baseline, their adolescents reported a greater improvement in anxiety when assigned to CATCH-IT. This finding, that CATCH-IT is associated with better outcomes for teens when parents report high-level depressive symptoms, contrasts with prior research suggesting that parental depressive symptoms are associated with *poorer* intervention outcomes for children with internalizing symptoms [69,70]. Our findings are consistent, however, with research reporting better youth intervention outcomes when parents report symptoms of anxiety [71–73], and may reflect the additional motivation symptomatic parents feel to support their children's engagement in the CATCH-IT intervention. It is also possible that parents with depressive symptoms were more engaged in the CATCH-IT parent intervention, and that their use of the on-line parent modules, as well as the motivational interviews focusing on their goals for supporting their child in completing CATCH-IT, improved their child's long-term outcomes. In fact, Legerstee and colleagues [71] suggested that anxious mothers may have benefitted from the parent intervention that accompanied their adolescent's intervention, and therefore were able to support their teen's engagement in treatment, leading to better outcomes over time. Unfortunately, baseline parental anxiety was not measured in this trial, but adolescents with elevated symptoms of depression at baseline were found to benefit more from CATCH-IT than non-symptomatic adolescents [12].

Additionally, the adolescent's relationship with their primary care physician moderated the trajectory of anxiety symptoms in adolescents assigned to CATCH-IT relative to HE. Adolescents who reported a weak connection to their primary care physician experienced a greater improvement in anxiety when they were assigned to HE rather than CATCH-IT. The benefits adolescents received from the HE intervention are likely a function of the non-specific factors associated with study involvement (e.g., recruitment, assessments, check-in phone calls, sense of achievement from completing modules), and perhaps these non-specific factors were more motivating for adolescents in the absence of a close connection with their primary care physician.

Secondary analyses also revealed some interesting moderating effects of adolescents' externalizing behaviors on their depressive symptoms across the 24-month follow-up interval, such that, when adolescents reported more symptoms of attentional and oppositional behaviors, they experienced a greater improvement in depressive symptoms if they were assigned to the HE group. By extension, this finding suggests that the CATCH-IT intervention, relative to HE, may be less helpful to adolescents who are struggling with externalizing concerns, perhaps due to its high reading demand, and its demand for attention, homework completion, and compliance. Solanto [74] suggests that the self-management challenges for adolescents with ADHD may interfere with their response to cognitive-behavioral and self-directed interventions. Nevertheless, given the overall low mean score for this sample on the DBD, the measure of externalizing behaviors used in this trial, these moderating effects must be interpreted with caution. Similar to our findings on symptoms of anxiety, depressive symptoms decreased more across the 24 months for adolescents in HE than in CATCH-IT when they reported a weak connection to their primary care physician.

There are several limitations associated with this study. We experienced attrition in the sample over the 24-month study period, particularly among adolescents with fewer resources (e.g., Chicago site, higher depressed mood, lower parental education). It is noteworthy that, to our knowledge, this is the only Internet-based intervention trial for youth with a 2-year follow-up, and such attrition is to be expected when such a long interval follows an intervention with relatively minimal face-to-face interaction. It is also noteworthy that attrition was higher for adolescents assigned to CATCH-IT versus HE, despite the presence of physician contact through motivational interviews in the CATCH-IT condition only. It is difficult to account for this finding, but it is possible that adolescents who benefitted most from the CATCH-IT intervention were less likely to feel a need to remain connected with the study throughout the follow-up interval. To address attrition in our sample, we chose to use mixed effect models, which are thought to be robust to missing data. The use of a second, potentially active internet-based intervention as a control is another limitation to the study. While the content of HE was not focused on mental health (only a single module towards the end of the intervention addressed mental health concerns), the program did present information on other health behaviors. It is possible that teens assigned to the HE condition received benefit above what they would have in an inactive or waitlist control. In addition, the examination of very long-term intervention effects (24 months) is necessarily constrained by the possibility of intervening environmental factors (e.g., natural disasters, family disruption) that may limit the ability to draw conclusions regarding causality.

5. Conclusions

Despite these limitations, the current study demonstrates long-term reductions in symptoms of depression in both intervention groups (HE and CATCH-IT). Additionally, participants assigned to CATCH-IT were found to have cross-over effects as seen in a reduction of anxiety symptoms, demonstrating that it is possible to develop preventive interventions for adolescent depression that target transdiagnostic factors representing shared underlying mechanisms for both disorders. Similarly, moderation results of depression and anxiety symptoms reported here, in addition to earlier moderation results of depressive disorder outcomes [48], suggest that CATCH-IT is beneficial when certain conditions are present (i.e., no significant externalizing symptoms (depressed mood), no significant hopelessness (depressive episodes), a supportive relationship with a physician (anxiety and depressive symptoms), heightened parental symptoms (anxiety), and adequate paternal monitoring (depressive episodes)). That is, pre-conditions (current depressed mood), lack of substantial co-morbidity, and supportive environmental factors may be necessary for adolescents to benefit from this largely self-directed model. Given that comorbid presentations of depression and anxiety are common and are associated with poor long-term outcomes, the discovery of a single preventive intervention that targets both disorders has significant implications for youth mental health promotion. These findings, along with the ability to implement the program across multiple primary care clinics, demonstrates the value of CATCH-IT as a feasible, online, population-based depression prevention intervention for at-risk adolescents.

Supplementary Materials: The following are available online at http://www.mdpi.com/1660-4601/17/21/7736/s1, Table S1: Predictors of missing 24-month SCARED, all participants, Table S2: Predictors of missing 24-month CES-D$_{10}$, all participants, Table S3: SCARED Moderator: Between-Group Comparisons: difference between CATCH-IT and HE simple slopes for time at selected levels of Parent CES-D^a, Table S4: SCARED Moderator: Between-Group Comparisons: difference between CATCH-IT and HE simple slopes for time at selected levels of PRPC, Table S5: CES-D$_{10}$ Moderator: Between-Group Comparisons: difference between CATCH-IT and HE simple slopes for time at selected levels of ADHD, Table S6: CES-D$_{10}$ Moderator: Between-Group Comparisons: difference between CATCH-IT and HE simple slopes for time at selected levels of ODCD, and Table S7: CES-D10 Moderator: Between-Group Comparisons: difference between CATCH-IT and HE simple slopes for time at selected levels of PRPC1.

Author Contributions: Conceptualization, T.G., K.R.B., L.S., M.L., and B.W.V.V.; methodology, T.G., K.R.B., L.S., M.F., and B.W.V.V.; validation, T.G., K.R.B., L.S., M.F., and B.W.V.V.; formal analysis, L.S.; investigation, T.G. and B.W.V.V.; data curation, L.S.; writing—original draft preparation, T.G. and K.R.B.; writing—review and editing, T.G., K.R.B., M.F., M.L., L.S., and B.W.V.V.; supervision, T.G. and B.W.V.V.; project administration, M.L.; funding acquisition, T.G. and B.W.V.V. All authors have read and agreed to the published version of the manuscript.

Funding: This research was funded The National Institute of Mental Health of the National Institutes of Health, grant number R01MH090035. Clinical Trial Registry (clinicaltrials.gov): NCT01893749.

Acknowledgments: Content is solely the responsibility of the authors and does not necessarily represent the official views of the National Institutes of Health. Ethical bodies that approved this study include: Wellesley College Institutional Review Board (IRB), University of Illinois at Chicago IRB, Advocate Health Care IRB, Franciscan St. Mary IRB, Northwestern IRB and NorthShore University Health Systems IRB. Methods developed under Robert Wood Johnson (Project Curb "Chicago Urban Resiliency Building": Reducing Life Course Disparities in Depression Outcomes in Urban Youth Through Early Preventive Intervention) supported and informed the implementation process. Thank you to Brady Goodwin, Joselyn Williams, Hendricks Brown, David A. Aaby, Mark Reinecke, Joshua Fogel, Emily Sykes, William R. Beardslee, Amy Kane, and Sophia Rintell for their contributions. B.W.V.V. would like to acknowledge the interest of Asok K. Ray, MD FRCS (Edin), Purnima Ray and Malika Ray in this research is appreciated.

Conflicts of Interest: Benjamin W. Van Voorhees has served as a consultant to Prevail Health Solutions, Inc., Mevident Inc., San Francisco and Social Kinetics, Palo Alto, CA, and the Hong Kong University to develop Internet-based interventions. The funders had no role in the design of the study; in the collection, analyses, or interpretation of data; in the writing of the manuscript, or in the decision to publish the results.

References

1. Rushton Jerry, L.; Michelle, F.; Schectman Robin, M. Epidemiology of depressive symptoms in the National Longitudinal Study of Adolescent Health. *J. Am. Acad. Child Adolesc. Psychiatry* **2002**, *41*, 199–205. [CrossRef] [PubMed]
2. Lewinsohn, P.M.; Rohde, P.; Klein, D.N.; Seeley, J.R. Natural course of adolescent major depressive disorder: I. Continuity into young adulthood. *J. Am. Acad. Child Adolesc. Psychiatry* **1999**, *38*, 56. [CrossRef] [PubMed]
3. Weissman, M.M.; Wolk, S.; Goldstein, R.B.; Moreau, D.; Adams, P.; Greenwald, S.; Klier, C.M.; Ryan, N.D.; Dahl, R.E.; Wickramaratne, P. Depressed adolescents grown up. *JAMA* **1999**, *281*, 1707. [CrossRef] [PubMed]
4. Birmaher, B.; Ryan, N.D.; Williamson, D.E.; Brent, D.A.; Kaufman, J.; Dahl, R.E.; Perel, J.; Nelson, B. Childhood and adolescent depression: A review of the past 10 years. Part I. *J. Am. Acad. Child Adolesc. Psychiatry* **1996**, *35*, 1427. [CrossRef]

5. Pine, D.S.; Goldstein, R.B.; Wolk, S.; Weissman, M.M. The Association Between Childhood Depression and Adulthood Body Mass Index. *Pediatrics* **2001**, *107*, 1049–1056. [CrossRef]
6. Balázs, J.; Miklósi, M.; Keresztény, Á.; Hoven, C.W.; Carli, V.; Wasserman, C.; Apter, A.; Bobes, J.; Brunner, R.; Cosman, D.; et al. Adolescent subthreshold-depression and anxiety: Psychopathology, functional impairment and increased suicide risk. *J. Child Psychol. Psychiatry* **2013**, *54*, 670–677. [CrossRef]
7. Georgiades, K.; Lewinsohn, P.M.; Monroe, S.M.; Seeley, J.R. Major depressive disorder in adolescence: The role of subthreshold symptoms. *J. Am. Acad. Child Adolesc. Psychiatry* **2006**, *45*, 936–944. [CrossRef]
8. Birmaher, B.; Ryan, N.D.; Williamson, D.E.; Brent, D.A.; Kaufman, J. Childhood and adolescent depression: A review of the past 10 years. Part II. *J. Am. Acad. Child Adolesc. Psychiatry* **1996**, *35*, 1575. [CrossRef]
9. Buntrock, C.; Berking, M.; Smit, F.; Lehr, D.; Nobis, S.; Riper, H.; Cuijpers, P.; Ebert, D. Preventing depression in adults with subthreshold depression: Health-economic evaluation alongside a pragmatic randomized controlled trial of a web-based intervention. *J. Med. Internet Res.* **2017**, *19*, e5. [CrossRef]
10. Hetrick, S.E.; Cox, G.R.; Witt, K.G.; Bir, J.J.; Merry, S.N. Cognitive behavioural therapy (CBT), third-wave CBT and interpersonal therapy (IPT) based interventions for preventing depression in children and adolescents. *Cochrane Database Syst. Rev.* **2016**. [CrossRef]
11. Brown, C.H.; Brincks, A.; Huang, S.; Perrino, T.; Cruden, G.; Pantin, H.; Howe, G.; Young, J.F.; Beardslee, W.; Montag, S. Two-year impact of prevention programs on adolescent depression: An integrative data analysis approach. *Prev. Sci.* **2018**, *19*, 74–94. [CrossRef]
12. Gladstone, T.; Terrizzi, D.; Stinson, A.; Nidetz, J.; Canel, J.; Ching, E.; Berry, A.; Cantorna, J.; Fogel, J.; Eder, M.; et al. Effect of Internet-based Cognitive Behavioral Humanistic and Interpersonal Training vs. Internet-based General Health Education on Adolescent Depression in Primary Care: A Randomized Clinical Trial. *JAMA Netw. Open* **2018**, *1*, e184278. [CrossRef]
13. Saulsberry, A.; Marko-Holguin, M.; Blomeke, K.; Hinkle, C.; Fogel, J.; Gladstone, T.; Bell, C.; Reinecke, M.; Corden, M.; Van Voorhees, B.W. Randomized Clinical Trial of a Primary Care Internet-based Intervention to Prevent Adolescent Depression: One-year Outcomes. *J. Can. Acad. Child Adolesc. Psychiatry* **2013**, *22*, 106–117. [PubMed]
14. Conejo-Cerón, S.; Moreno-Peral, P.; Rodríguez-Morejón, A.; Motrico, E.; Navas-Campaña, D.; Rigabert, A.; Martín-Pérez, C.; Rodríguez-Bayón, A.; Ballesta-Rodríguez, M.I.; Luna, J.d.D.; et al. Effectiveness of Psychological and Educational Interventions to Prevent Depression in Primary Care: A Systematic Review and Meta-Analysis. *Ann. Fam. Med.* **2017**, *15*, 262–271. [CrossRef] [PubMed]
15. Garber, J.; Clarke, G.N.; Weersing, V.R.; Beardslee, W.R.; Brent, D.A.; Gladstone, T.R.G.; DeBar, L.L.; Lynch, F.L.; D'Angelo, E.; Hollon, S.D.; et al. Prevention of depression in at-risk adolescents: A randomized controlled trial. *JAMA* **2009**, *301*, 2215. [CrossRef]
16. Beardslee, W.R.; Brent, D.A.; Weersing, V.R.; Clarke, G.N.; Porta, G.; Hollon, S.D.; Gladstone, T.R.G.; Gallop, R.; Lynch, F.L.; Iyengar, S.; et al. Prevention of depression in at-risk adolescents: Longer-term effects. *JAMA Psychiatry* **2013**, *70*, 1161. [CrossRef]
17. Gillham, J.E.; Hamilton, J.; Freres, D.R.; Patton, K.; Gallop, R. Preventing Depression Among Early Adolescents in the Primary Care Setting: A Randomized Controlled Study of the Penn Resiliency Program. *J. Abnorm. Child Psychol.* **2006**, *34*, 195–211. [CrossRef]
18. Merikangas, K.R.; He, J.-P.; Burstein, M.; Swanson, S.A.; Avenevoli, S.; Cui, L.; Benjet, C.; Georgiades, K.; Swendsen, J. Lifetime prevalence of mental disorders in U.S. adolescents: Results from the National Comorbidity Survey Replication—Adolescent Supplement (NCS-A). *J. Am. Acad. Child Adolesc. Psychiatry* **2010**, *49*, 980. [CrossRef] [PubMed]
19. Merikangas, K.R.; Nakamura, E.F.; Kessler, R.C. Epidemiology of mental disorders in children and adolescents. *Dialogues Clin. Neurosci.* **2009**, *11*, 7–20. [PubMed]
20. Kessler, R.C.; Berglund, P.; Demler, O.; Jin, R.; Merikangas, K.R.; Walters, E.E. Lifetime prevalence and age-of-onset distributions of DSM-IV disorders in the National Comorbidity Survey Replication. *Arch. Gen. Psychiatry* **2005**, *62*, 593–602. [CrossRef]
21. Kessler, R.; Avenevoli, S.; McLaughlin, K.; Green, J.; Lakoma, M.; Petukhova, M.; Pine, D.; Sampson, N.; Zaslavsky, A.; Merikangas, K. Lifetime co-morbidity of DSM-IV disorders in the US national comorbidity survey replication adolescent supplement (NCS-A). *Psychol. Med.* **2012**, *42*, 1997–2010. [CrossRef] [PubMed]

22. Keenan, K.; Feng, X.; Hipwell, A.; Klostermann, S. Depression begets depression: Comparing the predictive utility of depression and anxiety symptoms to later depression. *J. Child Psychol. Psychiatry* **2009**, *50*, 1167–1175. [CrossRef]
23. Snyder, J.; Bullard, L.; Wagener, A.; Leong, P.K. Childhood Anxiety and Depressive Symptoms: Trajectories, Relationship, and Association with Subsequent Depression. *J. Clin. Child Adolesc. Psychol.* **2009**, *38*, 837. [CrossRef]
24. Hale III, W.W.; Raaijmakers, Q.A.; Muris, P.; Van Hoof, A.; Meeus, W.H. One factor or two parallel processes? Comorbidity and development of adolescent anxiety and depressive disorder symptoms. *J. Child Psychol. Psychiatry* **2009**, *50*, 1218–1226. [CrossRef] [PubMed]
25. Lavigne, J.V.; Lavigne, J.V.; Hopkins, J.; Hopkins, J.; Gouze, K.R.; Gouze, K.R.; Bryant, F.B.; Bryant, F.B. Bidirectional Influences of Anxiety and Depression in Young Children. *J. Abnorm. Child Psychol.* **2015**, *43*, 163–176. [CrossRef] [PubMed]
26. Merikangas, K.R.; Avenevoli, S. Epidemiology of mood and anxiety disorders in children and adolescents. In *Textbook in Psychiatric Epidemiology*; Wiley-Liss: Hoboken, NJ, USA, 2002.
27. Copeland, W.E.; Wolke, D.; Shanahan, L.; Costello, E.J. Adult functional outcomes of common childhood psychiatric problems: A prospective, longitudinal study. *JAMA Psychiatry* **2015**, *72*, 892–899. [CrossRef] [PubMed]
28. Copeland, W.E.; Alaie, I.; Jonsson, U.; Shanahan, L. Associations of Childhood and Adolescent Depression With Adult Psychiatric and Functional Outcomes. *J. Am. Acad. Child Adolesc. Psychiatry* **2020**. [CrossRef]
29. Weller, B.E.; Blanford, K.L.; Butler, A.M. Estimated Prevalence of Psychiatric Comorbidities in U.S. Adolescents With Depression by Race/Ethnicity, 2011–2012. *J. Adolesc. Health* **2018**, *62*, 716–721. [CrossRef]
30. Costello, E.J.; Mustillo, S.; Erkanli, A.; Keeler, G. Prevalence and development of psychiatric disorders in childhood and adolescence. *Arch. Gen. Psychiatry* **2003**, *60*, 837–844. [CrossRef]
31. Melton, T.; Croarkin, P.; Strawn, J.; Mcclintock, S. Comorbid Anxiety and Depressive Symptoms in Children and Adolescents: A Systematic Review and Analysis. *J. Psychiatr. Pract.* **2016**, *22*, 84–98. [CrossRef]
32. Avenevoli, S.; Swendsen, J.; He, J.-P.; Burstein, M.; Merikangas, K.R. Major depression in the national comorbidity survey-adolescent supplement: Prevalence, correlates, and treatment. *J. Am. Acad. Child Adolesc. Psychiatry* **2015**, *54*, 37. [CrossRef]
33. Angold, A.; Costello, E.J. Depressive comorbidity in children and adolescents. *Am. J. Psychiatry* **1993**, *150*, 1779–1791. [PubMed]
34. Garber, J.; Weersing, V.R. Comorbidity of Anxiety and Depression in Youth: Implications for Treatment and Prevention. *Clin. Psychol.* **2010**, *17*, 293–306. [CrossRef] [PubMed]
35. Clark, L.A.; Watson, D. Tripartite model of anxiety and depression: Psychometric evidence and taxonomic implications. *J. Abnorm. Psychol.* **1991**, *100*, 316. [CrossRef] [PubMed]
36. Dozois, D.J.; Beck, A.T. Cognitive schemas, beliefs and assumptions. In *Risk Factors in Depression*; Elsevier: Amsterdam, The Netherlands, 2008; pp. 119–143.
37. Kranzler, A.; Young, J.F.; Hankin, B.L.; Abela, J.R.; Elias, M.J.; Selby, E.A. Emotional awareness: A transdiagnostic predictor of depression and anxiety for children and adolescents. *J. Clin. Child Adolesc. Psychol.* **2016**, *45*, 262–269. [CrossRef]
38. Schäfer, J.Ö.; Naumann, E.; Holmes, E.A.; Tuschen-Caffier, B.; Samson, A.C. Emotion regulation strategies in depressive and anxiety symptoms in youth: A meta-analytic review. *J. Youth Adolesc.* **2017**, *46*, 261–276. [CrossRef]
39. Ehrenreich, J.T.; Goldstein, C.R.; Wright, L.R.; Barlow, D.H. Development of a Unified Protocol for the Treatment of Emotional Disorders in Youth. *Child Fam. Behav. Ther.* **2009**, *31*, 20–37. [CrossRef]
40. Barlow, D.H.; Allen, L.B.; Choate, M.L. Toward a unified treatment for emotional disorders. *Behav. Ther.* **2004**, *35*, 205–230. [CrossRef]
41. Garber, J.; Brunwasser, S.M.; Zerr, A.A.; Schwartz, K.T.; Sova, K.; Weersing, V.R. Treatment and prevention of depression and anxiety in youth: Test of cross-over effects. *Depress. Anxiety* **2016**, *33*, 939–959. [CrossRef]
42. Van Voorhees, B.W.; Watson, N.; Bridges, J.F.P.; Fogel, J.; Galas, J.; Kramer, C.; Connery, M.; McGill, A.; Marko, M.; Cardenas, A.; et al. Development and pilot study of a marketing strategy for primary care/internet-based depression prevention intervention for adolescents (the CATCH-IT intervention). *Prim. Care Companion J. Clin. Psychiatry* **2010**, *12*, PCC.09m00791. [CrossRef]

43. Gladstone, T.G.; Marko-Holguin, M.; Rothberg, P.; Nidetz, J.; Diehl, A.; DeFrino, D.T.; Harris, M.; Ching, E.; Eder, M.; Canel, J.; et al. An internet-based adolescent depression preventive intervention: Study protocol for a randomized control trial. *Trials* **2015**, *16*, 203. [CrossRef] [PubMed]
44. Van Voorhees, B.W.; Fogel, J.; Reinecke, M.A.; Gladstone, T.; Stuart, S.; Gollan, J.; Bradford, N.; Domanico, R.; Fagan, B.; Ross, R.; et al. Randomized clinical trial of an Internet-based depression prevention program for adolescents (Project CATCH-IT) in primary care: 12-week outcomes. *J. Dev. Behav. Pediatrics* **2009**, *30*, 23–37. [CrossRef] [PubMed]
45. Richards, K.; Marko-Holguin, M.; Fogel, J.; Anker, L.; Ronayne, J.; Van Voorhees, B.W. Randomized clinical trial of an internet-based intervention to prevent adolescent depression in a primary care setting (Catch-It): 2.5-year outcomes. *J. Evid. Based Psychother.* **2016**, *16*, 113. [PubMed]
46. Christensen, H.; Griffiths, K.M. The prevention of depression using the Internet. *Med. J. Aust.* **2002**, *177*, S122–S125. [CrossRef] [PubMed]
47. Ip, P.; Chim, D.; Chan, K.L.; Li, T.M.; Ho, F.K.W.; Van Voorhees, B.W.; Tiwari, A.; Tsang, A.; Chan, C.W.L.; Ho, M. Effectiveness of a culturally attuned Internet-based depression prevention program for Chinese adolescents: A randomized controlled trial. *Depress. Anxiety* **2016**, *33*, 1123–1131. [CrossRef] [PubMed]
48. Van Voorhees, B.G.T.; Sobowale, K.; Brown, C.H.; Aaby, D.; Terrizzi, P.; Canel, J.; Ching, E.; Berry, A.; Cantorna, J. 24-Month Outcomes of Primary Care Web-Based Depression Prevention Intervention in Adolescents: Randomized Clinical Trial. *J. Med. Internet Res.* **2020**, *22*. [CrossRef]
49. Curran, G.M.; Bauer, M.; Mittman, B.; Pyne, J.M.; Stetler, C. Effectiveness-implementation hybrid designs: Combining elements of clinical effectiveness and implementation research to enhance public health impact. *Med. Care* **2012**, *50*, 217. [CrossRef]
50. Mahoney, N.; Gladstone, T.; DeFrino, D.; Stinson, A.; Nidetz, J.; Canel, J.; Ching, E.; Berry, A.; Cantorna, J.; Fogel, J.; et al. Prevention of Adolescent Depression in Primary Care: Barriers and Relational Work Solutions. *Calif. J. Health Promot.* **2017**, *15*, 1–12. [CrossRef]
51. Stuart, S.; Robertson, M. *Interpersonal Psychotherapy: A Clinician's Guide*; Oxford University Press: New York, NY, USA, 2003.
52. Jacobson, N.S.; Martell, C.R.; Dimidjian, S. Behavioral activation treatment for depression: Returning to contextual roots. *Clin. Psychol.* **2001**, *8*, 255–270. [CrossRef]
53. Gagne, R.M.; Briggs, L.J.; Wagner, W. *Principles of Instructional Design*; HBJ College: Fort Worth, TX, USA, 1992.
54. Van Voorhees, B.W.; Gladstone, T.; Cordel, S.; Marko-Holguin, M.; Beardslee, W.; Kuwabara, S.; Kaplan, M.A.; Fogel, J.; Diehl, A.; Hansen, C.; et al. Development of a technology-based behavioral vaccine to prevent adolescent depression: A health system integration model. *Internet Interv.* **2015**, *2*, 303–313. [CrossRef]
55. Kaufman, J.; Birmaher, B.; Brent, D.; Rao, U.; Flynn, C.; Moreci, P.; Williamson, D.; Ryan, N. Schedule for affective disorders and schizophrenia for school-age children-present and lifetime version (K-SADS-PL): Initial reliability and validity data. *J. Am. Acad. Child Adolesc. Psychiatry* **1997**, *36*, 980–988. [CrossRef] [PubMed]
56. Radloff, L.S. The use of the Center for Epidemiologic Studies Depression Scale in adolescents and young adults. *J. Youth Adolesc.* **1991**, *20*, 149–166. [CrossRef] [PubMed]
57. Birmaher, B.; Khetarpal, S.; Brent, D.; Cully, M.; Balach, L.; Kaufman, J.; Neer, S.M. The screen for child anxiety related emotional disorders (SCARED): Scale construction and psychometric characteristics. *J. Am. Acad. Child Adolesc. Psychiatry* **1997**, *36*, 545–553. [CrossRef] [PubMed]
58. Silva, R.R.; Alpert, M.; Pouget, E.; Silva, V.; Trosper, S.; Reyes, K.; Dummit, S. A rating scale for disruptive behavior disorders, based on the DSM-IV item pool. *Psychiatr. Q.* **2005**, *76*, 327–339. [CrossRef] [PubMed]
59. Weissman, M.M.; Orvaschel, H.; Padian, N. Children's symptom and social functioning: Self-report scales. *J. Nerv. Ment. Disord.* **1980**, *168*, 736–740. [CrossRef]
60. Beck, A.T.; Weissman, A.; Lester, D.; Trexler, L. The measurement of pessimism: The hopelessness scale. *J. Consult. Clin. Psychol.* **1974**, *42*, 861. [CrossRef]
61. Schaefer, E.S. A configurational analysis of children's reports of parent behavior. *J. Consult. Psychol.* **1965**, *29*, 552. [CrossRef]
62. Armitage, C.J.; Conner, M. Efficacy of the theory of planned behaviour: A meta-analytic review. *Br. J. Soc. Psychol.* **2001**, *40*, 471–499. [CrossRef]
63. Prochaska, J.O.; Velicer, W.F.; DiClemente, C.C.; Fava, J. Measuring processes of change: Applications to the cessation of smoking. *J. Consult. Clin. Psychol.* **1988**, *56*, 520. [CrossRef]

64. Hankin, B.L.; Abramson, L.Y. Measuring cognitive vulnerability to depression in adolescence: Reliability, validity, and gender differences. *J. Clin. Child Adolesc. Psychol.* **2002**, *31*, 491–504. [CrossRef]
65. Van Voorhees, B.W.; Vanderplough-Booth, K.; Fogel, J.; Gladstone, T.; Bell, C.; Stuart, S.; Gollan, J.; Bradford, N.; Domanico, R.; Fagan, B. Integrative internet-based depression prevention for adolescents: A randomized clinical trial in primary care for vulnerability and protective factors. *J. Can. Acad. Child Adolesc. Psychiatry* **2008**, *17*, 184. [PubMed]
66. Compton, S.N.; March, J.S.; Brent, D.; Albano, A.M.; Weersing, V.R.; Curry, J. Cognitive-behavioral psychotherapy for anxiety and depressive disorders in children and adolescents: An evidence-based medicine review. *J. Am. Acad. Child Adolesc. Psychiatry* **2004**, *43*, 930–959. [CrossRef] [PubMed]
67. Hudson, J.L.; Rapee, R.M.; Deveney, C.; Schniering, C.A.; Lyneham, H.J.; Bovopoulos, N. Cognitive-behavioral treatment versus an active control for children and adolescents with anxiety disorders: A randomized trial. *J. Am. Acad. Child Adolesc. Psychiatry* **2009**, *48*, 533–544. [CrossRef] [PubMed]
68. Martin, F.; Oliver, T. Behavioural activation for children and young people: A systematic review of progress and promise. *Eur. Child Adolesc. Psychiatry* **2019**, *28*, 427–441. [CrossRef] [PubMed]
69. Gladstone, T.R.; Diehl, A.; Thomann, L.O.; Beardslee, W.R. The Association Between Parental Depression and Child Psychosocial Intervention Outcomes: Directions for Future Research. *Harv. Rev. Psychiatry* **2019**, *27*, 241–253. [CrossRef] [PubMed]
70. Eckshtain, D.; Marchette, L.K.; Schleider, J.; Weisz, J.R. Parental depressive symptoms as a predictor of outcome in the treatment of child depression. *J. Abnorm. Child Psychol.* **2018**, *46*, 825–837. [CrossRef] [PubMed]
71. Legerstee, J.; Huizink, A.; Van Gastel, W.; Liber, J.M.; Treffers, P.; Verhulst, F.C.; Utens, E. Maternal anxiety predicts favourable treatment outcomes in anxiety-disordered adolescents. *Acta Psychiatr. Scand.* **2008**, *117*, 289–298. [CrossRef]
72. Toren, P.; Wolmer, L.; Rosental, B.; Eldar, S.; Koren, S.; Lask, M.; Weizman, R.; Laor, N. Case series: Brief parent-child group therapy for childhood anxiety disorders using a manual-based cognitive-behavioral technique. *J. Am. Acad. Child Adolesc. Psychiatry* **2000**, *39*, 1309–1312. [CrossRef]
73. Gordon, M.; Antshel, K.M.; Lewandowski, L. Predictors of treatment outcome in a child and adolescent psychiatry clinic: A naturalistic exploration. *Child. Youth Serv. Rev.* **2012**, *34*, 213–217. [CrossRef]
74. Solanto, M.V. Commentary: Development of a new, much-needed, cognitive-behavioral intervention for adolescents with ADHD–a reflection on Sprich et al.(2016). *J. Child Psychol. Psychiatry* **2016**, *57*, 1227–1228. [CrossRef]

Publisher's Note: MDPI stays neutral with regard to jurisdictional claims in published maps and institutional affiliations.

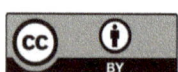

© 2020 by the authors. Licensee MDPI, Basel, Switzerland. This article is an open access article distributed under the terms and conditions of the Creative Commons Attribution (CC BY) license (http://creativecommons.org/licenses/by/4.0/).

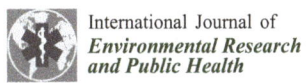

Article

Clinical Utility of an Internet-Delivered Version of the Unified Protocol for Transdiagnostic Treatment of Emotional Disorders in Adolescents (iUP-A): A Pilot Open Trial

Bonifacio Sandín, Julia García-Escalera, Rosa M. Valiente *, Victoria Espinosa and Paloma Chorot

Facultad de Psicología, Universidad Nacional de Educación a Distancia (UNED), 20040 Madrid, Spain; bsandin@psi.uned.es (B.S.); jgarciaescalera@psi.uned.es (J.G.-E.); vespinosa36@alumno.uned.es (V.E.); pchorot@psi.uned.es (P.C.)
* Correspondence: rmvalien@psi.uned.es

Received: 30 September 2020; Accepted: 6 November 2020; Published: 10 November 2020

Abstract: The Unified Protocol for Transdiagnostic Treatment of Emotional Disorders in Adolescents (UP-A) has been shown to be effective for reducing symptoms of anxiety and depression in adolescents with emotional disorders. Internet-delivered psychological treatments have great potential to improve access to evidence-based psychological therapy since they are associated with reduced human and economic costs and less social stigma. Recently, our group developed an online version of the UP-A (the iUP-A) for the treatment of emotional disorders in adolescents. The aim of this pilot trial was to test the clinical utility of the iUP-A in a small sample ($n = 12$) of adolescents with elevated anxiety and/or depressive symptoms. Intention-to-treat and completer analyses revealed pre- to post-intervention self-reported decreases of anxiety and depressive symptoms, anxiety sensitivity, emotional avoidance, panic disorder symptoms, panic disorder severity, generalized anxiety disorder symptoms, pathological worry, and major depressive disorder symptoms. We found high feasibility and acceptability of the program with all participants and responsible parents reporting an improvement in the adolescents' ability to cope with emotions. Results suggest that the iUP-A may provide a new approach to improve access to treatment for anxious and depressive adolescents in Spain; however, further research must be conducted before firm conclusions can be drawn.

Keywords: transdiagnostic; iUP-A; i-CBT; AMTE; anxiety; depression; adolescents; online therapy

1. Introduction

Anxiety and depression in youth represent a growing public health concern. Epidemiological studies indicate that as many as 32.4% and 10.6% of adolescents have lifetime prevalence rates of anxiety and depressive disorders, respectively [1]. Anxiety and depression have been associated with severe impairment and increased risk for future psychopathological problems [2]. Subclinical symptoms of anxiety and depression are also very prevalent (32% and 29.2%, respectively) and have been related to functional impairment and suicidality [3]. In addition to the high prevalence of these emotional disorders, anxiety and depression are overlapping conditions throughout the lifespan, with rates of comorbidity as high as 75% in clinical samples [4]. Children and adolescents with anxiety and mood disorders also share a number of underlying vulnerability and maintenance factors, such as temperament (e.g., negative affect), difficulty regulating affect across emotions (e.g., behavioral avoidance), and clinical dispositions to experiment negative reactions to emotions (e.g., anxiety sensitivity) [5,6].

Evidence-based cognitive-behavioral therapy (CBT) for anxiety and depressive disorders has traditionally been disorder-specific, i.e., focused on treating one disorder at a time without paying therapeutic attention to comorbid conditions. In contrast, the transdiagnostic approach tries to address this limitation by focusing on the shared features of anxiety and depressive disorders rather than on the symptoms specific to each of these disorders [7]. In line with this perspective, transdiagnostic CBT (T-CBT) for emotional disorders has emerged as a new therapeutic approach that targets psychopathological processes common to both anxiety and depression. Addressing emotional disorders' risk and maintenance factors during adolescence may also help prevent the development of anxiety and depression later in life. The efficacy of T-CBT for emotional disorders has been found to be high and comparable to disorder-specific CBT treatments' efficacy in recent meta-analyses [8–10].

The Unified Protocols for Transdiagnostic Treatment of Emotional Disorders in Children (UP-C) and Adolescents (UP-A) are recent manualized treatments developed by Ehrenreich-May et al. [11] to address a broad array of emotional disorders' symptoms in children and adolescents. Both protocols take a transdiagnostic approach by focusing on a set of core change principles including prevention of emotional avoidance (effortful engagement in experiencing intense emotions), enhancement of cognitive flexibility (evaluation of potentially problematic cognitions), and change of maladaptive action tendencies (encouraging youth to alter problematic behavioral patterns related to their emotional symptoms). These protocols place particular emphasis on emotion regulation since a goal of these treatments is to help patients to learn how to experience uncomfortable emotions and how to respond to them in more adaptive and non-avoidant ways. The UP-C and UP-A are flexible administered treatment protocols designed to improve emotion reactivity and emotion regulation and to ameliorate anxiety and depressive symptoms by means of an array of evidence-based treatment techniques (e.g., psychoeducation, behavioral activation, cognitive restructuring, etc.) that are applied to a range of emotions including fear, anxiety, sadness, and anger.

The UP-A has a growing body of data supporting its efficacy in treating anxiety and depressive disorders and symptoms in adolescent samples [8–15]. In a multiple-baseline trial with three adolescents, all participants experienced a reduction in the severity of their principal anxiety or depression diagnosis at post-treatment [12]. The study of Trosper et al. [15], an open trial with 12 adolescents, found significant reductions in the principal disorders' severity from pre- to post-treatment, as well as improvements in adolescents' emotion regulation according to parent ratings. In a most recent study, Ehrenreich et al. [13] demonstrated the efficacy of the UP-A in a randomized, waitlist-controlled trial including 51 adolescents with a primary diagnosis of an anxiety or depressive disorder. According to the authors, the UP-A outperformed the waitlist condition since significant treatment effects were found in favor of the UP-A on all outcome measures. Additionally, at post-treatment participants in the UP-A condition showed lower diagnostic severity and greater improvements according to clinician-rated measures compared to those in the waitlist condition.

Recently, our group has reported data concerning the Spanish validation of the UP-A adapted as a universal school-based prevention program of anxiety and depression [16,17]. In an open-trial including 28 adolescents, significant self-reported decreases from pre- to post-intervention were found in anxiety outcome measures [17]; in addition, this study also provided support for the acceptability and feasibility of the Spanish version of the UP-A. In a more recent publication using the Spanish UP-A, results of a randomized waitlist-controlled trial including 151 school adolescents revealed that those participants with greater baseline emotional symptoms in the UP-A group trended toward significantly greater decreases in depression symptoms compared to the control group [16].

Internet-delivered psychological treatments represent an emerging model of service delivery with the potential to improve access to evidence-based treatments for anxiety and depressive disorders [18]. It has been suggested that internet-based treatments have several advantages compared with traditional face-to-face interventions, including improved access to evidence-based treatments and cost-effectiveness [19]. As these authors suggested, the fact that patients can return to the program at their convenience to access treatment information may facilitate learning and retention. Additionally, patients in internet interventions may receive therapist support faster than they would in traditional face-to-face treatments and may feel less stigma than when attending traditional psychological therapy. Several reviews and meta-analyses have shown comparable reductions in anxiety and depression symptoms from internet-based CBT (iCBT) and face-to-face CBT in adults [18,20,21], children, and adolescents [22].

A transdiagnostic iCBT treatment (T-iCBT) was recently developed by Titov's group to treat anxiety and depression [18]. In a similar vein, Botella's group developed a T-iCBT protocol based on Barlow's UP [23] designed to treat emotional disorders in adults [24]. Several meta-analyses have shown that T-iCBT protocols could be effective in the reduction of anxious and depressive symptomatology [9,25]. Recently, our group has developed an internet-based version of the UP-A (i.e., the iUP-A) [26]. As far as we know, this is the first T-iCBT treatment that targets anxiety and depression in adolescents, as well as the first adaptation of the UP-A into a web-based or online format.

The aim of this pilot trial was to test the clinical utility, feasibility, and acceptability of the iUP-A in a small sample of adolescents living in Spain. We hypothesized to find a significant change from pre- to post-treatment in: (a) primary outcome measures (general levels of anxiety and depression), (b) transdiagnostic variables (positive and negative affect, anxiety sensitivity, and emotional avoidance), and (c) disorder-specific measures (symptoms of anxiety and depressive disorders, panic disorder severity, pathological worry, and symptoms of social anxiety). Specifically, we hypothesized that participants would evidence a significant reduction in all outcome measures at posttreatment compared to pretreatment levels, except for positive affect where we expected to find a significant increase. A second aim of the study was to examine the feasibility and acceptability of the iUP-A and of the web platform that implements it, called Learn to Manage your Emotions (Aprende a Manejar tus Emociones; AMTE).

2. Materials and Methods

2.1. Participants

Families were recruited through information posted by the Universidad Nacional de Educación a Distancia (UNED) on Twitter and on the UNED's website as well as through school counselors' referrals. The inclusion criteria for the adolescents were: (a) 12 to 18 years of age; (b) meeting diagnostic criteria for any anxiety and/or depressive disorder or having subthreshold anxiety and/or depression symptoms based on the Mini International Neuropsychiatric Interview (MINI) [27,28] at assessment; (c) having an e-mail address and daily access to the internet through a computer or electronic tablet; (d) stability of psychotropic medications (if any) for at least three months; (e) Spanish proficiency.

Exclusion criteria were: (a) a diagnosis of a severe psychopathology such as psychotic disorder, bipolar disorder, severe depressive disorder, intellectual disability, severe learning disability, autism spectrum disorder, or substance dependence; (b) being at moderate or severe risk for suicide (based on the MINI); (c) on-going psychological treatment; (d) no informed consent.

A total of 23 families were screened by telephone for eligibility. Participant flow through the study is presented in Figure 1. Post-treatment data were available for eight participants, all of whom completed the eight modules of the iUP-A. A total of four adolescents dropped out of the study, three reported being dissatisfied with the program whereas one reported a lack of time for the intervention. Of these four adolescents, two finished the first module, one finished the first four modules and one finished the first five modules.

A total of 12 adolescents met the inclusion criteria and were included in the study. There were eight girls (67%) and four boys (M age = 15.58 years old; SD = 1.73; range = 13 to 18). All adolescents were Spanish residents. Regarding the living situation, 10 adolescents (83.3%) were living with both of their parents whereas two were living with their mother and siblings due to parents' divorce. In all cases (100%), the gender of the parent responsible for treatment was female.

None of the enrolled participants were taking psychotropic medication and only one had previously received psychological treatment (for a total of 10 sessions). Lastly, five adolescents (41.7%) were waiting for an appointment in the mental health department of the Spanish public healthcare system after being referred by their general practitioner or family doctor.

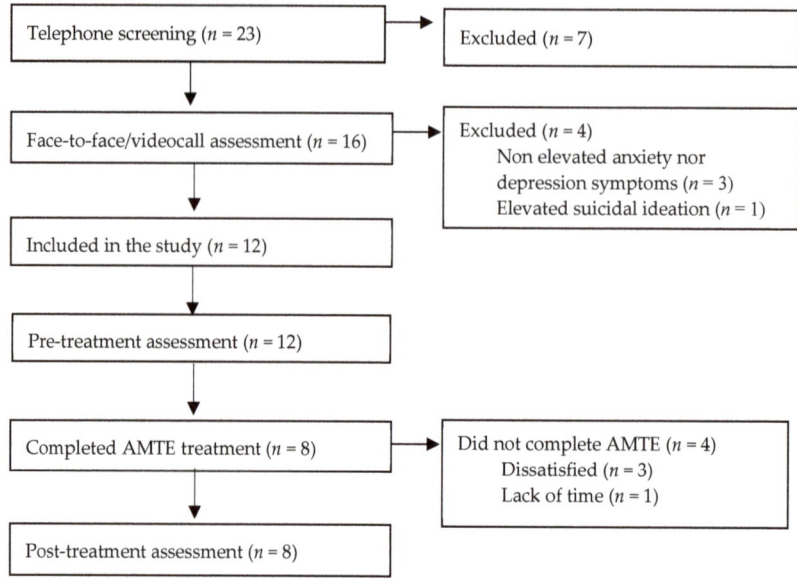

Figure 1. Participant flow through the study.

Regarding participants' diagnoses, nine participants (75%) were diagnosed with some clinical disorder whereas three showed subthreshold anxiety and/or depressive symptoms (see Table 1).

Table 1. Diagnoses or symptoms of the 12 participants.

Principal Diagnosis/Symptoms	Comorbid Diagnoses/Symptoms
Social phobia	Depressive symptoms
Bulimia	Major depressive disorder
Anxiety and depressive symptoms	—
Social phobia	—
Major depressive disorder	Generalized anxiety disorder
Panic disorder with agoraphobia	Obsessive-compulsive disorder
Anxiety symptoms	—
Hypomanic episode–current and past	Separation anxiety disorder; Obsessive-compulsive disorder; Oppositional defiant disorder
Depressive symptoms	—
Panic disorder without agoraphobia	—
Major depressive disorder	Posttraumatic stress disorder
Posttraumatic stress disorder	Agoraphobia; Social phobia; Obsessive-compulsive disorder; Transient TIC Disorder

2.2. Procedure and Design

This study employed an uncontrolled pre-post open trial design. It was granted ethical approval from the Research Ethics Committee of the UNED and was registered on Clinicaltrials.gov (Identifier NCT04182061). The TREND Statement guidelines for nonrandomized interventions [29] were followed when reporting the trial. No incentives were provided to the adolescents or parents for participating in this trial.

Recruitment was carried out in two steps: a telephone screening with the responsible parent and a face-to-face or video call assessment. Once the telephone screening had been made and the informed consent had been signed and returned, potential participants and their parents were invited to an assessment session that was conducted either face-to-face or through video call. In this session, a clinical psychologist conducted a full diagnostic interview with the adolescent and briefly talked with the parent(s) to gain insight regarding their concerns about the adolescents' main problems and symptoms.

Following the assessment session, the adolescents meeting inclusion criteria were included in the study and both the responsible parent and the adolescent received an e-mail to register on the web platform Aprende a Manejar tus Emociones (AMTE) (Learn to Manage your Emotions). Then, one week before the intervention started, the adolescents were invited to fill in the self-report measures (see the Instruments section) on the AMTE platform. A week after the intervention ended, the adolescents were also invited to fill in the same self-report measures on the AMTE platform.

2.3. Intervention

The internet UP-A (iUP-A) was delivered by means of the AMTE platform. The iUP-A was adapted from the Unified Protocol for Transdiagnostic Treatment of Emotional Disorders in Adolescents (UP-A) [30].

As does the UP-A, the iUP-A uses evidence-based treatment techniques that cut across disorder-specific CBT treatment manuals for adolescent anxiety and depression (e.g., psychoeducation, cognitive restructuring, exposure, behavioral activation, relapse prevention, etc.). It also includes motivational enhancement as well as mindfulness-based techniques. The AMTE program includes the same eight core modules of the UP-A and participants are advised to complete one module per week (except for module seven, which usually takes one more week to complete). Table 2 provides an overview of the structure and specific topics address in the eight treatment modules.

Table 2. Descriptions of the modules (M) included in the AMTE platform.

Module Title	Main Contents
[M1] Building motivation	Obtain three top problems, severity ratings, and a goal for each problem. Discover what motivates the adolescent to change.
[M2] Getting to know your emotions	Psychoeducation about emotions and their function. Understand the three parts of emotional experiences. Learn about emotional behaviors and the cycle of avoidance.
[M3] Enjoy positive activities	Psychoeducation about opposite action and behavioral experiments. Come up with a list of enjoyed activities. Engage the adolescent in behavioral experiments (behavioral activation) for sadness.
[M4] Awareness of your emotional experiences	Introduce the rationale for present-moment awareness and non-judgmental awareness. Practice body scanning. Practice awareness skills when exposed to non emotional and emotional triggers.
[M5] Learn to be flexible in your thinking	Learn about the concept of "thinking traps" (i.e., cognitive distortions), automatic thoughts, and alternative thoughts. Learn detective thinking and problem-solving skills.
[M6] Cope with your body sensations	Psychoeducation about body sensations, their relationship with intense emotions, and their harmlessness. Conduct exposures to body sensations to learn to tolerate uncomfortable physical feelings.
[M7] Cope with emotional situations	Review the cycle of avoidance and introduce situational emotion exposures. Create an Emotional Behaviors Form to identify relevant exposures. Assign exposures for home learning.
[M8] Maintain your gains	Review skills that have been most useful for each adolescent and make an individualized relapse prevention plan.

The intervention can be used on (laptop) computers and tablets. Parents log in to a separate section of the program and have access to a summary of each module as well as to information regarding the progress of their adolescent in treatment. The therapists log in to a therapists' section of the AMTE platform where they can monitor the progression of each adolescent in the treatment (last access to the platform, progression in the treatment modules, time spent on the platform, etc.) and see the adolescent's answers to the home learning assignments.

The treatment platform was designed with an age-appropriate appearance. The first time the adolescents log in, they personalize an avatar (virtual human) by changing its hair, skin color, clothing, and gender. The platform AMTE uses a narrator (called "Doctor") that presents treatment contents through written messages whereas the avatar presents encouraging written messages to the participant. The AMTE platform uses an island overarching theme (see Figure 2).

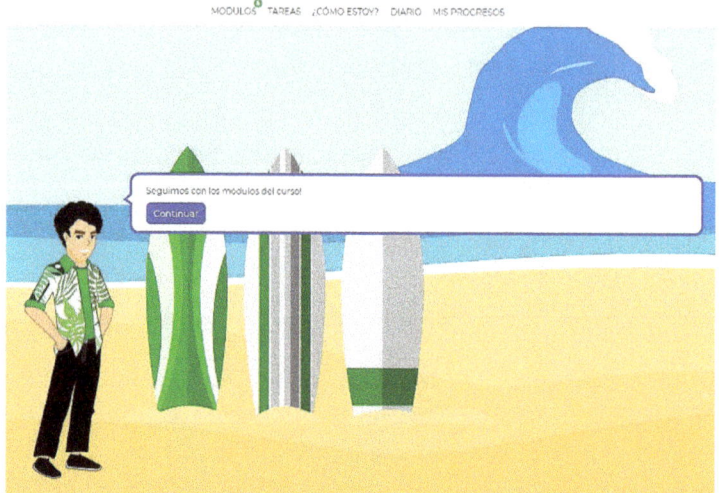

Figure 2. Screenshot of the AMTE homepage.

Each module contains written texts presented by the Doctor or the avatar, explanatory videos, exercises, home learning assignments, and downloadable PDFs (with the exercises, the home learning assignments, and summaries of each module). The expected time to complete each module (contents, exercises, and home learning assignments) is approximately 50 min. The AMTE platform is interactive with responses to home learning assignments being directly entered into the program and saved so that the therapist can immediately review the adolescent's progress. Participants may also initiate contact with the therapists by sending messages via the AMTE platform whenever they have questions or want to discuss any aspects of the treatment.

During the treatment period, both the adolescent and the treatment responsible parent had weekly telephone contact with their assigned clinical psychologist, the same one that did the face-to-face or videocall assessment. The psychologist called the responsible parent's cell phone, spoke for about 10 min with the parent (to check on the parent's main concerns regarding the adolescent and address any problems that may have arisen) and for another 10 min or so with the adolescent (to review the participant's responses to the home learning assignments and support the adolescent in using the program).

2.4. Instruments

The clinical diagnoses were conducted by means of the MINI [27,28]. The questionnaires EAN [31], CDN [31], and the total score on the RCADS-30 [32] were used as primary outcome measures. To assess transdiagnostic constructs the questionnaires PANASN [33], CASI [34,35], and EASI-A [36,37] were used. Disorder-specific symptoms of anxiety and depressive disorders were assessed through the RCADS-30 subscales [32], and the questionnaires PSWQ-11 [38], SASC-R [39,40], and PDSS-SR [39–42].

Finally, the Feasibility and Acceptability Questionnaire (FAQ) was used to assess the experiences of the adolescents and parents with the program.

Mini International Neuropsychiatric Interview for Children and Adolescents (MINI-KID) [27,28]. The MINI-KID is a structured diagnostic interview for people aged 6 to 17 years. It is based on DSM-IV and ICD-10 criteria for psychiatric disorders. The reliability and validity of MINI-KID has been demonstrated [43].

Revised Child Anxiety and Depression Scale–30 (RCADS-30) [32]. The RCADS-30 is a 30-item self-report scale comprised of the following subscales derived from the Diagnostic and Statistical Manual of Mental Disorders (DSM-IV/5) criteria: (1) social phobia (Soc.P), (2) generalized anxiety disorder (GAD), (3) obsessive-compulsive disorder (OCD), (4) panic disorder (PD), (5) separation anxiety disorder (SAD), and (6) major depressive disorder (MDD). This scale has previously demonstrated good psychometric properties [7]. Each item is scored from zero ("never") to three ("always"), with higher scores representing more severe symptoms.

Anxiety Scale for Children (Escala de Ansiedad para Niños, EAN) [31]. The EAN is a 10-item self-report scale that assesses anxiety symptoms in children and adolescents. It has shown good psychometric properties [16]. The participants are instructed to indicate how frequently they have experienced general anxiety symptoms (cognitive, physiological, etc.) on a four-point, Likert-type scale, ranging from zero ("never or almost never") to three ("always or almost always").

Depression Questionnaire for Children (Cuestionario de Depresión para Niños; CDN) [31]. The CDN scale is a 16-item, self-report questionnaire designed to assess symptoms of major depressive disorder and dysthymic disorder (according to DSM-IV/5 criteria) in children and adolescents. Participants rate each item on a four-point, Likert-type scale, ranging from zero ("never or almost never") to three ("always or almost always"). The CDN has demonstrated good psychometric properties [16,32].

Positive and Negative Affect Schedule for Children and Adolescents (Escalas PANAS de Afecto Positivo y Negativo para Niños y Adolescentes; PANASN) [33]. The PANASN provides scores for two subscales of 10 items each measuring positive and negative affect. Participants are asked to rate items according to how they usually feel from one ("never or almost never") to three ("a lot of the time"). This self-report scale has demonstrated adequate psychometric properties [32].

Childhood Anxiety Sensitivity Index (CASI) [34,35]. The CASI is an 18-item self-report questionnaire measuring anxiety sensitivity in children and adolescents, that is, distress reactions to symptoms of anxiety. Participants rate the frequency with which they experience each item using a three-point, Likert-type scale from one ("never") to three ("a lot of the time"). The Spanish adaptation of the CASI used in the present study has demonstrated good psychometric properties in previous studies [44].

Emotional Avoidance Strategy Inventory for Adolescents (EASI-A) [36,37]. The EASI-A is a 17-item self-report questionnaire in which respondents are instructed to indicate the degree to which each statement is true using a five-point, Likert-type scale ranging from zero ("never or almost never") to four ("always or almost always").

PSWQ-11 questionnaire for children and adolescents (PSWQN-11) [38]. It is an age-downward version of the 11-item Penn State Worry Questionnaire [45]. This 11-item self-report questionnaire assesses pathological worry. Respondents are instructed to indicate the degree to which they agree with each statement using a five-point Likert-type scale from one ("Totally disagree") to five ("totally agree").

Social Anxiety Scale for Children-Revised (SASC-R) [39,40]. The SASC-R is an 18-item self-report questionnaire in which respondents are instructed to indicate the frequency with which they experience each symptom of social anxiety using a four-point Likert-type scale from one ("never") to three ("a lot of the time").

Panic Disorder Severity Scale—Self-Report (PDSS—SR) [41]. The abbreviated adapted version by Sandin (2010) [42] was used. The PDSS—SR is a seven-item self-report questionnaire that assesses the severity of the panic disorder in the last month. Using a five-point Likert-type scale from zero ("not at all") to four ("very much"), participants rate the distress associated with panic attacks, anticipatory anxiety regarding new attacks, and interoceptive and situational avoidance. This scale has demonstrated adequate psychometric properties in adult samples [46].

Feasibility and Acceptability Questionnaire (FAQ) [47]. This questionnaire includes a version for the adolescents and a version for the parents. Both versions include three separate sections (subscales) each comprised of six items: (1) experience with the online platform, (2) satisfaction with the program, and (3) therapeutic alliance. All items are assessed on an 11-point scale from 0 ("totally disagree") to 10 ("totally agree"). The parents' version includes an additional section that assesses the experience of the treatment responsible parent with the parents' section of the online platform. This section includes two items. The satisfaction with the program section of the FAQ includes the six questions from the satisfaction questionnaire of Rapee et al. (2006) [48].

2.5. Statistical Analysis

All statistical analyses were done with the SPSS v.24 software program (IBM Corp., Armonk, NY, USA). For the completer sample ($n = 8$), changes in the outcome scores between pre- and post-treatment were examined using the Wilcoxon signed-rank test, a nonparametric alternative to paired samples t-test. In addition to the completer analyses, calculations were repeated with the total sample ($n = 12$) after replacing missing values for the dropout cases with their last observation carried forward (LOCF). To gain further insight into the statistical significance of the improvements, effect sizes were calculated for all outcome measures using Cohen's d (meanpre-meanpost/pooled SD) [49]. Before the statistical analysis of the data, we computed the statistical power (with an alpha error of 0.05, one-tailed) of the Wilcoxon signed-rank test (matched pairs) using the G*Power 3.1.9.7 [50]. The statistical power ranged from 75% to 100% (average = 96.7%) for the statistically significant outcome measures (described in Tables 3 and 4); the power was 57% for the two marginally significant variables (SAD subscale of the RCADAS-30) and 87% PANASN-Positive Affect.

Table 3. Means (M), standard deviations (SD), Wilcoxon tests, and effect sizes (Cohen's d) for primary (CDN, EAN, and RCADS-30 total score) and disorder-specific (subscales of the RCADS-30) outcome measures.

Measures	Pre-Treatment $n = 12$		Post-Treatment $n = 8$		Completer Sample Analyses $n = 8$		Intention-to-Treat Analyses [b] $n = 12$
	M	SD	M	SD	Z [a]	d	d
CDN	19.17	11.50	15.25	8.92	1.47	1.14	0.66
EAN	14.50	8.58	10.88	5.82	2.38 **	2.36	1.43
RCADS-30							
Total	32.58	18.43	24.25	9.68	2.38 **	4.14	2.58
MDD	6.42	4.08	4.88	3.23	2.05 *	0.96	0.58
PD	4.83	5.11	1.75	1.98	1.99 *	2.54	1.75
Soc.P	8.58	4.40	8.25	3.49	1.06	0.88	0.52
SAD	1.25	1.54	0.88	1.13	1.84 +	0.74	0.52
GAD	7.33	3.80	5.88	2.10	2.21 *	2.27	1.25
OCD	4.17	4.59	2.63	1.85	1.10	1.32	0.93

Note. [a] Z Wilcoxon test based on positive ranks (exact signification, one-tailed). [b] Z values are identical to those of the completer sample. CDN = Depression Questionnaire for Children; EAN = Anxiety Scale for Children; GAD = generalized anxiety disorder; MDD = major depressive disorder; OCD = obsessive compulsive disorder; PD = panic disorder; RCADS-30 = Revised Child Anxiety and Depression Scale-30; SAD = separation anxiety disorder; Soc.P = social phobia. + $p < 0.10$; * $p < 0.05$; ** $p < 0.01$.

Table 4. Means (M), standard deviations (SD), Wilcoxon test and effect sizes (Cohen's d) for transdiagnostic (PANAS, CASI and EASI) and disorder-specific (PDSS-SR, PSWQ-N, and SASC-R) outcome measures.

Measures	Pre-Treatment n = 12		Post-Treatment n = 8		Completer Sample Analyses n = 8		Intention-to-Treat Analyses [b] n = 12
	M	SD	M	SD	Z [a]	d	d
PANASN-NA	21.08	2.91	20.75	2.66	0.50	0.53	0.35
PANASN-PA	20.50	3.80	23.38	4.27	1.47 +	−1.13	−0.73
CASI	31.92	8.52	29.00	4.66	2.22 *	2.87	1.74
EASI-A	37.25	16.24	32.13	12.91	1.82 *	2.97	1.19
PDSS-SR	10.58	8.03	2.75	3.49	2.52 **	4.82	2.59
PSWQ-N	32.92	12.92	27.25	5.42	2.39 **	3.40	2.30
SASC-R	37.67	10.82	40.88	5.79	0.42	0.67	0.37

Note. [a] Z Wilcoxon test based on positive ranks (exact signification, 1-tailed) (for PANAS-PA, the Z score was based on negative ranks). [b] Z values are identical to those of the completer sample. CASI = Childhood Anxiety Sensitivity Index; EASI-A = Emotional Avoidance Strategy Inventory for Adolescents; FNE = Fear of Negative Evaluation; PANASN-NA = Negative Affect scale of the Positive and Negative Affect Schedule for Children and Adolescents; PANASN-PA = Positive Affect scale of the Positive and Negative Affect Schedule for Children and Adolescents; PDSS-SR = Panic Disorder Severity Scale—Self-Report; PSWQ-N = PSWQ-11 questionnaire for children and adolescents; SASC-R = Social Anxiety Scale for Children—Revised. + $p < 0.10$; * $p < 0.05$; ** $p < 0.01$.

3. Results

3.1. Intervention Effects

A Wilcoxon matched-pairs signed-rank test including the completer sample, i.e., all the adolescents that finished the intervention ($n = 8$), showed a significant decrease in anxiety symptoms (EAN, $p = 0.008$) associated with a large effect size. Likewise, there were significant reductions in the RCADS-30 total score ($p = 0.008$), associated with a very large effect size. There were also significant reductions associated to several subscales of the RCADS-30: major depressive disorder ($p = 0.031$), panic disorder ($p = 0.031$), and generalized anxiety disorder ($p = 0.016$). Due to the small sample size, we also took into account marginally significant results ($p < 0.10$), which were found for the separation anxiety disorder subscale of the RCADS-30 ($p = 0.063$). Identical results were obtained including the intent-to-treat sample ($n = 12$); see Table 3.

Wilcoxon tests including the adolescents that finished the intervention ($n = 8$) showed significant reductions on the transdiagnostic outcome measures of anxiety sensitivity (CASI; $p = 0.016$) and emotional avoidance (EASI-A; $p = 0.039$), both associated with large effect sizes. Also, there were significant reductions in panic disorder severity (PDDSS-SR; $p = 0.004$) and pathological worry (PSWQ-N; $p = 0.008$), both associated with large within-group effect sizes. We also found that an increase in PANASN-PA from pre- to post-treatment was marginally significant ($p = 0.094$). Identical results were obtained including the intent-to-treat sample ($n = 12$); see Table 4.

3.2. Feasibility and Acceptability

3.2.1. Adolescent Report

The FAQ was completed by eight adolescents (66.66% of those who participated in the program) on a scale from 0 to 10 (see Table 5). In relation to the questions assessing experience with the program, mean ratings ranged between 7.25 and 9.38. Regarding the satisfaction with the program, the mean ratings of the first four questions ranged between 8.50 and 9.38. In addition, all adolescents reported that their ability to cope with emotions had improved significantly (mean improvement from 4.13 to 8.25). Finally, ratings on the therapeutic alliance were high with mean ratings ranging from 8.88 to 9.88.

Table 5. Descriptive statistics for the items of the FAQ (adolescent version) (n = 8).

Experience with the Online Platform (Range: 0–10)	M	SD
How easy has it been for you to use the AMTE online platform?	9.00	1.20
How easy has it been for you to understand what the videos and Dr. AMTE were telling you?	8.50	1.77
How useful has it been for you what Dr. AMTE and the different videos were teaching you?	9.38	0.92
How easy has it been for you to include the AMTE program in your daily routine?	8.50	1.60
To what degree have you been able to do the exercises and home learning assignments without technical or computer problems?	7.25	1.58
To what extent have you applied what you have learned with AMTE to your real life?	8.50	0.93
Satisfaction with the Program (Range: 0–10)	**M**	**SD**
How much did you learn in this program?	8.75	1.58
How effective was this program in helping you cope with your problems?	8.86	1.07
How much did you enjoy doing this program?	8.50	1.20
To what extent would you recommend the program to other adolescents?	9.38	0.74
What was your ability to cope with emotions before the program?	4.13	1.64
What was your ability to cope with emotions after the program?	8.25	1.39
Ability to cope with emotions after the program minus ability before	4.13	1.96
Therapeutic Alliance (Range: 0–10)	**M**	**SD**
How much has your therapist helped you deal with your top problems?	8.88	1.46
How appreciated by your therapist have you felt?	9.50	0.76
To what extent have you felt that you and your therapist respected each other?	9.88	0.35
To what extent have you agreed with your therapist on what things were important for you to work to overcome?	9.50	1.07
To what extent have you felt that your therapist cared about you?	9.38	0.92
How correct do you think the way you and your therapist have worked to solve your problems has been?	9.38	0.92

3.2.2. Parents Report

The FAQ (parent version) was also completed by eight mothers (the mothers of the eight adolescents that finished the intervention) on a scale from 0 to 10 (see Table 6). In relation to the questions assessing the experience of the adolescent with the program according to the perception of the parent, mean ratings ranged between 8.38 and 9.25. Likewise, seven mothers (out of eight) reported having logged in to the family section of the platform at least once with the mean satisfaction with the platform being 7.29. Regarding the parent perception of satisfaction of the adolescents with the program, the mean ratings of the first four questions ranged between 8 and 9.75. Also, all mothers reported that the ability of their child to cope with emotions had significantly improved (mean improvement from 4.63 to 8.00). Finally, ratings on the therapeutic alliance were very high with mean ratings ranging from 9.38 to 9.88.

Table 6. Descriptive statistics for the items of the FAQ (parent version) (n = 8).

Experience of the Adolescent with the Online Platform (Range: 0–10)	M	SD
How easy has it been for your son/daughter to use the AMTE online platform?	8.50	1.31
How easy has it been for your child to understand what the videos and Dr. AMTE were telling them?	9.25	1.04
How useful has it been for your child what Dr. AMTE and the different videos were teaching them?	8.88	1.36
How easy has it been for your child to include the AMTE program in their daily routine?	8.63	1.41
To what degree has your child been able to do the exercises and home learning assignments without technical or computer problems?	8.63	1.06
To what extent has your child applied what he/she has learned with AMTE to their real life?	8.38	1.60
Experience with the Parent's Section of the Online Platform	**n (%) [yes]**	
Have you ever logged in to the parent's section of the AMTE platform?	7 (87.50%)	
To what extent has the parent's section of the platform helped you to help your son/daughter during treatment? (range: 0–10)	7.29	2.81

Table 6. *Cont.*

Satisfaction with the Program (Range: 0–10)	M	SD
How much has your child learned in this program?	9.14	0.69
How effective was this program in helping your child cope with their problems?	9.14	1.07
How much has your child enjoyed doing this program?	8.00	2.27
To what extent would you recommend the program to other adolescents?	9.75	0.71
What was the ability of your child to cope with emotions before the program?	4.63	2.00
What was the ability of your child to cope with their emotions after the program?	8.00	1.51
Ability to cope with emotions after the program minus ability before	3.38	1.51
Therapeutic Alliance (Range: 0–10)	**M**	**SD**
How much has the therapist helped your child deal with their top problems?	9.38	0.92
How appreciated by the therapist has your child felt?	9.88	0.35
To what extent have you felt that you and the therapist respected each other?	9.88	0.35
To what extent have you agreed with the therapist on what things were important for your son/daughter to work to overcome?	9.75	0.46
To what extent have you felt that the therapist cared about your child?	9.88	0.35
How correct do you think the AMTE's approach to solving your child problems has been?	9.75	0.46

4. Discussion

The purpose of the current study was to examine the clinical utility of the UP-A adapted to an internet-delivered program (i.e., the iUP-A). We explored whether the iUP-A would significantly decrease, from pretreatment to posttreatment, the levels of (a) general measures of anxiety and depression, (b) transdiagnostic constructs (positive and negative affect, anxiety sensitivity, and emotional avoidance), and (c) disorder-specific measures (anxiety and depressive disorder symptoms, panic disorder severity, pathological worry, and social anxiety). We also examined the acceptability and feasibility of the iUP-A. As far as we know, this is the first study that examines the clinical utility of an online T-CBT program for the treatment of anxiety and depression in adolescents; thus, this is also the first evaluation of the UP-A implemented as a web-based intervention.

Consistent with our hypotheses, the participants of this study reported improvements in general symptoms of anxiety and depression, transdiagnostic measures, and disorder-specific symptomatology. According to the effect sizes' estimates, the magnitude of the changes were medium (for positive affect and symptoms of MDD, social phobia, and separation anxiety disorder), large (for anxiety sensitivity, emotional avoidance and symptoms of general anxiety, panic disorder, GAD, and OCD), and very large (for panic disorder severity, pathological worry, and general symptomatology of anxiety and depression measured by RCADS-total score). Overall, we found significant or marginally significant improvements in all variables except for general symptoms of depression (questionnaire CDN), negative affect, social anxiety, and symptoms of OCD and social phobia. One surprising finding was the lack of significant effects on positive and negative affect. Although, according to the descriptive statistics, these temperamental variables changed from pretreatment to posttreatment as expected (the positive affect increased whereas the negative affect decreased), such changes did not reach the level of statistical significance.

The findings of this open trial are particularly noteworthy because the iUP-A appears to be effective at managing the three kinds of main variables examined (general symptoms of anxiety and depression, transdiagnostic measures, and specific symptoms of several anxiety and depressive disorders). Most of these positive effects were associated with large and very large effect sizes, which is consistent with results of the UP-A reported by Ehrenreich-May's group [12,13,15], as well as with findings of our group related to the Spanish version of the UP-A [16,17]. These data are also consistent with the results reported by authors who administered Super Skills for Life, a T-CBT protocol that has been applied as an indicated prevention program for adolescents [51] and children [52] at risk of developing anxiety disorders.

The fact that the iUP-A was able to modify two major transdiagnostic variables (i.e., anxiety sensitivity and emotional avoidance) is an important strength of the present study. The core treatment modules of the UP-A, like the UP's core modules [23], were designed to explicitly target aversive reactions to emotions (e.g., anxiety sensitivity) and the subsequent emotional avoidance. These are core transdiagnostic underlying processes related to the vulnerability and maintenance of emotional disorders and, therefore, processes shared by individuals with anxiety and depression. Surprisingly, there is a lack of evidence in the literature concerning the efficacy and clinical utility of the UP and UP-A reducing the levels of these main transdiagnostic mechanisms [10]. To our knowledge, this is the first study that provides empirical evidence of the UP-A's ability to modify high levels of anxiety sensitivity and emotional avoidance in youth. The study of Calear et al. [53] used the same scale we used to measure anxiety sensitivity (i.e., the CASI) but did not obtain significant results. Concerning affectivity, although some studies have shown the ability of the UP to produce changes in negative affect (or neuroticism) and positive affect (or extraversion) [10,54] we did not find such an effect.

This is the first trial that examines the feasibility and acceptability of an internet-based version of the UP-A. Regarding feasibility, the attrition rate in this study was 33.33%, a percentage comparable to studies that have evaluated face-to-face transdiagnostic treatments for anxiety and depressive disorders in adults [55], children [56], and adolescents [13]. Other authors have reported lower rates of adherence in studies based on computerized treatments. For example, Stallard et al. [57] reported an adherence rate of 60% for a computerized CBT intervention for anxiety and depression in a sample of children and adolescents. In addition, eight participants in our study completed the post-treatment assessment and had also finished all treatment modules, whereas in other studies with adolescent samples, e.g., Tillfors et al. [58], the average number of completed modules was only 2.9 out of a total of 10 modules. The good adherence shown by participants of the present study may be related to the fact that our treatment included a weekly call from the therapist; the study of Carlbring et al. [59] found that weekly calls increased by 93% the number of participants who finished all modules.

The second aspect of feasibility is the usability, which is the degree to which the participants had a positive experience with the web platform. This was assessed by means of the subscale "experience with the online platform". Both the adolescents and parents reported a very positive experience with the platform (e.g., mean ratings ranged from 7.25 to 9.38 on a 0 to 10 Likert scale). The third indicator of feasibility is the alliance with the therapist. This was highly rated both by the adolescents (mean ratings ranged from 8.88 to 9.88) and by the parents (mean ratings ranged from 9.38 to 9.88). The levels of therapeutic alliance found in the present study are rather higher than the ones reported by other studies of internet-CBT [60].

Regarding acceptability, the iUP-A and AMTE platform were very positively evaluated by the adolescents and their parents. Users' satisfaction scores ranged from 8.50 to 9.38 (Likert scale 0 to 10) whereas parents' satisfaction with the program was also very high, with mean scores ranging from 8 to 9.75 (strong endorsement). These ratings were higher than the ones of similar studies [48]. The participants reported an increase in their coping skills, enjoyment of the program, and reported that they would recommend the program to other adolescents. It is worth noting that a good acceptability is an important issue because expectations about the treatment may affect treatment outcomes.

5. Limitations and Future Research

The strengths of this study include performing a comprehensive assessment of feasibility and acceptability, as well as including relevant outcomes in several important domains (general symptoms of anxiety and depression, transdiagnostic constructs, and disorder-specific anxiety and depression symptoms). However, as a preliminary investigation of the iUP-A, it also has several limitations. The first limitation is that the sample size of the current study was too small and may have limited our ability to detect effects of the treatment; however, most of the outcome measures' effect sizes were large. A second limitation is the lack of a control group since this limits the possibility of establishing causal inferences between the treatment and the changes in the dependent variables. Due to this, it is difficult to determine whether the large effects associated with the treatment may partially reflect a spontaneous improvement over time. Thirdly, the present study did not include follow-up assessments, thereby reducing our ability to draw firm conclusions about the long-term efficacy of the iUP-A. Finally, the current investigation relied on self-report outcome measures.

Although the results are promising, they are very preliminary. These limitations preclude from drawing firm conclusions concerning the efficacy of the iUP-A in the treatment of anxiety and depressive disorders in adolescents. Future research on the efficacy of the iUP-A should address these shortcomings including (a) larger sample size and control conditions in order to be able to establish causal inferences regarding the effect of the intervention vs. the effect due to the passage of time, (b) follow-up assessments to examine if the effect of the treatment is sustained over time, and (c) clinical-rated outcome measures in addition to self-report measures. New research on the efficacy of the iUP-A has important implications for clinical psychology related to the treatment and prevention of anxiety and depression in youth since the UP-A is a consolidated transdiagnostic program for the treatment of emotional disorders. On the other hand, the iUP-A has the advantages of an internet-delivered intervention, thus being a particularly promising intervention program to be applied in the current situation of social isolation linked to COVID-19.

6. Conclusions

Overall, the results of the present study suggest that the UP-A delivered via the internet (i.e., the iUP-A) is a promising transdiagnostic CBT program for the treatment of anxiety and depressive disorders in adolescents. Importantly, the iUP-A was not only potentially efficacious but also feasible and acceptable to the participants and their parents. The present study provides preliminary empirical evidence in support of the clinical utility of a Spanish, web-based version of the UP-A (i.e., the iUP-A). This is the first study that provides empirical evidence of the clinical utility of an internet-based version of the UP-A. We found improvements in outcomes associated with several important domains (i.e., anxiety and depression symptoms, as well as vulnerability transdiagnostic constructs), suggesting that the iUP-A is an efficacious treatment reducing general comorbidity of anxiety and depression across emotional disorders (anxiety and depressive disorders). This study also provides empirical evidence concerning the ability of the iUP-A to ameliorate the disorder-specific symptomatology related to anxiety disorders. An innovative contribution of this investigation was to empirically test the effect of the iUP-A on core mechanisms underlying emotional disorders (positive and negative affectivity, anxiety sensitivity, and emotional avoidance). We found that the iUP-A was able to significantly reduce the levels of anxiety sensitivity and emotional avoidance (effect sizes = 1.74 and 1.19, respectively). Finally, the data concerning adherence, usability, therapeutic alliance, and satisfaction with the web platform suggest that the adolescents perceived the treatment as feasible and were highly satisfied with it. We conclude that the iUP-A is feasible and acceptable, as well as potentially efficacious in reducing symptoms (comorbid and disorder-specific) of anxiety and depression as well as underlying vulnerability and maintenance processes.

Author Contributions: B.S., R.M.V. and P.C. development of the iUP-A protocol and the web platform, conceptualization and design of the study, study coordination, preparation of the pre-posttreatment assessment protocol, original draft preparation, writing review and editing, and interpretation of data. B.S. statistical analysis. J.G.-E. data collection, diagnostic interviews, initial screening, clinical support, preparation of database, statistical analysis, interpretation of data, original draft preparation, writing review and editing, and study coordination. V.E. data collection, diagnostic interviews, and clinical support. All authors have read and agreed to the published version of the manuscript.

Funding: This work is supported by the Spanish Ministry of Economy and Competitiveness (grant number PSI2013-44480-P) awarded to authors B.S., P.C. and R.M.V. and by the European Social Fund and the Community of Madrid (grant number: PEJD-2019-POST/SOC-16746) awarded to author J.G.-E.

Conflicts of Interest: The authors declare no conflict of interest.

References

1. Kessler, R.C.; Petukhova, M.; Sampson, N.A.; Zaslavsky, A.M.; Wittchen, H. Twelve-month and lifetime prevalence and lifetime morbid risk of anxiety and mood disorders in the United States. *Int. J. Methods Psychiatry. Res.* **2012**, *21*, 169–184. [CrossRef]
2. Ahlen, J.; Lenhard, F.; Ghaderi, A. Universal prevention for anxiety and depressive symptoms in children: A meta-analysis of randomized and cluster-randomized trials. *J. Prim. Prev.* **2015**, *36*, 387–403. [CrossRef]
3. Balázs, J.; Miklósi, M.; Keresztény, Á.; Hoven, C.W.; Carli, V.; Wasserman, C.; Apter, A.; Bobes, J.; Brunner, R.; Cosman, D. Adolescent subthreshold-depression and anxiety: Psychopathology, functional impairment and increased suicide risk. *J. Child. Psychol. Psychiatry* **2013**, *54*, 670–677. [CrossRef]
4. Weersing, V.R.; Gonzalez, A.; Campo, J.V.; Lucas, A.N. Brief behavioral therapy for pediatric anxiety and depression: Piloting an integrated treatment approach. *Cogn. Behav. Pract.* **2008**, *15*, 126–139. [CrossRef]
5. Ehrenreich-May, J.; Bilek, E.L.; Queen, A.H.; Hernandez Rodriguez, J. A unified protocol for the group treatment of childhood anxiety and depression. *Rev. Psicopatol. Psicol. Clin.* **2012**, *17*, 219–236. [CrossRef]
6. Sandín, B.; Chorot, P.; Valiente, R.M. Psicopatología de la ansiedad y trastornos de ansiedad: Hacia un enfoque transdiagnóstico [*Psychopathology of anxiety and the anxiety disorders: Towards a transdignostic perspective*]. In *Manual de Psicopatología*, 3rd ed.; Belloch, A., Sandín, B., Ramos, F., Eds.; McGraw-Hill: Madrid, Spain, 2020; Volume 2, pp. 3–34.
7. Sandín, B.; Chorot, P.; Valiente, R.M. Transdiagnóstico: Nueva frontera en psicología clínica [*Transdiagnostic: A new frontier in clinical psychology*]. *Rev. Psicopatol. Psicol. Clin.* **2012**, *17*, 185–203. [CrossRef]
8. Andersen, P.; Toner, P.; Bland, M.; McMillan, D. Effectiveness of transdiagnostic cognitive behaviour therapy for anxiety and depression in adults: A systematic review and meta-analysis. *Behav. Cogn. Psychother.* **2016**, *44*, 673–690. [CrossRef] [PubMed]
9. García-Escalera, J.; Chorot, P.; Valiente, R.M.; Reales, J.M.; Sandín, B. Efficacy of transdiagnostic cognitive-behavioral therapy for anxiety and depression in adults, children and adolescents: A meta-analysis. *Rev. Psicopatol. Psicol. Clin.* **2016**, *21*, 147–175. [CrossRef]
10. Sakiris, N.; Berle, D. A systematic review and meta-analysis of the unified protocol as a transdiagnostic emotion regulation based intervention. *Clin. Psychol. Rev.* **2019**, *72*, 1–13. [CrossRef]
11. Ehrenreich-May, J.; Kennedy, S.M.; Sherman, J.A.; Bilek, L.B.; Buzzella, B.A.; Bennett, S.M.; Barlow, D.H. *Unified Protocols for Transdiagnostic Treatment of Emotional Disorders in Children and Adolescents*; Oxford University Press: New York, NY, USA, 2018.
12. Ehrenreich, J.T.; Goldstein, C.R.; Wright, L.R.; Barlow, D.H. Development of a unified protocol for the treatment of emotional disorders in youth. *Child. Fam. Behav. Ther.* **2009**, *31*, 20–37. [CrossRef]
13. Ehrenreich-May, J.; Rosenfield, D.; Queen, A.H.; Kennedy, S.M.; Remmes, C.S.; Barlow, D.H. An initial waitlist-controlled trial of the unified protocol for the treatment of emotional disorders in adolescents. *J. Anxiety Disord.* **2017**, *46*, 46–55. [CrossRef] [PubMed]
14. Osma, J. *Aplicaciones del Protocolo Unificado Para el Tratamiento Transdiagnóstico de la Disregulación Emocional*; Alianza Editorial: Madrid, Spain, 2019.
15. Trosper, S.E.; Buzzella, B.A.; Bennett, S.M.; Ehrenreich, J.T. Emotion regulation in youth with emotional disorders: Implications for a unified treatment approach. *Clin. Child. Fam. Psychol. Rev.* **2009**, *12*, 234–254. [CrossRef] [PubMed]
16. García-Escalera, J.; Valiente, R.M.; Sandín, B.; Ehrenreich-May, J.; Prieto, A.; Chorot, P. The unified protocol for transdiagnostic treatment of emotional disorders in adolescents (UP-A) adapted as a school-based anxiety and depression prevention program: An initial cluster randomized wait-list-controlled trial. *Behav. Ther.* **2020**, *51*, 461–473. [CrossRef] [PubMed]
17. García-Escalera, J.; Chorot, P.; Sandín, B.; Ehrenreich-May, J.; Prieto, A.; Valiente, R.M. An open trial applying the unified protocol for transdiagnostic treatment of emotional disorders in adolescents (UP-A) adapted as a school-based prevention program. *Child. Youth Care Forum* **2019**, *48*, 29–53. [CrossRef]
18. Titov, N.; Dear, B.F.; Johnston, L.; Terides, M. Transdiagnostic internet treatment for anxiety and depression. *Rev. Psicopatol. Psicol. Clin.* **2012**, *17*, 237–260. [CrossRef]
19. Andersson, G.; Titov, N. Advantages and limitations of internet-based interventions for common mental disorders. *World Psychiatry* **2014**, *13*, 4–11. [CrossRef]

20. Carlbring, P.; Andersson, G.; Cuijpers, P.; Riper, H.; Hedman-Lagerlöf, E. Internet-based vs. face-to-face cognitive behavior therapy for psychiatric and somatic disorders: An updated systematic review and meta-analysis. *Cogn. Behav. Ther.* **2018**, *47*, 1–18. [CrossRef]
21. Etzelmueller, A.; Vis, C.; Karyotaki, E.; Baumeister, H.; Titov, N.; Berking, M.; Cuijpers, P.; Riper, H.; Ebert, D.D. Effects of internet-based cognitive behavioral therapy in routine care for adults in treatment for depression and anxiety: Systematic review and meta-analysis. *JMIR* **2020**, *22*, 1–27. [CrossRef]
22. Vigerland, S.; Lenhard, F.; Bonnert, M.; Lalouni, M.; Hedman, E.; Ahlen, J.; Olén, O.; Serlachius, E.; Ljótsson, B. Internet-delivered cognitive behavior therapy for children and adolescents: A systematic review and meta-analysis. *Clin. Psychol. Rev.* **2016**, *50*, 1–10. [CrossRef]
23. Barlow, D.H.; Farchione, T.J.; Sauer-Zavala, S.; Latin, H.M.; Ellard, K.K.; Bullis, J.R.; Bentley, K.H.; Boettcher, H.T.; Cassiello-Robbins, C. *Unified Protocol for Transdiagnostic Treatment of Emotional Disorders: Therapist Guide*; Oxford University Press: New York, NY, USA, 2018.
24. Gonzalez-Robles, A.; Garcia-Palacios, A.; Baños, R.; Riera, A.; Llorca, G.; Traver, F.; Haro, G.; Palop, V.; Lera, G.; Romeu, J.E.; et al. Effectiveness of a transdiagnostic internet-based protocol for the treatment of emotional disorders versus treatment as usual in specialized care: Study protocol for a randomized controlled trial. *Trials* **2015**, *16*, 488–493. [CrossRef]
25. Păsărelu, C.R.; Andersson, G.; Bergman Nordgren, L.; Dobrean, A. Internet-delivered transdiagnostic and tailored cognitive behavioral therapy for anxiety and depression: A systematic review and meta-analysis of randomized controlled trials. *Cogn. Behav. Ther.* **2017**, *46*, 1–28. [CrossRef] [PubMed]
26. Sandín, B.; Valiente, R.M.; García-Escalera, J.; Pineda, D.; Espinosa, V.; Magaz, A.M.; Chorot, P. Protocolo unificado para el tratamiento transdiagnóstico de los trastornos emocionales en adolescentes a través de internet (iUP-A): Aplicación web y protocolo de un ensayo controlado aleatorizado [*Internet-delivered unified protocol for transdiagnostic treatment of emotional disorders in adolescents (iUP-A): Web application and study protocol for a randomized controlled trial*]. *Rev. Psicopatol. Psicol. Clin.* **2019**, *24*, 197–215. [CrossRef]
27. Sheehan, D.V.; Lecrubier, Y.; Sheehan, K.H.; Amorim, P.; Janavs, J.; Weiller, E.; Hergueta, T.; Baker, R.; Dunbar, G.C. The Mini-International Neuropsychiatric Interview (MINI): The development and validation of a structured diagnostic psychiatric interview for DSM-IV and ICD-10. *J. Clin. Psychiatry* **1998**, *59*, 22–33. [CrossRef] [PubMed]
28. Colón-Soto, M.; Díaz, V.; Soto, O.; Santana, C. *Mini International Neuropsychiatric Interview Para Niños y Adolescentes (MINI-KID) Versión en Español*; Medical Outcome Symptoms: Tampa, FL, USA, 2005.
29. Des Jarlais, D.C.; Lyles, C.; Crepaz, N. TREND Group Improving the reporting quality of nonrandomized evaluations of behavioral and public health interventions: The TREND statement. *Am. J. Public Health* **2004**, *94*, 361–366. [CrossRef] [PubMed]
30. Ehrenreich-May, J.; Queen, A.H.; Bilek, E.L.; Remmes, C.S.; Kristen, K.M. The Unified Protocols for the Treatment of Emotional Disorders in Children and Adolescents. In *Transdiagnostic Treatments for Children and Adolescents: Principles and Practice*; Ehrenreich-May, J., Chu, B.C., Eds.; Guilford Press: New York, NY, USA, 2014; pp. 267–292.
31. Sandín, B.; Chorot, P.; Valiente, R.M. *TCC de los Trastornos de Ansiedad: Innovaciones en Niños y Adolescentes [CBT for Anxiety Disorders: Innovations for Children and Adolescents]*; Klinik: Madrid, Spain, 2016.
32. Sandín, B.; Chorot, P.; Valiente, R.M.; Chorpita, B.F. Development of a 30-item version of the Revised Child Anxiety and Depression Scale. *Rev. Psicopatol. Psicol. Clin.* **2010**, *15*, 165–178. [CrossRef]
33. Sandín, B. Escalas PANAS de afecto positivo y negativo para niños y adolescentes (PANASN) [*The PANAS scales of positive and negative affect for children and adolescents (PANASN)*]. *Rev. Psicopatol. Psicol. Clin.* **2003**, *8*, 173–182. [CrossRef]
34. Silverman, W.K.; Fleisig, W.; Rabian, B.; Peterson, R.A. Childhood anxiety sensitivity index. *J. Clin. Child. Adolesc. Psychol.* **1991**, *20*, 162–168. [CrossRef]
35. Sandín, B.; Chorot, P.; Santed, M.A.; Valiente, R.M. Análisis factorial confirmatorio del Índice de Sensibilidad a la Ansiedad para Niños [*A confirmatory factor analysis of the Childhood Anxiety Sensitivity Index*]. *Psicothema* **2002**, *14*, 333–339.
36. Kennedy, S.M.; Ehrenreich-May, J. Assessment of emotional avoidance in adolescents: Psychometric properties of a new multidimensional measure. *J. Psychopathol. Behav. Assess.* **2016**, *39*, 279–290. [CrossRef]

37. García-Escalera, J.; Chorot, P.; Valiente, R.; Sandín, B.; Tonarely, N.; Ehrenreich-May, J. *Spanish Version of the Emotional Avoidance Strategy Inventory for Adolescents (EASI-A)*; Universidad Nacional de Educación a Distancia: Madrid, Spain, 2016; Unpublished.
38. Sandín, B.; Chorot, P.; Valiente, R.M. *Cuestionario PSWQ para Niños y Adolescentes (PSWQN-11) [Questionnaire PSWQ for Children and Adolescents (PSWQ-11)]*; Universidad Nacional de Educación a Distancia: Madrid, Spain, 2010; Unpublished.
39. La Greca, A.M.; Stone, W.L. Social anxiety scale for children-revised: Factor structure and concurrent validity. *J. Clin. Child. Psychol.* **1993**, *22*, 17–27. [CrossRef]
40. Sandín, B. *Ansiedad, Miedos y Fobias en Niños y Adolescentes [Anxiety, Fears and Phobias in Children and Adolescents]*; Dykinson: Madrid, Spain, 1997.
41. Houck, P.R.; Spiegel, D.A.; Shear, M.K.; Rucci, P. Reliability of the self-report version of the panic disorder severity scale. *Depress. Anxiety* **2002**, *15*, 183–185. [CrossRef] [PubMed]
42. Sandín, B. Panic Disorder Severity Scale–Self Report (PDSS-SR) (Spanish version). In *Trastorno de Pánico*; Sandín, B., Ed.; UNED: Madrid, Spain, 2010.
43. Sheehan, D.V.; Sheehan, K.H.; Shytle, R.D.; Janavs, J.; Bannon, Y.; Rogers, J.E.; Milo, K.M.; Stock, S.L.; Wilkinson, B. Reliability and validity of the mini international neuropsychiatric interview for children and adolescents (MINI-KID). *J. Clin. Psychiatry* **2010**, *71*, 313–326. [CrossRef] [PubMed]
44. Valiente, R.M.; Sandín, B.; Chorot, P. Miedos comunes en niños y adolescentes: Relación con la sensibilidad a la ansiedad, el rasgo de ansiedad, la afectividad negativa y la depresión [Common fears in children and adolescents: Their relationship to anxiety sensitivity, trait anxiety, negative affectivity, and depression]. *Rev. Psicopatol. Psicol. Clin.* **2002**, *7*, 61–70. [CrossRef]
45. Sandín, B.; Chorot, P.; Valiente, R.M.; Lostao, L. Validación española del cuestionario de preocupación PSWQ: Estructura factorial y propiedades psicométricas [Spanish validation of the PSWQ: Factor structure and psychometric properties]. *Rev. Psicopatol. Psicol. Clin.* **2009**, *14*, 107–122. [CrossRef]
46. Sánchez-Arribas, C.; Chorot, P.; Valiente, R.M.; Sandín, B. Evaluación de factores cognitivos positivos y negativos relacionadas con el trastorno de pánico: Validación del CATP [Assessment of positive and negative cognitive factors related to panic disorder: Validation of the CATP]. *Rev. Psicopatol. Psicol. Clin.* **2015**, *20*, 85–100. [CrossRef]
47. Sandín, B.; Valiente, R.M.; García-Escalera, J.; Chorot, P. *Feasibility and Acceptability Questionnaire (FAQ)*; Universidad Nacional de Educación a Distancia: Madrid, Spain, 2020; Unpublished.
48. Rapee, R.M.; Wignall, A.; Sheffield, J.; Kowalenko, N.; Davis, A.; McLoone, J.; Spence, S.H. Adolescents' reactions to universal and indicated prevention programs for depression: Perceived stigma and consumer satisfaction. *Prevent. Sci.* **2006**, *7*, 167–177. [CrossRef]
49. Cohen, J. A power primer. *Psychol. Bull.* **1992**, *112*, 155. [CrossRef]
50. Faul, F.; Erdfelder, E.; Lang, A.-G.; Buchner, A. G*Power 3: A flexible statistical power analysis program for the social, behavioral, and biomedical sciences. *Behav. Res. Methods* **2007**, *39*, 175–191. [CrossRef]
51. De la Torre-Luque, A.; Fiol-Veny, A.; Essau, C.A.; Balle, M.; Bornas, X. Effects of a transdiagnostic cognitive behaviour therapy-based programme on the natural course of anxiety symptoms in adolescence. *J. Affect. Disord.* **2020**, *264*, 474–482. [CrossRef]
52. Fernández-Martínez, I.; Orgilés, M.; Morales, A.; Espada, J.P.; Essau, C.A. One-Year follow-up effects of a cognitive behavior therapy-based transdiagnostic program for emotional problems in young children: A school-based cluster-randomized controlled trial. *J. Affect. Disord.* **2020**, *262*, 258–266. [CrossRef]
53. Calear, A.L.; Batterham, P.J.; Poyser, C.T.; Mackinnon, A.J.; Griffiths, K.M.; Christensen, H. Cluster randomised controlled trial of the e-couch Anxiety and Worry program in schools. *J. Affect. Disord.* **2016**, *196*, 210–217. [CrossRef] [PubMed]
54. González-Robles, A.; Díaz-García, A.; García-Palacios, A.; Roca, P.; Ramos-Quiroga, J.A.; Botella, C. Effectiveness of a Transdiagnostic Guided Internet-Delivered Protocol for Emotional Disorders Versus Treatment as Usual in Specialized Care: Randomized Controlled Trial. *J. Med. Internet Res.* **2020**, *22*, 1–23. [CrossRef] [PubMed]
55. Ellard, K.K.; Bernstein, E.E.; Hearing, C.; Baek, J.H.; Sylvia, L.G.; Nierenberg, A.A.; Barlow, D.H.; Deckersbach, T. Transdiagnostic treatment of bipolar disorder and comorbid anxiety using the Unified Protocol for Emotional Disorders: A pilot feasibility and acceptability trial. *J. Affect. Disord.* **2017**, *219*, 209–221. [CrossRef] [PubMed]

56. Bilek, E.L.; Ehrenreich-May, J. An open trial investigation of a transdiagnostic group treatment for children with anxiety and depressive symptoms. *Behav. Ther.* **2012**, *43*, 887–897. [CrossRef]
57. Stallard, P.; Richardson, T.; Velleman, S.; Attwood, M. Computerized CBT (Think, Feel, Do) for depression and anxiety in children and adolescents: Outcomes and feedback from a pilot randomized controlled trial. *Behav. Cogn. Psychother.* **2011**, *39*, 273. [CrossRef]
58. Tillfors, M.; Andersson, G.; Ekselius, L.; Furmark, T.; Lewenhaupt, S.; Karlsson, A.; Carlbring, P. A randomized trial of internet-delivered treatment for social anxiety disorder in high school students. *Cogn. Behav. Ther.* **2011**, *40*, 147–157. [CrossRef] [PubMed]
59. Carlbring, P.; Gunnarsdóttir, M.; Hedensjö, L.; Andersson, G.; Ekselius, L.; Furmark, T. Treatment of social phobia: Randomised trial of internet-delivered cognitive-behavioural therapy with telephone support. *Br. J. Psychiatry* **2007**, *190*, 123–128. [CrossRef]
60. Andersson, G.; Paxling, B.; Wiwe, M.; Vernmark, K.; Felix, C.B.; Lundborg, L.; Furmark, T.; Cuijpers, P.; Carlbring, P. Therapeutic alliance in guided internet-delivered cognitive behavioural treatment of depression, generalized anxiety disorder and social anxiety disorder. *Behav. Res. Ther.* **2012**, *50*, 544–550. [CrossRef]

Publisher's Note: MDPI stays neutral with regard to jurisdictional claims in published maps and institutional affiliations.

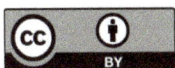

© 2020 by the authors. Licensee MDPI, Basel, Switzerland. This article is an open access article distributed under the terms and conditions of the Creative Commons Attribution (CC BY) license (http://creativecommons.org/licenses/by/4.0/).

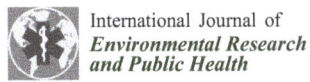

Article

Brief Psychological Intervention Through Mobile App and Conference Calls for the Prevention of Depression in Non-Professional Caregivers: A Pilot Study

Patricia Otero [1],*, Isabel Hita [2], Ángela J. Torres [3] and Fernando L. Vázquez [2]

1. Department of Psychology, University of A Coruña, 15071 A Coruña, Spain
2. Department of Clinical Psychology and Psychobiology, University of Santiago de Compostela, 15782 Santiago de Compostela, Spain; isabel.hita@usc.es (I.H.); fernandolino.vazquez@usc.es (F.L.V.)
3. Department of Psychiatry, Radiology and Public Health, University of Santiago de Compostela, 15782 Santiago de Compostela, Spain; angelajuana.torres@usc.es
* Correspondence: patricia.otero.otero@udc.es; Tel.: +34-881014683

Received: 3 June 2020; Accepted: 24 June 2020; Published: 25 June 2020

Abstract: Despite its potential, no intervention aimed at non-professional caregivers administered through a smartphone app has been proven to prevent depression. The objective of this pilot study was to evaluate the efficacy and feasibility of an indicated depression-prevention intervention for non-professional caregivers administered through an app with the addition of conference-call contact. The intervention was administered to 31 caregivers (Mean age = 54.0 years, 93.5% women). An independent evaluation determined the incidence of depression, depressive symptoms, risk of developing depression, and the variables in the theoretical model (positive environmental reinforcement, negative automatic thoughts) at the pre-intervention and post-intervention, as well as the one- and three-month follow-ups. The incidence of depression at 3 months of follow-up was 6.5%. There was a significant reduction in depressive symptoms ($p < 0.001$) and in the risk of developing depression ($p < 0.001$) at the post-intervention and at the one- and three-month follow-ups. The model's variables improved significantly after the intervention and were associated with post-intervention depressive symptoms. The intervention was more effective in caregivers who had a lower level of depressive symptoms at the pre-intervention. Adherence and satisfaction with the intervention were high. The results encourage future research using a randomized controlled clinical trial.

Keywords: depression; nonprofessional caregiver; prevention; cognitive; behavioral; telephone; app

1. Introduction

Caregivers for dependent family members perform a job that requires them to meet many demands and cope with difficult situations, oftentimes over a long period of time [1], such as looking for a diagnosis, learning to care for their family member, financial matters [2], decreased environmental reinforcement [3], insomnia or low-quality sleep [4,5], or a decrease in capabilities of the family member [6]. Therefore, caregivers' quality of life is affected [7–9], and these risk factors can increase their vulnerability to mental health disorders, especially depression [10]. In fact, a systematic review and meta-analysis on ten studies with a total of 790 caregivers [11] found a relative risk ranging from 2.80 to 38.68 for suffering from a depressive disorder in caregivers compared to non-caregivers. Specifically, previous research has found that 8.9% of caregivers meet the criteria for an episode of major depression [12], which is nearly fivefold higher than the 1.8% prevalence of major depression in the general population [13]. These figures are quite important because major depression is highly disabling and constitutes the third-leading cause of years lived with disabilities [14]. In addition, it is recurrent in 27% to 42% of people who experienced one major depressive episode and symptoms are chronic in 12% to 16% of those who have developed clinical depression [15–17]. Likewise, it entails enormous socioeconomic costs, resulting in billions of dollars annually [18]. Furthermore, in the case of caregivers, it can interfere with the proper performance of their tasks in caring for the dependent person [19].

Therefore, given the prevalence and serious repercussions of depression, its prevention among the caregiver population is critical. Among preventive strategies, indicated prevention interventions are particularly interesting. These are interventions aimed at individuals with subclinical symptoms who do not meet the diagnostic criteria for a major depressive episode [20]. The goal is to reduce the progression of these symptoms and to prevent their worsening into major depression [21].

There are only three previous studies on the indicated prevention of depression in non-professional caregivers providing care for dependent family members. The first evaluated the efficacy of a five-session problem-solving intervention using a group face-to-face format (about five participants per group) compared to a usual-care control group. It found a lower incidence of depression (4.5% vs. 13.1%) and fewer depressive symptoms ($d = 1.54$) after the intervention [22] and at the 12-month [23] and eight-year follow-up [24]. The second evaluated the efficacy of a five-session cognitive-behavioral face-to-face group intervention (about five participants per group) compared to a usual-care control group. It found a lower incidence of depression (1.1% vs. 12.2%) and fewer depressive symptoms ($d = 1.05$) after the intervention [25] and at the 12-month follow-up [26]. The therapeutic changes found were clinically significant [27]. However, these interventions were conducted using a traditional face-to-face format, which could compromise their accessibility. Caregivers often have barriers that make it difficult for them to attend face-to-face interventions, including lack of time, a lack of a substitute caregiver in their absence, a shortage of mental health services, travel and cost concerns, and fear of stigmatization.

The use of communication technologies available to practically all caregivers, such as the telephone, reduces these barriers. The telephone offers travel savings, anonymity, lower cost, and accessibility to the most remote communities [28], in addition to solving specific barriers in the caregiver population, such as lack of time and difficulties in finding a substitute caregiver. Therefore, in the third study of indicated depression prevention aimed at caregivers, Vázquez et al. (2020) [29], took a cognitive-behavioral depression-indicated prevention intervention that had previously been tested in a face-to-face format and adapted it into a five-session conference call format. The study also examined the efficacy of its components using a dismantling strategy. They found that the incidence of depression was lower in the group that received either the complete conference call intervention or the behavioral activation component only, compared to the control group (1.5% and 1.4% vs. 8.8%), and depressive symptoms were significantly lower in both intervention groups compared to the control group ($d = 1.16$ and $d = 1.29$), with no differences between them.

Although these results were very promising, the prevention intervention for depression could be optimized by utilizing a smartphone app. Currently, it is estimated that more than five billion people worldwide have mobile devices and more than half of these connections are smartphones. Furthermore, 80% of adults in Spain own a smartphone or use apps [30]. The smartphone app allows the caregiver greater mobility and accessibility by allowing access wherever and whenever they want 24 h a day. It increases the flexibility of program participation and can be adapted to caregivers' personal routines without wait times, having to make appointments, or attend sessions at a fixed time. Users can also review the materials as many times as they want and interact and receive feedback immediately [31,32].

However, given its novelty, there are only two previous studies evaluating apps for the treatment of depression [33,34], and neither of them are aimed at preventing depression or are aimed at caregivers of dependent family members. In particular, Arean et al. (2016) [33] found no significant difference at the post-intervention time point and the one-month follow-up between a cognitive training intervention, another problem-based intervention, and an attention control group in which participants received therapeutically inactive information on health. At the three-month follow-up, participants in both interventions showed higher remission rates compared to controls (50% and 49% vs. 32%), but only those with moderate depressive symptoms who participated in the problem-solving group showed fewer depressive symptoms than the control group ($d = 0.76$). In addition, Ly et al. (2014) [34] found no post-intervention differences between a program based on behavioral activation and another based on mindfulness. At the six-month follow-up, the behavioral activation intervention was more effective for patients with greater initial severity of depression ($d = 0.47$), while the mindfulness intervention was more effective for patients with lower severity ($d = 0.98$).

However, lack of adherence is one of the main limitations of interventions that do not use a face-to-face format. Dropout rates for interventions using apps were high, reaching 31.6%, and the level of compliance with tasks between sessions is unknown [33]. These problems are critical, because when evaluating the efficacy of interventions, high dropout rates can lead to bias and limit the generalizability of the results [35]. Furthermore, task completion is a significant predictor of therapy outcomes in depression prevention interventions among the caregiver population [36]. One way to reduce drop-out rates in interventions that are not conducted in an in-person format would be to establish telephone contact [31]. In addition, using the positive and corrective feedback technique, which consists of reinforcing the correct performance of a behavior and providing instructions to change behaviors that have been conducted incorrectly [37], could increase the effectiveness of interventions and strengthen caregivers' commitment to completing the homework tasks.

The objective of this study was to evaluate the efficacy and feasibility of an indicated depression-prevention intervention for non-professional caregivers with depressive symptoms administered through a smartphone app together with positive and corrective feedback through a telephone conference call.

2. Materials and Methods

2.1. Participants

A pretest–posttest design with a 1- and 3-month follow-up without a comparison group was used. Participants were recruited from the population of officially recognized (by the Administration) non-professional caregivers providing care for people in situations of dependency in the Autonomous Community of Galicia. To obtain a sample with similar characteristics to that of a future large-scale randomized controlled trial, the sample was selected by random stratified sampling following the following steps: (1) we contacted 11 regional and national associations related to caregivers via email and telephone, explained the purpose of the pilot study and obtained their cooperation; (2) every association made a list of all the non-professional caregivers they had, assigning a sequential number to each participant (e.g., 1, 2, 3, ...); (3) a random number generator was used to select the sample, taking 10 participants per association (i.e., 110 random numbers were generated). The staff of every association contacted the randomly selected caregivers personally and put them in contact with the research team, who explained to them the purpose of the study and answered all their questions.

To participate in the study, they had to meet the following criteria: (a) be a non-professional caregiver for a family member in a dependent situation; (b) the dependent family member was officially recognized by the competent public bodies in Spain; (c) have a smartphone; (d) be at risk for depression, defined as a score equal to or greater than 16 on the Center for Epidemiologic Studies Depression Scale (CES-D; [38]; Spanish version [39]); (e) not meet the DSM-5 diagnostic criteria for a major depressive episode (American Psychiatric Association [40]); and (f) agree to participate in all evaluations. Exclusion criteria were: (a) having received psychological or psychopharmacological treatment in the last two months prior to study entry; (b) presenting with other disorders that could act as confounding variables (e.g., symptoms due to substance use); (c) presenting with serious mental health or medical disorders that require immediate intervention (e.g., suicidal ideation) or that make the study impossible (e.g., significant cognitive impairment, severe visual deficit); (d) the dependent family member had a very poor prognosis for the next 6 months; and (e) the caregiver anticipated a change of address or institutionalization of the dependent family member.

Of the 110 caregivers contacted, 101 agreed to take the eligibility assessment. Of these, a total of 33 (32.7%) met the eligibility criteria and were invited to participate in the study, and 2 (6.1%) of these refused to participate due to personal issues and difficulty handling the smartphone (93.9% participated in the pilot study). The final sample consisted of 31 caregivers (93.5% women with a mean age of 54.0 years); no dropout occurred. There were no differences between participants and those who refuse participation on sex ($p = 1.000$, Fisher exact test), age ($U = 24.00$; $z = -0.529$; $p = 0.597$), marital status ($p = 0.216$, Fisher–Freeman–Halton test), social class ($p = 0.557$, Fisher–Freeman–Halton test), monthly household income ($p = 0.097$, Fisher–Freeman–Halton test), level of education ($p = 1.000$, Fisher–Freeman–Halton test), primary activity ($p = 0.432$, Fisher–Freeman–Halton test), care recipient sex ($p = 0.489$, Fisher exact test), care recipient age ($U = 16.50$; $z = -1.094$; $p = 0.274$), relationship to caregiver ($p = 0.424$, Fisher–Freeman–Halton test), care recipient diagnosis ($p = 0.318$, Fisher–Freeman–Halton test), daily hours of care ($U = 20.50$; $z = -0.814$; $p = 0.416$), care duration ($U = 11.50$; $z = -1.477$; $p = 0.140$), depressive symptoms ($U = 20.50$; $z = -0.796$; $p = 0.426$), positive environmental reinforcement ($U = 29.50$; $z = -0.114$; $p = 0.909$), or negative automatic thoughts ($U = 29.00$; $z = -0.151$; $p = 0.880$).

Participation was voluntary and no financial or other incentives were provided. The confidentiality of the participants was guaranteed and all gave their informed consent. The investigation was conducted following the principles of the Declaration of Helsinki and was approved by the Bioethics Committee of the University of Santiago de Compostela (Code number 07/09/2016).

2.2. Instruments

The participants were evaluated at the pre- and post-intervention time points and the 1- and 3-month follow-ups. Data was collected through self-administered instruments through the smartphone app by the participants, and by a structured clinical interview administered via telephone by two independent evaluators. These interviewers were previously trained specifically for this study by two experts with more than 25 years of experience in evaluation and were unaware of the purpose of the study and the administered intervention.

This study used an ad hoc questionnaire to evaluate the sociodemographic variables and the care situation. The Structured Clinical Interview for DSM-5—Clinician Version (SCID-5-CV; [41]) was used to evaluate episodes of major depression, which offers good test-retest reliability for psychiatric patients (kappa index > 0.80 for all disorders). CES-D was administered to assess depressive symptoms ([38]; Spanish version [39]), with an internal consistency of 0.89. In order to assess the variables in the theoretical model in which the intervention was based, we used the Environmental Reward Observation Scale (EROS; [42]; Spanish version [43]), which evaluates positive reinforcement with an internal consistency of 0.86, and the Automatic Thoughts Questionnaire (ATQ; [44]; Spanish version [45]) which assess the frequency of negative automatic thoughts with an internal consistency of 0.96. The Client Satisfaction Questionnaire (CSQ-8; [46]; Spanish version [47]) was used to assess satisfaction with the intervention, with an internal consistency of 0.80.

Finally, to assess the acceptability of the interventions, data on attendance at sessions, and completion of assignments between sessions were collected through an ad hoc record worksheet prepared for this study.

2.3. Intervention

Before the study, a cognitive-behavioral intervention for indicated prevention of depression was adapted for application via a smartphone app. Previous studies had demonstrated that this intervention was effective in reducing the incidence of depression and depressive symptoms in the population of caregivers at short- and long-term when administered in a face-to-face group format [24,25] and in a conference call format [29]. This intervention is based on the Multifactorial Integrative Model of

Depression developed by Lewinsohn et al. [48]. The adaptations consisted of modifying the content for presentation on smartphone screens (summarization and simplification of the content and changes to the format), designing the app interface, developing a daily reminder system that sent notifications to the mobile phone, and recording of between sessions homework tasks. The app-based intervention consisted of five modules that participants downloaded on their mobile and were programmed to be completed one per week. Module 1 explained the concept of depression and the need for active coping with depressive symptoms, and participants were trained in an activation control strategy (controlled breathing technique), self-reinforcement, and daily mood monitoring. Module 2 focused on how pleasant activities affect mood, and participants made plans to introduce them into their day-to-day activities. Module 3 addressed how thoughts affect mood, and participants were trained in techniques to manage negative thoughts. Module 4 explained how social contacts affect mood, and participants were trained in assertive communication and how to increase social contacts. In Module 5, participants reviewed everything they had learned and preventing relapse was addressed (see Table 1). The app, called Happy, was developed by independent programmers using the Apache Cordova framework, thus achieving a hybrid application, which is internally based on HTML, Javascript and CSS. For its development, an agile development methodology was followed. It was available for both Android and iOS in one language (Spanish) at the Google Play Store and the Apple App Store respectively, and operative for Android devices 4.4 or greater and for iOS 9 or greater. After the installation in the participant's device, a user and password login previously facilitated by the research team was mandatory to access the app. The app offered participants the previously mentioned battery of questionnaires and, after being completed by the user, a notification with a summary of the results was sent. If the user met the eligibility criteria, they were invited to participate in the intervention by the research team. Every week, the app allowed access to the contents of the corresponding module, sending a message informing the participants that they could access the next module. Upon completion of the module, between-session tasks were assigned, and the app sent a daily notification to users reminding them to complete and record their intersessional homework tasks. The stored data was hosted on an internal server in a MySQL database protected under username/password, and which can only be accessed from an authorized host (only the research team, complying with all security and confidentiality guarantees).

Table 1. Contents of the brief intervention program.

Module	Content
Module 1	Presentation of group members Purpose of the program Information about depression and active coping of symptoms Mood rating Training in diaphragmatic breathing Self-reinforcement Homework: Mood rating, practice breathing control technique, self-reinforcement
Module 2	Explanation of the relationship between pleasant activities and mood Guidelines and strategies to increase pleasant activities Planning pleasant activities Behavioral contract Homework: Mood rating, practice breathing control technique, self-reinforcement, perform the planned pleasant activities
Module 3	Explanation of the relationship between thoughts and mood Thought management techniques (direct approach, priming, distraction) Planning pleasant activities Behavioral contract Homework: Mood rating, practice breathing control technique, self-reinforcement, perform the planned pleasant activities, practice the thought management techniques

Table 1. *Cont.*

Module	Content
Module 3	Explanation of the relationship between thoughts and mood Thought management techniques (direct approach, priming, distraction) Planning pleasant activities Behavioral contract Homework: Mood rating, practice breathing control technique, self-reinforcement, perform the planned pleasant activities, practice the thought management techniques
Module 4	Explanation of the relationship between social contact and mood Guidelines and strategies to increase and improve social relationships Planning pleasant and social activities Homework: Mood rating, practice breathing control technique, self-reinforcement, perform the planned pleasant activities, practice the thought management techniques, make social contacts
Module 5	Review of what was learned. Maintaining progress Relapse prevention Farewell and closure

In addition, a five-session intervention was manualized to establish telephone contact lasting approximately 30 min (1 session/week) with the participants in a group format (5–6 participants) using a conference call system. In these sessions, the group's rules were explained and positive or corrective feedback was administered following the guidelines of Miltenberger (2012) [37]. The positive feedback consisted of providing information on how to correctly perform the homework tasks and providing reinforcement, and corrective feedback consisted of identifying the tasks that were not completed properly, suggesting relevant changes to improve performance.

The conference call intervention was administered by a psychologist and a doctor of psychology previously trained by experts with more than 25 years of experience in cognitive-behavioral therapies applied in different formats (e.g., individual, group) and through different means (e.g., face-to-face, telephone, online). The sessions were recorded, and adherence to the protocol was evaluated, yielding a protocol adherence of 92%. There were no significant differences between therapists in the results of the intervention.

2.4. Statistical Analysis

The quantitative data were analyzed by intention-to-treat. The missing values were imputed using the Last Observation Carried Forward Method. The McNemar test for paired data was used to analyze the incidence of depression and the risk of depression. Depressive symptoms were analyzed using repeated measures analysis of variance (ANOVA) and post hoc pairwise tests with Bonferroni correction. Student's *t*-test for paired data was used to analyze the changes in depressive symptoms between the pre- and post-intervention time points and between pre-intervention and follow-ups, and changes in reinforcement and negative automatic thoughts at the pre- and post-intervention time points. The effect size was calculated using Cohen's *d* (small = 0.2, medium = 0.5 and large = 0.8; [49]). Pearson's correlation was used to analyze the association between positive environmental reinforcement, negative thoughts, and depressive symptoms at the post-intervention time point. Multiple linear regression analyses were performed to analyze variables that were predictive of a reduction in depressive symptoms, following the recommendations of Domenéch and Navarro (2006) [50]. Frequency analyses and descriptive statistics of sessions attended, tasks performed, and CSQ-8 scores were performed to analyze adherence and satisfaction with the intervention. The analyses were conducted using statistical package SPSS for Windows (version 22.0, IBMCorp., Armonk, NY, USA).

3. Results

3.1. Characteristics of the Sample

Table 2 presents the most relevant sociodemographic, care situation and clinical characteristics of the caregivers who participated in the study. The 93.5% of caregivers were women and the mean age of them was 54.0 years (range 41–71; Standard Deviation [SD] = 9.4). Of the caregivers, 93.5% lived with a partner; 58.1% declared that they belonged to a low/lower-middle social class; 58.1% had a monthly household income of between 1000 and 1999 Euros; 54.8% had a high school or university-level education; and 51.6% were not active members of the workforce (they were unemployed, did not work outside the home, or were retired).

Table 2. Sociodemographic, care situation and clinical characteristics for the sample.

Sociodemographic Variables	n = 31	%
Sex		
Men	2	6.5
Women	29	93.5
Age		
M	54	
SD	9.4	
Range	41–71	
Marital status		
With partner	29	93.5
No partner (single, separated, divorced, widowed)	2	6.5
Social class		
Low/lower middle	18	58.1
Middle/upper middle	13	41.9
Monthly household income		
Up to €999	7	22.6
Between 1000 and 1999 euros	18	58.1
€2000 or more	6	19.3
Level of education		
Up to primary school education	14	45.2
Secondary/University	17	54.8
Primary activity		
Active worker	15	48.4
Unemployed/retired/housework	16	51.6
Care situation variables		
Care recipient sex		
Male	16	51.6
Female	15	48.4
Care recipient age		
M	54	
SD	28.1	
Range	5–93	
Relationship to caregiver		
Son/daughter	12	38.7
Father/mother	9	29
Other family members	10	32.3
Care recipient diagnosis		
Mental/neurological disorders/brain damage	15	48.4
Diseases of the skeletomuscular/connective tissue/cardiovascular/respiratory systems	7	22.6
Chromosomal/congenital/perinatal abnormalities	5	16.1
Others	4	12.9
Daily hours of care		
M	15.7	
SD	7.6	

Table 2. Cont.

Sociodemographic Variables	n = 31	%
Care duration (years)		
M	15.9	
SD	11.9	
Clinical variables		
CES-D Score		
M	26.8	
SD	8.6	
EROS Score		
M	24.1	
SD	4.1	
ATQ Score		
M	70.7	
SD	19.9	

M = Mean; SD = Standard Deviation; CES-D: Centre for Epidemiologic Studies Depression Scale; EROS: The Environmental Reward Observation Scale; ATQ: Automatic Thoughts Questionnaire.

In 51.6% of the cases, the family members receiving care were men, with a mean age of 54.0 years (SD = 28.1), ranging from 5 to 93 years. Most caregivers provided care to a family member, with the largest percentage being parents providing care for a child (38.7%). The most common type of illness observed among family members receiving care were mental health disorders, neurological diseases, and brain damage (48.4%). The time spent caring for the loved one was intensive and continuous. In this sample, caregivers devoted an average of 15.7 h a day to caring for their family member and had done so for an average of 15.9 years.

The mean depressive symptoms score was 26.8 (SD = 8.6). The mean positive environmental reinforcement score was 24.1 (SD = 4.1). The mean score for automatic negative thoughts was 70.7 (SD = 19.9).

3.2. Incidence of Depression

No participant developed an episode of major depression at the post-intervention time point or the one-month follow-up. Only two participants (6.5%) developed an episode of major depression at the three-month follow-up. Of them, one was diagnosed with an episode of major depression according to the DSM-5 diagnostic criteria, and one received an imputed value indicating depression.

Furthermore, there were no significant differences in the incidence of depression between the pre-intervention and post-intervention time points or between the pre-intervention time point and the one- and three-month follow-ups.

3.3. Depressive Symptomatology

Figure 1 shows the progression of depressive symptom scores at the pre-intervention time point (Mean [M] = 26.8), post-intervention time point (M = 15.3), and one- and three-month follow-ups (M = 17.2 and M = 15.5, respectively). The repeated-measures ANOVA showed that changes in depressive symptom scores were statistically significant: $F(3, 90) = 24.434$, $p < 0.001$, $\eta^2 = 0.449$. Compared to the pre-intervention time point, depressive symptoms were significantly lower at the post-intervention time point and at the one- and three-month follow-ups, with large effect sizes (Cohen's d between 0.91 and 1.37; see Table 3).

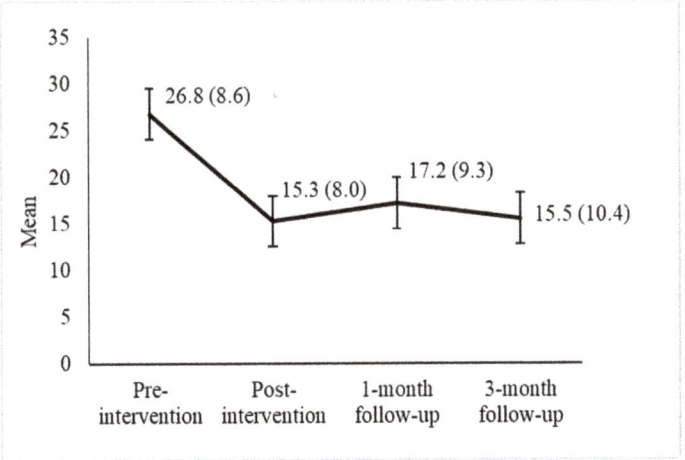

Figure 1. Depressive symptoms at the evaluation time points. The numbers indicate the mean Centre for Epidemiologic Studies Depression Scale (CES-D) score and the standard deviation is given in parentheses.

Table 3. Student-*t* and Cohen's *d* values between the pre-intervention and post-intervention scores, and at the one- and three-month follow-up measurements ($n = 31$).

Variables	*t*	*p*	*d*	95% CI Minimum	95% CI Maximum
Depressive symptomatology (CES-D)					
Pre-intervention vs. post-intervention	7.62	<0.001	1.37	0.87	1.86
Pre-intervention vs. one-month follow-up	5.09	<0.001	0.91	0.49	1.33
Pre-intervention vs. three-month follow-up	6.89	<0.001	1.24	0.76	1.7
Positive Environmental Reinforcement (EROS)					
Pre-intervention vs. post-intervention	−5.61	<0.001	1.01	0.57	1.43
Automatic negative thoughts (ATQ)					
Pre-intervention vs. post-intervention	3.47	<0.001	0.62	0.23	1

95% CI: 95% Confidence Interval; CES-D: Centre for Epidemiologic Studies Depression Scale; EROS: The Environmental Reward Observation Scale; ATQ: Automatic Thoughts Questionnaire.

In addition, 54.8% ($n = 17$) were not at risk of depression (i.e., CES-D score ≥ 16) at the post-intervention time point, 48.4% ($n = 15$) at the one-month follow-up, and 54.8% ($n = 17$) at the three-month follow-up. The decrease in the risk of depression between the pre-intervention and post-intervention time points was significant ($p < 0.001$), as was the difference between the pre-intervention time point and the one- and three-month follow-ups ($p < 0.001$ in both cases).

3.4. Variables for the Theoretical Model and Their Association with Depressive Symptoms

Figure 2 shows the progression of positive environmental reinforcement and negative thoughts scores at the pre-intervention time point ($M = 24.1$ and $M = 70.7$, respectively) and post-intervention time point ($M = 27.4$ and $M = 58.3$, respectively). After the intervention, the degree of positive environmental reinforcement from caregivers increased significantly: $t(30) = -5.61$, $p < 0.001$, with a large effect size ($d = 1.01$). The frequency of negative thoughts decreased significantly: $t(30) = 3.47$, $p < 0.001$, with a medium effect size ($d = 0.62$) (see Table 3).

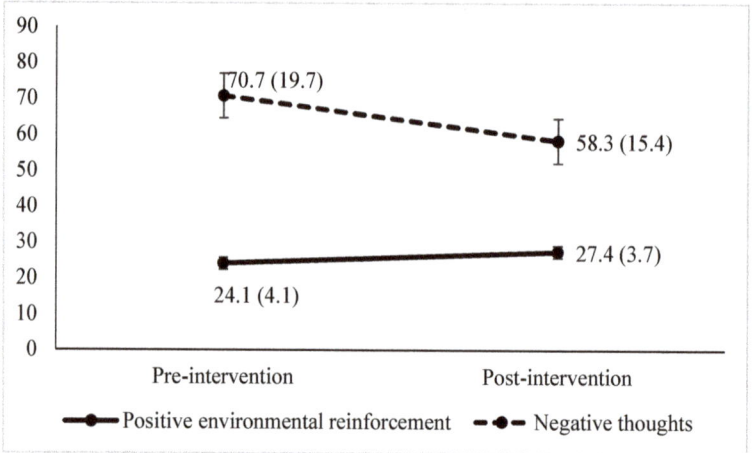

Figure 2. Positive environmental reinforcement and negative thoughts at the evaluation time points. The numbers indicate the mean scores and the standard deviations is given in parentheses.

Furthermore, a significant negative correlation was found between the degree of positive post-intervention environmental reinforcement and post-intervention depressive symptoms, $r(31) = -0.61$, $p < 0.001$. A positive correlation was also found between post-intervention negative automatic thoughts and post-intervention depressive symptomatology, $r(31) = 0.59$, $p = 0.001$.

3.5. Variables Predictive for the Results for Depressive Symptoms

The multiple linear regression analysis resulted in a significant model with an $R^2 = 0.295$ (ETS = 7.07), $F(3, 27) = 3760$, $p = 0.022$. The level of pre-intervention depressive symptomatology was a predictor of post-intervention depressive symptomatology, $\beta = 0.40$, $p = 0.033$, 95% CI [0.33, 0.702].

3.6. Adherence and Satisfaction with the Intervention

Caregivers attended a mean of 4.8 sessions out of the five sessions that comprised the intervention (SD = 0.9). In this sample, 93.5% of caregivers attended all sessions. Furthermore, caregivers performed an average of 14.2 tasks out of the 18 assigned during the intervention and had a high degree of satisfaction with the intervention, with a mean score of 28.1 (SD = 3.9) on the CSQ-8.

4. Discussion

The objective of this pilot study was to evaluate the efficacy and feasibility of an indicated depression-prevention intervention administered through a smartphone app with the addition of conference-call contact aimed at non-professional caregivers with depressive symptoms. It was found that the incidence of depression, depressive symptoms, and the risk of depression decreased after the intervention. Furthermore, these changes were maintained at the three-month follow-up.

Only two caregivers (6.5%) had developed depression at the three-month follow-up. Although this incidence of depression is slightly higher than that found at the three-month follow-up in the previous study that used the same intervention in a face-to-face format [26] and conference call format [51], the numbers are nevertheless encouraging. In fact, they are less than 15.5% and 15.9% found in the control groups at the same follow-up time in the studies by Vázquez et al. [24,26].

There was also a significant reduction in depressive symptoms after the intervention, which continued until the three-month follow-up, with a large effect size ($d = 1.37$), which was larger than the effect size at the three-month follow-up following the face-to-face intervention format ($d = 1.01$) [26], but less than the effect size for the conference call format ($d = 1.46$) [51].

The mean score was reduced to 15.5 points, slightly below the threshold for risk of developing clinical depression, which is considered to be a score of 16 or more. Although this is consistent with other depression-prevention interventions [52], the mean score at the three-month follow-up was higher than that found using the same intervention delivered in face-to-face and conference call format [26,51]. On the other hand, it led to a significantly lower percentage of participants being at risk of developing depression, a figure that went from 100% at the pre-intervention time point to 45.2% at the post-intervention time point, though this is not as low as when the intervention is delivered face-to-face (29.5%) [25] and group conference call (18%) [51]. One possible explanation for these findings may be that the baseline level of depressive symptoms was greater in this study ($M = 26.8$) than for the studies examining the face-to-face format ($M = 23.7$) [26] and the conference-call telephone format ($M = 22.4$) [51]. In addition, administering the intervention through an app could also have some impact. While the face-to-face intervention or conference call-only format is more interactive, the smartphone app format of the intervention depends to a great extent on the caregiver's self-determination and autonomy to read the texts with full attention and interpret them appropriately. Depending on their profile, certain caregivers may benefit more from the program if more human contact is added to the intervention program (such as reviewing the content read on the app during conference calls or increasing the duration of conference call sessions).

Regarding the variables in the theoretical model based on which the intervention was developed, a significant increase in positive environmental reinforcement was found after the intervention with a large effect size ($d = 1.01$), along with a significant decrease in negative thoughts with a medium effect size ($d = 0.62$). These results are consistent with the formulation of the multifactorial integrative model of depression developed by Lewinsohn et al. (1985) [48]. Furthermore, the correlations found between post-intervention positive environmental reinforcement, negative thoughts, and depressive symptoms suggest that there is a relationship between the variables in the theoretical model and depressive symptoms, consistent with the proposed model by Lewinsohn et al. (1985) [48]. However, these results should be taken with caution because the variable associations are not synonymous with causality. The changes in the variables from the theoretical model achieved with the intervention could have had an effect on depressive symptoms, but it is also possible that the change in depressive symptoms affected the variables from the theoretical model (positive environmental reinforcement and negative thoughts).

Those caregivers who had fewer depressive symptoms at the pre-intervention time point had better results after the intervention. One possible explanation is that the therapeutic change is more achievable when depressive symptoms are in their initial phase. Therefore, it is of utmost importance to administer preventive interventions in populations with the initial signs of depressive symptoms to prevent future depression.

Furthermore, adherence to the intervention was high. In this sample, 93.5% of caregivers attended all weekly conference call sessions. It is possible that telephone administration of the intervention, the short duration of the weekly telephone calls (only 30 min), the duration of the intervention (only five weeks), and adjusting to times that were convenient for them facilitated caregivers' attendance at these sessions. Caregivers performed an average of 14.2 homework tasks out of the 18 assigned during the intervention. Notifications to record tasks sent from the app itself to the caregiver's smartphone may have motivated and reminded the caregivers to complete and record the tasks. Lastly, satisfaction with the intervention was high, with a mean of 28.1 out of a maximum of 32 on the CSQ-8. Thus, participants rated the quality of the program very positively and indicated that it helped them better manage the difficulties that they experienced on a day-to-day basis.

This study has important implications for research and clinical practice. This is the first study on a psychological intervention for the indicated prevention of depression aimed at non-professional caregivers and administered through a smartphone app. Its innovative format and conference call delivery increases the accessibility of interventions and gives therapists new tools to reach more patients, following the recommendations of the National Institute of Mental Health Psychosocial

Intervention Development Workgroup (2002) [53] and the New Freedom Commission on Mental Health (2003) [54]. It allows caregivers to receive a psychological intervention program at the most convenient time and place for them. Its duration is short (only five weeks), and the non-face-to-face and group format of the conference calls makes the intervention more cost-efficient, enabling reduced waiting lists and lowering the cost to the healthcare system. In addition, this intervention could prevent the personal suffering associated with depression. If its long-term efficacy is demonstrated in a randomized controlled trial as in the previous face-to-face interventions [26], an intervention of just five modules (via application) could prevent (or at least delay) the onset of depression for 12 months. Later, if depressive symptoms of the caregiver increase, we recommend the caregiver to review the contents learned or conduct reinforcement sessions to refresh the learned skills. If a caregiver develops a major depressive episode, they could resort to appropriate individual treatment in the healthcare system, allowing a clinical step-by-step care [32].

However, the present study has some limitations, mainly its lack of a control group and the corresponding randomization of the participants to the treatment conditions, as well as its small sample size. Likewise, it should be noted that a three-month follow-up could be too soon to draw definitive conclusions on the prevention of depression. Therefore, additional extended follow-ups are recommended. Lastly, although the smartphone app intervention format offers many advantages thanks to its accessibility, we do not know under what conditions the participants interact with the app. We did not have information about how much attention they paid to the texts, if there were distractions while interacting with the app, or how they interpreted the contents of the program. Certain caregivers, depending on their profile, may benefit more from a program with the addition of more human contact.

Despite the limitations, and consistent with the methodological recommendations made by Muñoz et al. (1996) [55] for studies on the prevention of depression, this study included aspects that made it a rigorous scientific study, such as the following: defining the population for which the intervention was designed (inclusion and exclusion criteria; defining the symptoms or objective condition); using specific, replicable, and manualized interventions; assessing therapists' adherence to the protocol; using reliable and valid outcome measures; conducting multimodal evaluations; and blinding evaluation of results.

5. Conclusions

The results of the intervention considered here indicate a reduction in the incidence of depression and depressive symptoms, as well as a significant improvement of positive environmental reinforcement and negative automatic thoughts. Moreover, the high adherence and satisfaction with the intervention shows its acceptability and feasibility. The strengths of this intervention include its brief and innovative format via smartphone app and conference call, increasing its accessibility, flexibility and cost-efficiency, appealing to caregivers and therapists. This innovation could change the way in which psychological interventions are administered and reach a greater number of users, benefiting both caregivers from the present and the future. Taking into account the previously mentioned limitations (a lack of control group and a small sample size), these findings encourage future research of a randomized controlled trial with a larger sample size, and long-term follow-up to confirm the results of this study.

Author Contributions: Conceptualization, F.L.V., P.O., and Á.J.T.; methodology, P.O., F.L.V. and I.H.; validation, P.O., I.H., and F.L.V.; formal analysis, P.O., I.H.; investigation, P.O. and I.H.; writing—original draft preparation, P.O., I.H., and F.L.V.; writing—review and editing, P.O., F.L.V., I.H. and Á.J.T.; supervision, F.L.V. and Á.J.T.; project administration, F.L.V. and Á.J.T.; funding acquisition, F.L.V. and Á.J.T. All authors have read and agreed to the published version of the manuscript.

Funding: This research was funded by the Ministry of Economy, Industry and Competitiveness (Spain), grant number PSI2016-79041-P.

Acknowledgments: We want to thank the support of non-profit associations related to non-professional family caregivers of the Autonomous Region of Galicia, and the Ministry of Education, University and Professional Training and the Ministry of Economy, Employment and Industry, and the ESF Galicia 2014–2020 operational program (Xunta de Galicia).

Conflicts of Interest: The authors declare no conflict of interest. The funders had no role in the design of the study, the collection, analyses, or interpretation of data, the writing of the manuscript, or the decision to publish the results.

References

1. Triantafillou, J.; Naiditch, M.; Repkova, K.; Stiehr, K.; Carretero, S.; Emilsson, T.; Di Santo, P.; Bednarik, R.; Brichtova, L.; Ceruzzi, F.; et al. *Informal Care in the Long-Term Care System: European Overview Paper*; Interlinks: Athens, Vienna, 2010.
2. Palacios-Ceña, D.; Famoso-Pérez, P.; Salom-Moreno, J.; Carrasco-Garrido, P.; Pérez-Corrales, J.; Paras-Bravo, P.; Güeita-Rodriguez, J. "Living an Obstacle Course": A qualitative study examining the experiences of caregivers of children with Rett syndrome. *Int. J. Environ. Res. Public Health* **2019**, *16*, 41. [CrossRef]
3. Vázquez, F.L.; López, L.; Blanco, V.; Otero, P.; Torres, A.J.; Ferraces, M.J. The impact of decreased environmental reward in predicting depression severity in caregivers. *An. Psychol.* **2019**, *35*, 357–363.
4. Simón, M.A.; Bueno, A.; Otero, P.; Blanco, V.; Vázquez, F.L. Caregiver burden and sleep quality in dependent people's family caregivers. *J. Clin. Med.* **2019**, *8*, 1072. [CrossRef] [PubMed]
5. Simón, M.A.; Bueno, A.; Otero, P.; Blanco, V.; Vázquez, F.L. Insomnia in female family caregivers of totally dependent patients with dementia: An exploratory study. *Behav. Psychol.* **2019**, *27*, 107–119.
6. Meuser, T.M.; Marwit, S.J. A comprehensive, stage-sensitive model of grief in dementia caregiving. *Gerontologist* **2001**, *41*, 658–670. [CrossRef] [PubMed]
7. Madruga, M.; Gozalo, M.; Prieto, J.; Adsuar, J.C.; Gusi, N. Psychological symptomatology in informal caregivers of persons with dementia: Influences on health-related quality of life. *Int. J. Environ. Res. Public Health* **2020**, *17*, 1078. [CrossRef] [PubMed]
8. Perpiñá-Galvañ, J.; Orts-Beneito, N.; Fernández-Alcántara, M.; García-Sanjuán, S.; García-Caro, M.P.; Cabañero-Martínez, M.J. Level of burden and health-related quality of life in caregivers of palliative care patients. *Int. J. Environ. Res. Public Health* **2019**, *16*, 4806. [CrossRef]
9. Vázquez, F.L.; Otero, P.; Simón, M.A.; Bueno, A.M.; Blanco, V. Psychometric properties of the Spanish version of the Caregiver Burden Inventory. *Int. J. Environ. Res. Public Health* **2019**, *16*, 217. [CrossRef]
10. Schulz, R.; O'Brien, A.T.; Bookwala, J.; Fleissner, K. Psychiatric and physical morbidity effects of dementia caregiving: Prevalence, correlates, and causes. *Gerontologist* **1995**, *35*, 771–791. [CrossRef]
11. Cuijpers, P. Depressive disorders in caregivers of dementia patients: A systematic review. *Aging Ment. Health* **2005**, *9*, 325–330. [CrossRef]
12. Torres, Á.; Blanco, V.; Vázquez, F.L.; Díaz, O.; Otero, P.; Hermida, E. Prevalence of major depressive episodes in non-professional caregivers. *Psychiatry Res.* **2015**, *226*, 333–339. [CrossRef] [PubMed]
13. Ayuso-Mateos, J.L.; Vázquez-Barquero, J.L.; Dowrick, C.; Lehtinen, V.; Dalgard, O.S.; Casey, P.; Wilkinson, C.; Lasa, L.; Page, H.; Dunn, G.; et al. Depressive disorders in Europe: Prevalence figures from the ODIN study. *Br. J. Psychiatry* **2001**, *179*, 308–316. [CrossRef] [PubMed]
14. GBD 2017 Disease and Injury Incidence and Prevalence Collaborators. Global, regional, and national incidence, prevalence, and years lived with disability for 354 diseases and injuries for 195 countries and territories, 1990–2017: A systematic analysis for the Global Burden of Disease Study 2017. *Lancet* **2018**, *392*, 1789–1858. [CrossRef]
15. Hardeveld, F.; Spijker, J.; De Graaf, R.; Nolen, W.A.; Beekman, A.T.F. Recurrence of major depressive disorder and its predictors in the general population: Results from the Netherlands Mental Health Survey and Incidence Study (NEMESIS). *Psychol. Med.* **2013**, *43*, 39–48. [CrossRef]
16. Hoertel, N.; Blanco, C.; Oquendo, M.A.; Wall, M.M.; Olfson, M.; Falissard, B.; Franco, S.; Peyre, H.; Lemogne, C.; Limosin, F. A comprehensive model of predictors of persistence and recurrence in adults with major depression: Results from a national 3-year prospective study. *J. Psychiatr. Res.* **2017**, *95*, 19–27. [CrossRef]
17. ten Have, M.; de Graaf, R.; van Dorsselaer, S.; Tuithof, M.; Kleinjan, M.; Penninx, B.W.J.H. Recurrence and chronicity of major depressive disorder and their risk indicators in a population cohort. *Acta Psychiatr. Scand.* **2018**, *137*, 503–515. [CrossRef]
18. Greenberg, P.E.; Fournier, A.A.; Sisitsky, T.; Pike, C.T.; Kessler, R.C. The economic burden of adults with major depressive disorder in the United States (2005 and 2010). *J. Clin. Psychiatry* **2015**, *76*, 155–162. [CrossRef]

19. Williamson, G.M.; Shaffer, D.R. Relationship quality and potentially harmful behaviors by spousal caregivers: How we were then, how we are now. *Psychol. Aging* **2001**, *16*, 217–226. [CrossRef]
20. Institute of Medicine. *Reducing Risks for Mental Disorders: Frontiers for Preventive Intervention Research*; National Academic Press: Washington, DC, USA, 1994.
21. Muñoz, R.F.; Beardslee, W.R.; Leykin, Y. Major depression can be prevented. *Am. Psychol.* **2012**, *67*, 285–295. [CrossRef]
22. Vázquez, F.L.; Otero, P.; Torres, A.; Hermida, E.; Blanco, V.; Díaz, O. A brief problem-solving indicated-prevention intervention for prevention of depression in nonprofessional caregivers. *Psicothema* **2013**, *25*, 87–92.
23. Otero, P.; Smit, F.; Cuijpers, P.; Torres, A.; Blanco, V.; Vázquez, F.L. Long-term efficacy of indicated prevention of depression in non-professional caregivers: Randomized controlled trial. *Psychol. Med.* **2015**, *45*, 1401–1412. [CrossRef] [PubMed]
24. López, L.; Smit, F.; Cuijpers, P.; Otero, P.; Blanco, V.; Torres, Á.; Vázquez, F.L. Problem-solving intervention to prevent depression in non-professional caregivers: A randomized controlled trial with 8 years of follow-up. *Psychol. Med.* **2020**, *50*, 1002–1009. [CrossRef] [PubMed]
25. Vázquez, F.L.; Hermida, E.; Torres, A.; Otero, P.; Blanco, V.; Díaz, O. Eficacia de una intervención preventiva cognitivo conductual en cuidadoras con síntomas depresivos elevados. [Efficacy of a brief cognitive-behavioral intervention in female caregivers with high depressive symptoms]. *Behav. Psychol.* **2014**, *22*, 79–96.
26. Vázquez, F.L.; Torres, Á.; Blanco, V.; Otero, P.; Díaz, O.; Ferraces, M.J. Long-term follow-up of a randomized clinical trial assessing the efficacy of a brief cognitive-behavioral depression prevention intervention for caregivers with elevated depressive symptoms. *Am. J. Geriatr. Psychiatry* **2016**, *24*, 421–432. [CrossRef] [PubMed]
27. Blanco, V.; Otero, P.; López, L.; Torres, Á.; Vázquez, F.L. Predictores del cambio clínicamente significativo en una intervención de prevención de la depresión. [Clinically significant predictors of change in an intervention for the prevention of depression]. *Rev. Iberoam. Psicol. Salud.* **2017**, *8*, 9–20. [CrossRef]
28. Reese, R.J.; Conoley, C.W.; Brossart, D.F. The attractiveness of telephone counseling: An empirical investigation of client perceptions. *J. Couns. Dev.* **2006**, *84*, 54–60. [CrossRef]
29. Vázquez, F.L.; López, L.; Torres, Á.J.; Otero, P.; Blanco, V.; Díaz, O.; Páramo, M. Analysis of the components of a cognitive-behavioral intervention for the prevention of depression administered via conference call to nonprofessional caregivers: A randomized controlled trial. *Int. J. Environ. Res. Public Health* **2020**, *17*, 2067. [CrossRef]
30. Taylor, K.; Silver, L. *Smartphone Ownership is Growing Rapidly around the World, but not Always Equally*; Pew Research Center: Washington, DC, USA, 2019.
31. Andersson, G.; Cuijpers, P. Internet-based and other computerized psychological treatments for adult depression: A meta-analysis. *Cogn. Behav. Ther.* **2009**, *38*, 196–205. [CrossRef]
32. Nicholas, J.; Ringland, K.E.; Graham, A.K.; Knapp, A.A.; Lattie, E.G.; Kwasny, M.J.; Mohr, D.C. Stepping up: Predictors of 'stepping' within an iCBT stepped-care intervention for depression. *Int. J. Environ. Res. Public Health* **2019**, *16*, 4689. [CrossRef]
33. Arean, P.A.; Hallgren, K.A.; Jordan, J.T.; Gazzaley, A.; Atkins, D.C.; Heagerty, P.J.; Anguera, J.A. The use and effectiveness of mobile Apps for depression: Results from a fully remote clinical trial. *J. Med. Internet Res.* **2016**, *18*, e330. [CrossRef]
34. Ly, K.H.; Trüschel, A.; Jarl, L.; Magnusson, S.; Windahl, T.; Johansson, R.; Carlbring, P.; Andersson, G. Behavioural activation versus mindfulness-based guided self-help treatment administered through a smartphone application: A randomised controlled trial. *BMJ Open* **2014**, *4*, e003440. [CrossRef] [PubMed]
35. Swift, J.K.; Greenberg, R.P. Premature discontinuation in adult psychotherapy: A meta-analysis. *J. Consult. Clin. Psychol.* **2012**, *80*, 547–559. [CrossRef] [PubMed]
36. Otero, P.; Vázquez, F.L.; Hermida, E.; Díaz, O.; Torres, Á. Relationship of cognitive behavioral therapy effects and homework in an indicated prevention of depression intervention for non-professional caregivers. *Psychol. Rep.* **2015**, *116*, 841–854. [CrossRef] [PubMed]
37. Miltenberger, R.G. *Behavior Modification: Principles and Procedures*, 5th ed.; Wadsworth/Thomson Learning: Belmont, MA, USA, 2012.
38. Radloff, L.S. The CES-D Scale: A self-report depression scale for research in the general population. *Appl. Psychol. Meas.* **1977**, *1*, 385–401. [CrossRef]

39. Vázquez, F.L.; Blanco, V.; López, M. An adaptation of the Center for Epidemiologic Studies Depression Scale for use in non-psychiatric Spanish populations. *Psychiatry Res.* **2007**, *149*, 247–252. [CrossRef]
40. American Psychiatric Association. *Diagnostic and Statistical Manual of Mental Disorders*; American Psychiatric Association: Washington, DC, USA, 2013.
41. First, M.B.; Williams, J.B.W.; Karg, R.S.; Spitzer, R.L. *Structured Clinical Interview for DSM-5® Disorders—Clinician Version (SCID-5-CV)*; American Psychiatric Association Publishing: Arlington, VA, USA, 2015.
42. Armento, M.E.A.; Hopko, D.R. The Environmental Reward Observation Scale (EROS): Development, validity, and reliability. *Behav. Ther.* **2007**, *38*, 107–119. [CrossRef]
43. Barraca, J.; Pérez-Álvarez, M. Adaptación española del Environmental Reward Observation Scale (EROS) [Spanish adaptation of Environmental Reward Observation Scale (EROS)]. *Ansiedad Estrés* **2010**, *16*, 95–107.
44. Hollon, S.D.; Kendall, P.C. Cognitive self-statements in depression: Development of an automatic thoughts questionnaire. *Cognit. Ther. Res.* **1980**, *4*, 383–395. [CrossRef]
45. Otero, P.; Vázquez, F.L.; Blanco, V.; Torres, Á. Propiedades psicométricas del Cuestionario de Pensamientos Automáticos (ATQ) en la población de cuidadores familiares [Psychometric properties of the Automatic Thoughts Questionnaire (ATQ) in family caregivers]. *Behav. Psychol.* **2017**, *25*, 387–403.
46. Larsen, D.L.; Attkisson, C.C.; Hargreaves, W.A.; Nguyen, T.D. Assessment of client/patient satisfaction: Development of a general scale. *Eval. Program Plan.* **1979**, *2*, 197–207. [CrossRef]
47. Vázquez, F.L.; Torres, Á.; Otero, P.; Blanco, V.; Attkisson, C.C. Psychometric properties of the Castilian Spanish version of the Client Satisfaction Questionnaire (CSQ-8). *Curr. Psychol.* **2019**, *38*, 829–835. [CrossRef]
48. Lewinsohn, P.M.; Hoberman, H.; Teri, L.; Hautzinger, M. An integrative theory of depression. In *Theoretical Issues in Behaviour Therapy*; Reiss, S., Bootzin, R.R., Eds.; Academic Press: New York, NY, USA, 1985; pp. 313–359.
49. Cohen, J. *Statistical Power Analysis for the Behavioural Sciences*, 2nd ed.; Lawrence Erlbaum Associates, Inc.: Hillsdale, NJ, USA, 1988.
50. Domenéch, J.M.; Navarro, J.B. *Regresión Lineal Múltiple con Predictores Cuantitativos y Categóricos [Multiple Regression with Quantitative and Cathegorical Predictors]*; Signo: Barcelona, Spain, 2006.
51. Vázquez, F.L.; Otero, P.; López, L.; Blanco, V.; Torres, A.; Díaz, O. La prevención de la depresión en cuidadores a través de multiconferencia telefónica [Prevention of depression in caregivers through conference calls]. *Clin. Salud.* **2018**, *29*, 14–20. [CrossRef]
52. Muñoz, R.F.; Cuijpers, P.; Smit, F.; Barrera, A.Z.; Leykin, Y. Prevention of major depression. *Annu. Rev. Clin. Psychol.* **2010**, *6*, 181–212. [CrossRef] [PubMed]
53. Hollon, S.D.; Muñoz, R.F.; Barlow, D.H.; Beardslee, W.R.; Bell, C.C.; Bernal, G.; Clarke, G.N.; Franciosi, L.P.; Kazdin, A.E.; Kohn, L.; et al. Psychosocial intervention development for the prevention and treatment of depression: Promoting innovation and increasing access. *Biol. Psychiatry* **2002**, *52*, 610–630. [CrossRef]
54. New Freedom Commission on Mental Health. *Achieving the Promise: Transforming Mental Health Care in America*; DHHS: Rockville, MD, USA, 2003.
55. Muñoz, R.F.; Mrazek, P.J.; Haggerty, R.J. Institute of Medicine report on prevention of mental disorders: Summary and commentary. *Am. Psychol.* **1996**, *51*, 1116–1122. [CrossRef] [PubMed]

© 2020 by the authors. Licensee MDPI, Basel, Switzerland. This article is an open access article distributed under the terms and conditions of the Creative Commons Attribution (CC BY) license (http://creativecommons.org/licenses/by/4.0/).

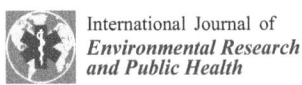 International Journal of
Environmental Research and Public Health

Article

A Low-Intensity Internet-Based Intervention Focused on the Promotion of Positive Affect for the Treatment of Depression in Spanish Primary Care: Secondary Analysis of a Randomized Controlled Trial

Mª Dolores Vara [1,2,*], Adriana Mira [3], Marta Miragall [2,3], Azucena García-Palacios [2,4], Cristina Botella [2,4], Margalida Gili [5,6,7], Pau Riera-Serra [5,6], Javier García-Campayo [7,8], Fermín Mayoral-Cleries [9] and Rosa Mª Baños [1,2,3]

[1] Polibienestar Research Institute, University of Valencia, 46022 Valencia, Spain; banos@uv.es
[2] CIBERObn Physiopathology of Obesity and Nutrition, Instituto de Salud Carlos III, 28029 Madrid, Spain; marta.miragall@uv.es (M.M.); azucena@uji.es (A.G.-P.); botella@uji.es (C.B.)
[3] Department of Personality, Evaluation and Psychological Treatment, Faculty of Psychology, University of Valencia, 46010 Valencia, Spain; adriana.mira@uv.es
[4] Department of Basic and Clinical Psychology and Psychobiology, Faculty of Health Sciences, Jaume I University, 12071 Castellon de la Plana, Spain
[5] Institut Universitari d'Investigació en Ciències de la Salut, University of Balearic Islands, E-07122 Palma de Mallorca, Spain; mgili@uib.es (M.G.); pau.riera@uib.es (P.R.-S.)
[6] Institut d'Investigació Sanitaria Illes Balears, 07120 Palma de Mallorca, Spain
[7] Primary Care Prevention and Health Promotion Research Network, RedIAPP, 28029 Madrid, Spain; jgarcamp@unizar.es
[8] Aragon Institute for Health Research (IIS Aragón), Miguel Servet Hospital, University of Zaragoza, 50009 Zaragoza, Spain
[9] Mental Health Unit, Hospital Regional of Malaga, Biomedicine Research Institute (IBIMA), 29010 Málaga, Spain; fermin.mayoral.sspa@juntadeandalucia.es
* Correspondence: m.dolores.vara@uv.es

Received: 26 September 2020; Accepted: 30 October 2020; Published: 3 November 2020

Abstract: *Background:* A large number of low-intensity Internet-based interventions (IBIs) for the treatment of depression have emerged in Primary Care; most of them focused on decreasing negative emotions. However, recent studies have highlighted the importance of addressing positive affect (PA) as well. This study is a secondary analysis of a randomized control trial. We examine the role of an IBI focused on promoting PA in patients with depression in Primary Care (PC). The specific objectives were to explore the profile of the patients who benefit the most and to analyze the change mechanisms that predict a significantly greater improvement in positive functioning measures. *Methods:* 56 patients were included. Measures of depression, affect, well-being, health-related quality of life, and health status were administered. *Results:* Participants who benefited the most were those who had lower incomes and education levels and worse mental health scores and well-being at baseline (7.9%–39.5% of explained variance). Improvements in depression severity and PA were significant predictors of long-term change in well-being, $F(3,55) = 17.78$, $p < 0.001$, $R^2 = 47.8\%$. *Conclusions:* This study highlights the importance of implementing IBIs in PC and the relevance of PA as a key target in Major Depressive Disorder treatment.

Keywords: depression; primary care; internet-based intervention; positive affect

1. Introduction

Major depressive disorder (MDD) is one of the most prevalent mental disorders worldwide, and it is associated with significant personal and social costs [1,2]. Specifically, the prevalence of depression in Spanish Primary Care (PC) is between 13.9 and 29% [3]. Even though there are effective treatments for this disorder (pharmacotherapy, psychotherapy, or both) [4,5], only half the people with depression receive adequate care [6], only two-thirds of patients respond to treatment, and only about one-third experience remission of their depressive symptoms [7,8]. Therefore, it is important to continue to explore different ways to improve these treatment outcomes.

Currently, there are evidence-based psychological treatments (e.g., cognitive-behavioral therapy, interpersonal therapy, problem-solving therapy) for depressive disorders in PC [9]. However, their therapeutic approaches have focused mainly on improving negative affect (NA) (e.g., depression, anxiety), paying less attention to the role of promoting positive affect (PA) and building positive resources (e.g., well-being, strengths) [10,11]. The literature indicates that MDD is related to low levels of positive emotions and that depression is more associated with low levels of PA than other emotional disorders [12]. Several studies point out the importance of promoting PA—as well as gratitude, resilience, and positive functioning—as core elements of interventions to facilitate recovery from depression [13,14].

A possible alternative in understanding MDD is to consider it a heterogeneous diagnostic construct with different underlying functional domains that may require different therapeutic strategies, as proposed in the Research Domain Criteria (RDoC) and transdiagnostic approaches [15]. Within this framework, MDD is proposed as resulting from alterations in two partly dissociable neurobiological dimensions: the upregulation of a negative valence system that promotes NA and leads to a pervasive depressed mood; and the downregulation of a positive valence system that guides the focus toward rewarding stimuli or PA, leading to loss of interest or pleasure (anhedonia) [16,17]. In the same vein, to effectively treat depression, research needs to propose psychotherapeutic interventions that include elements to downregulate NA and upregulate PA.

Several therapeutic approaches from the positive psychology (PP) field [18] are emerging with the aim of enhancing positive emotional human functioning (e.g., well-being, resilience, satisfaction with life), especially PA. Some reviews and meta-analyses show that PP interventions are effective in reducing depressive symptoms and increasing well-being [19–22], emphasizing their role alongside standard treatments for clinical depression [23].

One of the most important obstacles to integrating these treatments in PC settings is the lack of time and resources [24]. Many of the empirically validated treatments for MDD consist of 15–20 sessions requiring one hour per week [25,26]. Although this treatment length is considered quite brief compared to previous approaches, it has been argued that it is still too intense to be implemented in PC. One way to reduce the high costs of MDD treatment and overcome the limitations of traditional treatments in PC (e.g., logistical, geographical, and access difficulties) is to propose the use of brief or low-intensity psychological interventions for the treatment of MDD. Internet-based interventions (IBIs) are an example of low-intensity interventions that have been shown to be appropriate and cost-effective options within the stepped care model for the treatment of MDD [27]. Given the potential of IBIs as low-intensity interventions in PC, we conducted a randomized control trial (RCT) in a sample of patients diagnosed with MDD in different PC settings in Spain [28]. In this study, we examined the effectiveness of three low-intensity IBIs (PA promotion vs. healthy lifestyle vs. mindfulness) along with improved treatment as usual (iTAU), compared to iTAU alone, and the results were promising [29]. Specifically, healthy lifestyle and mindfulness interventions were effective in reducing depression severity, compared to iTAU, at post-treatment. Moreover, all the interventions were also effective in improving medium- and long-term quality of life. Finally, the PA promotion intervention was found to be effective in improving well-being at the six-month follow-up and NA at the 12-month follow-up, compared to iTAU.

The present study is a secondary analysis of the RCT carried out by Gili et al. [29]. More specifically, this study carries out an in-depth examination of the role of a specific IBI to promote PA as an adjunct therapy to iTAU in PC settings, given PA's potential as a strategy to improve well-being in MDD patients. Hence, the specific objectives are to determine: (1) which patient profile (i.e., sociodemographic and clinical baseline variables) predicts the improvement in depression severity and positive functioning in the post-treatment and follow-up sessions (Objective 1); and (2) which change mechanism predicts the greatest change in measures related to positive functioning in the post-treatment and follow-up sessions (Objective 2). The results on the efficacy of the PA intervention (vs. iTAU condition) can be found in Gili et al. [29]. Nevertheless, we will also analyze the changes in the primary and secondary outcomes from pre-treatment to post-treatment and at the 6- and 12-month follow-ups to provide a better understanding of the results of Objective 1 and 2. No specific hypotheses are proposed due to the exploratory nature of the analyses.

2. Materials and Methods

2.1. Study Design

This is a secondary analysis study of an RCT with repeated measures (baseline, post-treatment, 6-month and 12-month follow-ups) with four independent conditions: (a) PA promotion IBI + iTAU; (b) healthy lifestyle psychoeducational IBI + iTAU; (c) mindfulness IBI + iTAU; and (d) only iTAU group, in PC ([29]; Current Controlled Trials ISRCTN82388279). In the present study, we will only focus on the condition of the PA promotion IBI + iTAU.

2.2. Participants

In the original study, a total of 221 participants were recruited in PC settings from the Spanish regions of Aragon, Andalusia, and the Balearic Islands. The present study included 56 participants (78.6% women) who completed the PA intervention. Ages ranged between 19 and 68 years, with a mean of 44.14 years ($SD = 10.38$). In addition, 55.4% of the participants were married, 80.4% lived with family or a partner, 28.6% had higher education, 44.6% were employed, and 23.2% had an income below the national minimum wage. Regarding depression severity at baseline, the average on the Spanish Patient Health Questionnaire-9 (PHQ-9) was 15.79 ($SD = 6.21$).

Inclusion criteria were: (a) having mild or moderately severe depressive symptoms according to the Spanish Patient Health Questionnaire-9 (PHQ-9; [30]) (5–9 = Mild depression; 10–14 = moderate depression); (b) age between 18–65 years; (c) ability to use a computer; (d) having Internet and an email account; and (e) being able to read and understand Spanish. The Mini International Neuropsychiatric Interview (MINI) 5.0 [31,32] was used to assess different mental disorders and establish the diagnosis. Patients were excluded from the study if they had (a) severe depression (score ≥14 on the PHQ-9); (b) a severe Axis I psychiatric disorder (e.g., psychotic disorders, presence of suicidal ideation or plan, alcohol/substance abuse or dependence); (c) any disease that can affect the central nervous system (e.g., brain pathology, traumatic brain injury, dementia); or (d) if they were currently receiving psychological treatment.

Full information on the participant flow of the PA intervention is shown in Figure 1.

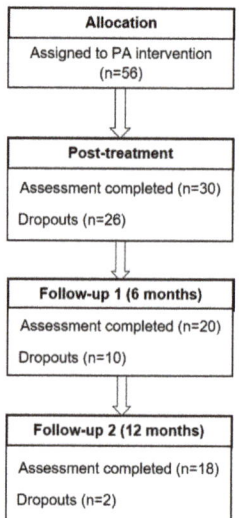

Figure 1. Patient flow diagram. PA: positive affect

2.3. Interventions

All the participants in the PA condition completed the low-intensity IBI and received iTAU from their general practitioner (GP).

2.3.1. Low-Intensity Internet-Based Computerized Intervention (IBI) Focused on the Promotion of PA

Before starting the online treatment, participants received a 90-min (3–5 patients) group face-to-face session conducted by a clinical psychologist. The objective of this session was to explain the program structure and the main components of the treatment, clarify the instructions for the use of the online platform, and motivate participants to change.

The online self-guided program consisted of four therapeutic modules (60 min per module approximately). The program duration could vary among the users, but it was usually completed in 4 to 8 weeks (maximum of 2 weeks per module). These modules contained multimedia elements (videos, images, texts) that provided information about MDD and coping strategies. These modules were sequential so that users could move step by step through the program. Moreover, users could review the module's contents after they had finished.

To enhance adherence, participants received two weekly automated mobile phone messages encouraging them to proceed with the program and reminding them of the importance of doing the homework tasks. In addition, the participants received automated emails encouraging them to continue with the modules if they had not accessed the program for a week.

Specifically, this intervention was based on PP techniques, and it was mainly designed to decrease depression severity and prevent relapse by promoting PA and subjective well-being. Table 1 shows each module, its objectives, and its specific content. For more information about the protocol for promoting PA, see García-Palacios, Mira, Mayoral, Baños, and Botella [33].

Table 1. Modules, objectives, and therapeutic content of Internet-Based Computerized Intervention (IBI).

Module	Objectives	Therapeutic Content
1. Learning to live	- Understanding the role of activity in mood regulation and our well-being. - Establishing and maintaining an adequate activity level and the relevance of choosing activities that are significant, with a personal meaning for the individual. - Learning the procedure to follow to schedule meaningful activities in daily life.	1. The role of activity in our well-being. 2. Things we should do and things we can do: meaningful activities. 3. The importance of daring, of getting involved with life. 4. Seeking social support. 5. Overcoming obstacles.
2. Learning to enjoy	- Learning about the effect of positive emotions in our lives. - Learning procedures to increase the likelihood of experiencing positive emotions, promoting the occurrence of pleasant activities to learn to enjoy the present moment.	1. Positive emotions, such as seeds or life anchors. 2. Satisfaction with the present. 3. Learning to generate good moments. 4. The importance of smiling. 5. Learn to identify, capture, and save good times.
3. Accepting to live	- Focusing on positive emotions related to the past (e.g., gratitude) or the future (such as optimism). - Identification and management of beliefs and behaviors that disturb the good moments.	1. Satisfaction with the past. 2. Satisfaction with the future. 3. Psychological well-being as a result of being active and practicing learned strategies.
4. Living and learning	- Understanding life as a continuous process of learning and personal growth. - Emphasizing the training in strategies to promote psychological strengths, resilience, and meaningful goals linked to important values.	1. Finding psychological well-being. 2. Potential, talents, and life goals. 3. Living with others, finding support in others. 4. What do I want my future to be like?

2.3.2. iTAU

The Treatment as Usual (TAU) in PC settings was improved. The participating GP received a training program on how to diagnose and treat depression in PC, based on the Spanish Guide for the Treatment of Depression in Primary Care [34]. Participants could receive medication for at least two months, and they had at least four visits with the GP that lasted an average of 30 min each. In cases with suicide risk, severe social dysfunction, or worsening of symptoms, the GP had to refer the patient to mental health facilities.

2.4. Measures

2.4.1. Primary Outcome Measure

Depression severity: The Patient Health Questionnaire-9 (PHQ-9; [35]) is a 9-item self-administered test for screening, diagnosing, monitoring, and measuring depression severity. Patients describe their state, taking into account the two weeks before the evaluation. Items are rated from 0 to 3, denoting "not at all", "several days", "more than half the days", and "nearly every day", respectively. Cut-off points of 5, 10, 15, and 20 represent mild, moderate, moderately severe, and severe depression

(DSM-IV-TR; [36]). The Spanish version has been shown to have good psychometric properties (for the diagnosis of any disorder, k = 0.74; overall accuracy, 88%; sensitivity, 87%; specificity, 88%) [30]. In the current study, the alpha coefficient was very satisfactory (α = 0.86).

2.4.2. Secondary Outcomes Measures

Affect: The Positive and Negative Affect Scale (PANAS; [37]) consists of 20 items that evaluate two independent dimensions: PA (10 items) and NA (10 items). The total score for each subscale ranges from 5 to 50, using a 5-point Likert-type scale (1 = very slightly or not at all, 5 = very much). The Spanish version by Sandín et al. [38] showed adequate internal consistency. In the current study, alpha coefficients were very satisfactory for both scales (αs = 0.87 and 0.86 for positive and negative subscales, respectively).

Well-being: The Pemberton Happiness Index (PHI; [39]) consists of 11 items related to different domains of remembered well-being (general, hedonic, eudaimonic, and social well-being), each with an 11-point Likert-type scale (0 = strongly disagree, 10 = strongly agree), and 10 items related to experienced well-being (positive and negative emotional events that may have happened the day before), with dichotomous response options (yes/no). The sum of the remembered and experienced well-being scores yields a combined well-being index (total well-being) ranging from 0 to 10. The validated Spanish version showed adequate psychometric properties [39]. In the current study, the alpha coefficient was very satisfactory (α = 0.86). In the current study, the alpha coefficient was very satisfactory (αs = 0.80).

Health-related quality of life: The Short Form 12 Health Survey (SF-12; [40]) is a 12-item questionnaire that measures aspects of health-related quality of life from the patient's perspective in two dimensions: physical health (general health, bodily pain, role-physical, physical functioning) and mental health (mental health, role-emotional, social-functioning, vitality). Scores > 50 represent better physical or mental health than the mean, and scores <50 represent worse physical or mental health than the mean. The Spanish version has been found to be a valid and reliable measure, showing good internal consistency [41]. In the current study, alpha coefficients were acceptable for both scales (αs = 0.80 for the physical health dimension and 0.66 for the mental health dimension, respectively).

Health status: The EuroQoL (EQ-5D; [42]) is a 5-item instrument to assess general health status (mobility, self-care, pain, usual activities, and psychological status) with three possible answers for each item (1 = no problem, 2 = moderate problem, 3 = severe problem). A summary index with a maximum score of 1 can be derived from these five dimensions using a conversion table [42]. The maximum score of 1 indicates the best health state, in contrast to the scores on individual questions, where higher scores indicate more severe or frequent problems. In addition to the descriptive system, the EQ-5D includes a visual analog scale (EQ VAS). The EQ VAS is a rating scale ranging from 0 (worst imaginable health state) to 100 (best imaginable health state), and it represents the evaluation of the patient's health state from his/her point of view. The validated Spanish version of the EQ-5D was used [42]. In this study, only the EQ VAS was taken into account.

2.4.3. Screening Related Measures

Sociodemographic data: Personal data that includes information such as age, sex, marital status, living alone or with others, educational level, employment, and income level.

Diagnostic interview: The MINI International Neuropsychiatric Interview version 5.0 (M.I.N.I. 5.0; [31]) is used in the screening to assess current depression and comorbid disorders. This measure is a structured diagnostic interview based on the DSM-IV and ICD-10 criteria. The Spanish version [32] was used for this study.

2.5. Procedure

Patients were recruited in Spanish PC settings from three different regions between March 2015 and March 2016. GPs detected possible participants with MDD using the PHQ-9. After a few days, an independent researcher used the MINI to assess the participants, taking into account the inclusion and exclusion criteria. Participants gave their signed written informed consent to be part of the study. Then, randomization was carried out by another independent researcher. All participants completed the pre-treatment assessment integrated into a web system (https://psicologiaytecnologia.labpsitec.es/). At the end of the treatment, they also completed the post-treatment and follow-up assessments through the website. The PHQ-9, PANAS, and SF-12 were administered at baseline, post-treatment, and 6-month and 12-month follow-ups. The PHI and EQ-5D were administered only at baseline and in the follow-up sessions. The Ethical Review Board of the regional health authority approved the study (Ref: IB 2144/13PI). More details about the study design, recruitment, and randomization methods are included in the protocol study by Castro et al. [28].

2.6. Data Analyses

All statistical analyses were performed using the SPSS v.26 (IBM Corp, Armonk, NY, USA). First, we implemented Multiple Imputation with Chained Equations (MICE) to replace the outcomes' missing values, performing 100 imputation models with 100 iterations per model [43].

Second, preliminary analyses were conducted to ensure that relevant assumptions of repeated-measures ANOVAs and multiple regression were met (i.e., normality, sphericity, and absence of multicollinearity). We tested normality, carrying out a visual inspection of the Q-Q (quantile-quantile) plots, verifying that the observed data was approximately closed to the expected data (i.e., the distance between the observed and expected data was not extreme). Hence, we assured that we met the normality assumption to carry out a repeated-measures ANOVA and multiple regression. Moreover, we tested the assumption of sphericity using Mauchly's test. If Mauchly's test statistic was significant (i.e., sphericity was not met), the degrees of freedom were adjusted using the Greenhouse–Geisser correction. Finally, we tested the absence of multicollinearity using the Variance Inflation Factor (VIF).

Third, seven repeated-measures ANOVA with time as within-factor—pre-treatment (Pre), post-treatment (Post), 6-month follow-up (FW6), and 12-month follow up (FW12)—were conducted to analyze the changes in each primary (i.e., PHQ-9) and secondary (i.e., PANAS-PA, PANAS-NA, PHI, SF-12 mental and physical health, EQ-5D) outcomes. Post-hoc analyses using Bonferroni corrections were carried out when significant effects were found. Within-group Cohen's d effect sizes with a 95% Confidence Interval were calculated.

Fourth, seven hierarchical multiple regression analyses with a stepwise selection of predictors within each block were conducted to explore which sociodemographic variables (i.e., sex, age, marital status, living alone or with others, educational level, employment, and income level) and pre-treatment scores on each primary and secondary outcome predicted the pre-post treatment, pre-FW6, and pre-FW12 change. The seven sociodemographic variables were entered in the first block, and six pre-treatment scores were entered in the second block to test the relevance of the extra explained variance of these variables in the dependent variables once the effects of the sociodemographic variables were controlled for. Given the small sample size to the number of predictors, a consideration of all predictors simultaneously in each regression was not tenable. Therefore, within each block, a statistical inclusion criterion for relevant predictors (stepwise method) was used. Creating two blocks in the regression analyses allowed us to test a lower number of predictors in each regression (i.e., seven instead of thirteen predictors).

To carry out correlation and regression analyses, categorical sociodemographic variables were transformed into recoded binary variables; that is, the correlation and regression analyses included: dichotomous variables (i.e., sex), continuous variables (i.e., age and scores in PHQ-9, PANAS-PA, PANAS-NA, PHI, SF-12 mental and physical health, EQ-5D) and recoded binary variables (i.e., ordinal or categorical variables were recoded into dichotomous variables with 0 and 1). Regarding the recoded binary variables, the categories were recategorized as follows: (a) marital status: 0 = not married (i.e., single, divorced, widowed); 1 = married or in a relationship; (b) *living alone or with others:* 0 = living alone; 1 = living with others (i.e., partner, sons, relatives, friends); (c) *educational level:* 0 = lower level (i.e., no education or primary school); 1 = higher level (i.e., secondary school or university studies); (d) *work status*: 0 = "not-working" (i.e., unemployed, retired, housekeeper, disability, student); 1 = employed; (e) *income level*: 0 = "lower than the minimum income (i.e., <641.40€); 1 = higher than the minimum income. We recoded into binary variables (instead of doing dummy variables) because the pair comparisons we constructed were theoretically appropriate, and a smaller number of predictors should be tested in the regression analyses. That is, if binary variables are used, only one predictor should be tested (e.g., 0 = "lower than the minimum income (i.e., <641.40€) vs. 1 = higher than the minimum income); however, if dummy variables are used, more than one predictor should be included in the regression equation (e.g., *dummy 1*: 0 = "lower than the minimum income < 641.40€ vs. 1 = between 1–2 minimum incomes; *dummy 2*: 0 = "lower than the minimum income < 641.40€ vs. 1 = between 2–4 minimum incomes). Moreover, the change in each primary and secondary outcome was calculated as follows: pre-post (post-treatment scores—pre-treatment scores), pre-FW6 (6-month follow up—pre-treatment scores), and pre-FW12 (12-month follow-up—pre-treatment scores). Negative values for the changes in PHQ and PANAS-NA meant improvements in these measures, whereas negative values for the changes in PANAS-PA, PHI, SF-12, and 5Q-5D meant a deterioration in these measures. The pairwise deletion method was used (i.e., whenever the variables of interest are present, they are analyzed) to deal with missing values and preserve all the data available in the regression analyses. The pre-treatment score on the corresponding dependent variable was not introduced in the equation regression model (e.g., the PHQ-9 pre score was not introduced as a predictor when the change in PHQ-9 was tested as a dependent variable).

Finally, four stepwise multiple regression analyses were conducted to analyze whether the changes in PHQ, PANAS-PA, or PANAS-NA were predictors of the change in PHI, SF-12 (mental and physical health), and EQ-5D. Changes in pre-post predictors were introduced for changes in pre-post dependent variables; changes in pre-post and pre-FW6 predictors were introduced for changes in pre-FW6 dependent variables; and changes in pre-post, pre-FW6, and pre-FW-12 predictors were introduced for changes in pre-FW12 dependent variables. All predictor variables were entered in the same block using the stepwise method.

It should be noted that the stepwise approach was used because we did not have an a priori hypotheses of which specific independent variables would predict the dependent variables, and consequently, we decided to identify the predictor variables relying on a statistical criterion.

3. Results

3.1. Sociodemographic Characteristics of the Sample

Table 2 shows a detailed description of the sociodemographic variables.

Table 2. Sociodemographic characteristics of the sample.

Sociodemographic Variables	%	n = 56
Sex		
Women	78.6%	44
Men	21.4%	12
Age (years)	44.14 (10.38) [a]	
Marital status		
Single	16.1% [b]	31
In a relationship/Married	55.4%	9
Divorced/Separated	16.1%	9
Widowed	1.8%	1
Income level		
Lower than the minimum income (<641,40€)	23.2%	13
Between 1–2 minimum incomes [c]	25.0%	14
Between 2–4 minimum incomes	21.4%	12

Table 2. Cont.

Sociodemographic Variables	%	n = 56
Work status		
Student	3.6%	2
Housekeeper	3.6%	2
Subsidized unemployed	5.4%	3
Unemployed with no subsidy	12.5%	7
Employee	44.6%	25
Sick leave	8.9%	5
Retired	3.6%	2
Disability	3.6%	2
Others	3.6%	2
Educational Level		
No education	5.4%	3
Primary school	16.1%	9
Secondary school	33.9%	19
University studies	28.6%	16
Living alone or with others		
Alone	8.9%	5
Living with partner	16.1%	9
Living with partner and children	53.6%	30
Living with relatives	8.9%	5
Living with friends or neighbors	1.8%	1

Note. [a] These values are the mean and standard deviation of age, which is a continuous variable. [b] Due to missing values, the sum of the percentages of the categories of the "marital status", "income level", "work status", "educational level", or "living alone or with others" are not 100%. That is, we do not have the 30.4% of the information regarding "income level" (n = 17); the 10.7% of the information regarding "marital status", "work status", and "living alone or with others" (n = 6); and the 16.1% of the information regarding the "educational level (n = 9). [c] Between "1–2 or "2–4" minimum incomes means that the minimum income level is equivalent to "641,40€ (641,40€× 1)–1282,80€ (641,40€× 2)" or "1282,80€ (641,40€× 2)–2.565,60€ (641,40€× 4)", respectively.

3.2. Primary and Secondary Outcome Scores at Pre-Treatment, Post-Treatment, and 6- and 12-Month Follow-Ups

Descriptive statistics, repeated-measures ANOVA results, and within-group effect sizes with 95% CI are shown in Table 3 for primary and secondary outcomes. The main effects of time were found for all the primary and secondary outcomes, with increases in the PANAS-PA, PHI, SF-12, and EQ-5D scores and decreases in the PHQ-9 and PANAS-NA scores.

Post-hoc analyses using the Bonferroni correction showed that there were significant differences from pre-treatment to post-treatment, FW6, and FW12 in depression severity (PHQ-9), PA (PANAS-PA), NA (PANAS-NA), and Mental Health (SF-12) ($p < 0.05$). Significant differences from pre-treatment to FW12 were found for Physical Health (SF-12), but not from pre-treatment to post-treatment or FW6. Finally, significant differences from baseline to the 6- and 12-month follow-ups were found for well-being (PHI) and health status (EQ-5D).

Table 3. Descriptive statistics and repeated-measures ANOVA results of the primary and secondary outcomes.

	PreM (SD)	PostM (SD)	FW6M (SD)	FW12M (SD)	F	Within-Group Effect Size, d [95% CI] Pre-Post	Within-Group Effect Size, d [95% CI] Pre-FW6	Within-Group Effect Size, d [95% CI] Pre-FW12
1. Depression Severity (PHQ-9)	15.79 (6.21)	10.57 (6.68)	8.63 (6.11)	9.75 (5.65)	$F(2.51, 137.89) = 33.15$, $MSE = 20.32$, $p < 0.001$	0.83 [0.55, 1.11]	1.14 [0.78, 1.49]	0.96 [0.61, 1.31]
2. Positive Affect (PANAS-PA)	17.63 (6.11)	20.75 (7.92)	22.27 (8.23)	22.95 (9.66)	$F(2.37, 130.09) = 9.61$, $MSE = 41.42$, $p < 0.001$	−0.50 [−0.78, −0.22]	−0.75 [−1.06, −0.43]	−0.86 [−1.15, −0.57]
3. Negative Affect (PANAS-NA)	26.82 (8.56)	22.23 (8.07)	21.21 (7.30)	22.02 (8.56)	$F(2.54, 139.72) = 11.37$, $MSE = 37.47$, $p < 0.001$	0.53 [0.28, 0.78]	0.65 [0.34, 0.96]	0.55 [0.25, 0.85]
4. Well-being (PHI)	4.21 (1.72)	-	5.70 (1.89)	5.59 (1.78)	$F(2110) = 33.48$, $MSE = 1.15$, $p < 0.001$	-	−0.85 [−1.12, −0.59]	−0.79 [−1.09, −0.49]
5. Mental Health (SF-12)	26.22 (8.08)	30.50 (10.43)	38.61 (10.83)	35.26 (13.42)	$F(2.53, 139.31) = 20.65$, $MSE = 94.52$, $p < 0.001$	−0.52 [−0.79, −0.26]	−1.51 [−1.98, −1.04]	−1.10 [−1.47, −0.74]
6. Physical Health (SF-12)	42.45 (9.83)	45.11 (11.32)	45.58 (10.15)	47.04 (10.66)	$F(3, 165) = 4.66$, $MSE = 44.02$, $p = 0.004$	−0.27 [−0.50, −0.03]	−0.31 [−0.59, −0.04]	−0.46 [−0.70, −0.22]
7. Health Status (EQ-5D)	47.86 (20.34)	-	62.68 (15.24)	66.57 (19.04)	$F(1.65, 90.64) = 24.68$, $MSE = 268.55$, $p < 0.001$	-	−0.72 [−1.00, −0.44]	−0.91 [−1.29, −0.53]

Notes. PHQ-9 = Patient Health Questionnaire-9; PANAS = The Positive and Negative Affect Scale; PHI = Pemberton Happiness Index; SF-12 = Short Form 12 Health Survey; EQ-5D = EuroQoL; PA = Positive affect; NA = Negative affect; Pre = Pre-treatment; Post = Post-treatment; FW6 = 6-month follow-up; FW12 = 12-month follow-up. MSE: Mean Squared Error.

3.3. Sociodemographic Variables and Pre-Treatment Scores as Predictors of the Changes in Primary and Secondary Outcomes in the PA Intervention

Point-Biserial and Pearson's correlations between potential predictors (sociodemographic and pre-treatment scores) are shown in Table 4. Positive significant relationships were found between age and educational level and income level; being married or in a relationship correlated positively with well-being (PHI) and with living with someone, and income level correlated positively with health status (5Q-5D). A negative significant relationship was found between age and physical health (SF-12). Negative significant relationships were found between depression severity (PHQ-9) and positive affect (PANAS), well-being (PHI), mental health and physical health (SF-12), and health status (5Q-5D). Finally, a positive significant relationship was found between depression severity (PHQ-9) and NA (PANAS).

Regarding hierarchical multiple regression analysis, coefficients of determination, unstandardized coefficients, standard errors, standard coefficients, and t-statistics are shown in Table 5. The statistical models for predicting the change in each primary and secondary outcome are described in the following paragraphs. Variance Inflation Factor ranged from 0.95 to 1.06 for all the regression analyses, indicating no problems with multicollinearity [44,45].

Models for predicting change in depression severity (PHQ). Level of income positively predicted the change from Pre-Post, $F(1,38) = 10.35$, $p = 0.003$, R^2 Adjusted = 19.7%; Level of income positively predicted the change from Pre-FW6, $F(1,38) = 5.50$, $p = 0.024$, R^2 Adjusted = 10.6%, and level of income positively predicted the change from Pre-FW12, $F(1,38) = 16.00$, $p < 001$, R^2 Adjusted = 28.3%. Once the sociodemographic variables were controlled, only well-being (PHI) positively predicted the change in PHQ from Pre-FW12, $F(2,38) = 13.39$, $p < 0.001$, R^2 Adjusted = 39.5%, which significantly increased the explained variance in 12.5% ($p = 0.008$). Lower level incomes predicted greater improvements in depression severity at post-treatment, and the 6- and 12-month follow-ups; and lower well-being predicted greater improvements in depression severity at the 12-month follow-up.

Models for predicting change in PA (PANAS). None of the variables entered predicted the Pre-Post, Pre-FW6, or Pre-FW12 change.

Models for predicting change in NA (PANAS). None of the variables entered predicted the Pre-Post, Pre-FW6, or Pre-FW12 change.

Models for predicting change in well-being (PHI). Mental health (SF-12) negatively predicted the change Pre-FW6 change, $F(1,38) = 4.27$, $p = 0.046$, R^2 Adjusted = 7.9%. None of the variables entered predicted the Pre-FW12 change. Lower mental health predicted greater improvements in well-being at the 6-month follow-up.

Models for predicting change in mental health (SF-12). Level of income negatively predicted the Pre-FW6 change, $F(1,38) = 5.71$, $p = 0.022$, R^2 Adjusted = 11.0%. None of the variables entered predicted the Pre-FW12 change. Lower income levels predicted greater improvements in mental health at the 6-month follow-up.

Models for predicting change in physical health (SF-12). Educational level predicted negatively the change from Pre-Post, $F(1,38) = 4.33$, $p = 0.044$, R^2 Adjusted = 8.1%; Pre-FW6, $F(1,38) = 8.23$, $p = 0.007$, R^2 Adjusted = 16.0%, and Pre-FW12, $F(1,38) = 9.04$, $p = 0.005$, R^2 Adjusted = 17.5%. Lower levels of education predicted greater improvements in physical health at post-treatment and 6- and 12-month follow-ups.

Models for predicting change in health status (EQ-5D). Level of income negatively predicted the Pre-FW6 change, $F(1,38) = 10.20$, $p = 0.003$, R^2 Adjusted = 19.5%. None of the variables entered predicted the Pre-FW12 change. Lower income levels predicted greater improvements in health status at the 6-month follow-up.

Table 4. Point-Biserial and Pearson's correlations between proposed predictor variables.

Sociodemographic Variables and Pre-Treatment Scores	1	2	3	4	5	6	7	8	9	10	11	12	13	14
1. Sex	—													
2. Age	−0.13	—												
3. Marital status (binary variable)	−0.05	0.03	—											
4. Living alone or not (binary variable)	0.13	−0.04	0.29 *	—										
5. Educational level (binary variable)	−0.19	0.33 *	0.04	−0.04	—									
6. Work status (binary variable)	−0.17	0.03	0.02	−0.14	0.02	—								
7. Income level (binary variable)	−0.13	0.50 **	0.26	0.05	0.21	0.22	—							
8. Depression Severity (PHQ-9)	0.02	−0.09	−0.23	0.05	−0.20	−0.12	−0.24	—						
9. Positive Affect (PANAS-PA)	−0.03	0.04	0.07	0.08	0.08	0.15	0.25	−0.33 *	—					
10. Negative Affect (PANAS-NA)	−0.05	−0.20	0.04	0.26	−0.16	0.04	−0.14	0.55 ***	−0.33 *	—				
11. Well-being (PHI)	0.04	0.10	0.33 *	−0.15	0.13	0.15	0.23	−0.51 ***	0.50 ***	−0.40 **	—			
12. Mental Health (SF-12)	0.13	0.08	0.26	0.11	0.09	0.05	0.28	−0.43 **	0.50 ***	−0.21	0.53 ***	—		
13. Physical Health (SF-12)	−0.05	−0.30 *	0.15	0.15	0.23	0.22	0.08	−0.36 **	0.15	−0.25	0.09	−0.09	—	
14. Health Status (EQ-5D)	−0.03	−0.12	0.20	0.07	0.15	0.26	0.44 **	−0.43 **	0.36 **	−0.16	0.42 **	0.26	0.40 **	—

Notes. PHQ-9 = Patient Health Questionnaire-9; PANAS = The Positive and Negative Affect Scale; PHI = Pemberton Happiness Index; SF-12 = Short Form 12 Health Survey; EQ-5D = EuroQoL; PA = Positive affect; NA = Negative affect. Point-Biserial's correlations were carried out among dichotomous and recoded binary variables and between dichotomous/recoded binary variables and continuous variables. Pearson's correlations were carried out among continuous variables. * $p < 0.05$, ** $p < 0.01$, *** $p < 0.001$.

Table 5. Models for sociodemographic variables and pre-treatment scores as predictors of change in primary and secondary outcomes.

Outcomes	Predictors	R	Adjusted R^2	R^2 Change	B	SE	β	t
Change in PHQ								
Pre-Post	Constant	0.47	0.20	0.22	−8.93	1.41		6.32 ***
	Level of incomes (binary variable)				5.57	1.73	0.47	3.22 **
Pre-FW6	Constant	0.36	0.11	0.13	−10.49	1.74		6.04 ***
	Level of incomes (binary variable)				4.99	2.13	0.36	2.35 *
Pre-FW12	Constant	0.55	0.28	0.30	−16.40	2.36		6.95 ***
	Level of incomes (binary variable)	0.65	0.40	0.13	6.57	1.83	0.47	3.60 **
	PHI				1.42	0.51	0.36	2.80 **
Change in PANAS positive								
Pre-Post		—	—	—	—	—	—	—
Pre-FW6		—	—	—	—	—	—	—

Table 5. Cont.

Outcomes	Predictors	R	Adjusted R²	R² Change	B	SE	β	t
Pre-FW12	-	-	-	-	-	-	-	-
Change in PANAS negative								
Pre-Post	-	-	-	-	-	-	-	-
Pre-FW6	-	-	-	-	-	-	-	-
Pre-FW12	-	-	-	-	-	-	-	-
Change in PHI								
Pre-FW6	Constant	0.32	0.08	0.10	2.97	0.75	-	3.97 ***
	SF-12 (Mental Health)				−0.06	0.03	−0.32	2.07 *
Pre-FW12	-	-	-	-	-	-	-	-
Change in SF-12 (Mental Health)								
Pre-Post	-	-	-	-	-	-	-	-
Pre-FW6	Constant	0.37	0.11	0.13	19.23	3.51	-	5.48 ***
	Level of incomes (binary variable)				−10.26	4.29	−0.37	2.39 *
Pre-FW12	-	-	-	-	-	-	-	-
Change in SF-12 (Physical Health)								
Pre-Post	Constant	0.32	0.08	0.11	7.77	2.85	-	2.73 *
	Education level (binary variable)				−6.87	3.30	−0.32	2.08 *
Pre-FW6	Constant	0.43	0.16	0.18	10.58	3.010	-	3.52 **
	Education level (binary variable)				−10.01	3.490	−0.43	2.87 **
Pre-FW12	Constant	0.44	0.18	0.20	11.11	2.51	-	4.42 ***
	Education level (binary variable)				−8.76	2.91	−0.44	3.01 **
Change in EQ-5D								
Pre-FW6	Constant	0.47	0.20	0.22	26.30	4.40	-	5.98 ***
	Level of incomes (binary variable)				−17.21	5.39	−0.47	3.19 **
Pre-FW12	-	-	-	-	-	-	-	-

Notes. * $p < 0.05$; ** $p < 0.01$; *** $p < 0.001$. PHQ-9 = Patient Health Questionnaire-9; PANAS = The Positive and Negative Affect Scale; PHI = Pemberton Happiness Index; SF-12 = Short Form 12 Health Survey; EQ-5D = EuroQoL; PA = Positive affect; NA = Negative affect; Pre = Pre-treatment; Post = Post-treatment; FW6 = 6-month follow-up; FW12 = 12-month follow-up.

3.4. Change in Depression Severity and PA and NA as Predictors of Change in Well-Being, Mental and Physical Health, and Health Status

Coefficients of determination, unstandardized coefficients, standard errors, standard coefficients, and t-statistics for each stepwise multiple regression analysis are shown in Table 6. The statistical models to explain the changes in well-being, mental and physical health and health status are described in the following paragraphs. Variance Inflation Factor ranged from 1.01 to 2.37 for all the regression analyses, indicating no problems with multicollinearity.

Models for predicting change in well-being (PHI). The Pre–Post change in depression severity (PHQ-9) negatively predicted the Pre-FW6 change in well-being, $F(1,55) = 6.60$, $p = 0.013$, R^2 Adjusted = 9.2%. The Pre-12FW change in depression severity (PHQ-9) and PA (PANAS-PA), and the Pre-6FW change in depression severity (PHQ-9) (negatively, positively and negatively -respectively-) predicted the Pre-FW12 change in well-being, $F(3,55) = 17.78$, $p < 0.001$, R^2 Adjusted = 47.8%. Greater improvements in depression severity at post-treatment predicted greater improvements in well-being at the 6-month follow-up and greater improvements in depression severity and PA at the 12-month follow-up, and greater improvements in depression severity at the 6-month follow-up predicted greater improvements in well-being at the 12-month follow-up.

Models for predicting change in mental health (SF-12). The Pre-FW6 change in depression severity (PHQ-9) negatively predicted the Pre-FW6 change in mental health, $F(1,55) = 7.37$, $p = 0.009$, R^2 Adjusted = 10.4%. Greater improvements in depression severity at the 6-month follow-up predicted greater improvements in mental health at the 6-month follow-up.

Models for predicting change in physical health (SF-12). Changes in Pre-Post treatment scores for depression severity (PHQ-9) and NA (PANAS-NA) negatively predicted the Pre-Post change in physical health, $F(1,55) = 5.19$, $p = 0.009$, R^2 Adjusted = 13.2%. Greater improvements in depression severity and NA at post-treatment predicted greater improvements in physical health at post-treatment.

Models for predicting change in health status (EQ-5D). The Pre-FW12 change in depression severity (PHQ-9) negatively predicted the Pre-FW12 change in health status, $F(1,55) = 5.91$ $p = 0.018$, R^2 Adjusted = 8.2%. Greater improvements in depression severity at the 12-month follow-up predicted greater improvements in health status at the 12-month follow-up.

Table 6. Models for changes in depression severity (PHQ-9) and affect (PANAS) as predictors of change in well-being (PHI), health-related quality of life (SF-12), and health status (EQ-5D).

Outcomes	Predictors	R	Adjusted R^2	R^2 Change	B	SE	β	t
Change in PHI								
Pre-FW6	Constant	0.33	0.09	0.11	1.06	0.25	-	4.33 ***
	Change in PHQ-9 Pre-Post				−0.08	0.03	−0.33	2.57 *
Pre-FW12	Constant	0.50	0.24	0.25	0.57	0.27	-	2.14 *
	Change in PHQ-9 Pre-FW12	0.63	0.37	0.14	−0.22	0.04	−0.88	5.84 ***
	Change in PANAS-PA Pre-FW12	0.71	0.48	0.12	0.08	0.02	0.37	3.73 ***
	Change in PHQ Pre-FW6				0.14	0.04	0.52	3.50 **
Change in SF-12 (Mental Health)								
Pre-Post	-	-	-	-	-	-	-	-
Pre-FW6	Constant	0.35	0.10	0.12	7.37	2.51	-	2.94 **
	Change in PHQ-9 Pre-FW6				−0.70	0.26	−0.35	2.72 **
Pre-FW12	-	-	-	-	-	-	-	-
Change in SF-12 (Physical Health)								
Pre-Post	Constant	0.31	0.08	0.10	−1.18	1.68	-	0.70
	Change in PHQ-9 Pre-Post	0.41	0.13	0.07	−0.44	0.21	−0.27	2.10 *
	Change in PANAS-NA Pre-Post				−0.34	0.17	−0.26	2.04 *
Pre-FW6	-	-	-	-	-	-	-	-
Pre-FW12	-	-	-	-	-	-	-	-
Change in EQ-5D								
Pre-FW6	-	-	-	-	-	-	-	-
Pre-FW12	Constant	0.31	0.08	0.10	11.56	4.39	-	2.64 *
	Change in PHQ-9 Pre-FW12				−1.19	0.49	−0.31	2.43 *

Notes. * $p < 0.05$; ** $p < 0.01$; *** $p < 0.001$. PHQ-9 = Patient Health Questionnaire-9; PANAS = The Positive and Negative Affect Scale; PHI = Pemberton Happiness Index; SF-12 = Short Form 12 Health Survey; EQ-5D = EuroQoL; PA = Positive affect; NA = Negative affect; Pre = Pre-treatment; Post = Post-treatment; FW6 = 6-month follow-up; FW12 = 12-month follow-up.

4. Discussion

The purpose of this study was to shed light on the *patient profiles* (Objective 1) and *change mechanisms* (e.g., PA or NA) (Objective 2) that predicted a significantly greater improvement in depressive severity and positive functioning variables in an IBI focused on promoting PA, along with iTAU, in patients with MDD.

The efficacy of this intervention was tested in Gili et al. [29], where the PA intervention is compared to other interventions and a control group. However, in this study, we analyzed the change in the primary and secondary treatment outcomes to contextualize the secondary analyses of the present study. The results showed that participants improved on all the variables evaluated from pre- to post-treatment (depression, NA, PA, and mental health) significantly, except physical health, and the improvements were maintained until the follow-ups. The same thing occurred with the variables evaluated at pre-treatment and the 6- and 12-month follow-ups (well-being and general health status) because both variables improved significantly from pre to follow-ups. Hence, it is important to highlight that the PA intervention was not only able to decrease negative functioning measures significantly (PHQ-9 and PANAS-NA) but also to increase the positive functioning variables (PANAS-PA, quality of life, and well-being).

Our results showed that PP-based strategies focusing especially on the promotion of PA might have an impact on the decline in clinical symptomatology and the increase in positive functioning variables, which is consistent with other studies [46,47]. These results emphasize the benefits of including PP exercises and techniques in conventional treatments to promote positive emotions and positive functioning measures [19,20]. Recent studies suggest the importance of directly working on the promotion of positive emotions to improve depressive symptoms and achieve greater changes in positive emotion outcomes [48–50]. Nevertheless, the role of PP in interventions for depression has been poorly studied. The majority of the interventions for depression focus on reducing distress and negative emotions; however, it is has been recognized that well-being and the increase in positive emotions and behaviors contribute to mitigating negative emotions in life [51] and help to reduce stress reactivity [52,53]. Depression is characterized by high levels of NA. However, patients suffering from depression also have low PA, which, if not addressed, increases the consequences of the problem [11,54,55]. Moreover, PA has been found to contribute to better physical and psychological health and well-being [56], and so its improvement should be considered a core element of depression treatment. Our results show that depression can be addressed effectively not only by managing negative symptoms but also by increasing positive emotions [57,58].

Regarding the profile of patients who benefited more from this kind of intervention, sociodemographic variables and baseline scores on specific psychological measures were predictors of the changes in the primary and secondary outcomes. Overall, patients with lower income levels (i.e., under the minimum income level), lower educational levels (i.e., no education or only primary school), and worse scores on mental health and well-being before starting the intervention benefited more from the intervention. More specifically, *lower income levels* predicted greater improvements in depression severity at post-treatment (19.7% of variance), 6-month follow-up (10.6% of variance), and 12-month follow-up (28.3% of variance), as well as greater improvements in mental health and health status at the 6-month follow-up (11.0% and 21.6% of variance, respectively); *worse mental health* predicted greater improvements in well-being at the 6-month follow-up (7.9% of variance); *lower well-being* predicted greater improvements in depression severity at the 12-month follow-up (11.2% of variance); and finally, *lower education levels* predicted greater improvements in physical health at post-treatment (8.1% of variance), 6-month follow-up (16.0% of variance), and 12-month follow-up (19.6% of variance).

Regarding the education and income levels, our results pointed out that these variables were associated with intervention efficacy. In addition, we should highlight that this PA intervention was implemented in public PC contexts, where health status, education level, and income level are usually lower than in other psychological treatment settings. Thus, this study suggests that a brief self-guided

IBI could help people in more disadvantaged situations. None of the other sociodemographic variables examined predicted treatment outcomes. This means that the PA intervention is equally useful for people of different ages, marital status, work status, and sexes, which supports its dissemination. This result is in line with previous studies that found no sociodemographic variables that moderated the results of IBIs for depression [59].

Regarding mental health and well-being status, our findings are congruent with the results obtained by an Individual Patient Data (IPD) meta-analysis of low-intensity interventions for depression [60]. This study found that higher severity of depressive symptoms at baseline was associated with a greater decrease after the completion of the treatment. Nevertheless, because the effect was relatively small, the authors remarked that it is more cautious to conclude that low-intensity interventions work similarly across all the ranges of depression severity. By contrast, another recent IPD meta-analysis found that baseline depressive symptom scores did not moderate treatment outcomes [59]. This finding does not agree with our results because it suggests that characteristics of the intervention (e.g., focused only on PA) or the participants (e.g., patients from public PC settings) could explain these differences. More research with larger samples and different IBIs is needed to draw firm conclusions.

Regarding the mechanism of change, the improvement in depression severity was the most common predictor of the change in quality of life (mental and physical), well-being, and health status. More specifically, greater improvements in *depression severity and NA at post-treatment* predicted greater improvements in physical health at post-treatment (8.2% and 5% of variance, respectively); greater improvements in *depression severity at the 6-month follow-up* predicted greater improvements in mental health and well-being at the 6-month follow-up (10.4% and 9.2% of variance, respectively) and well-being at the 12-month follow-up (11.1% of variance); greater improvements in *depression severity at the 12-month follow-up* predicted greater improvements in well-being and health status at the 12-month follow-up (23.9% and 8.2% of variance, respectively). Furthermore, the increase in PA was also a relevant variable in increasing well-being in the long term. Specifically, greater improvements in *PA at the 12-month follow-up* predicted greater improvements in well-being at the 12-month follow-up (12.8% of variance). Hence, our results point out two important mechanisms of change in well-being in the long term (12-month follow-up): the improvement in depressive symptoms (PHQ-9) and the improvement in PA. These findings suggest that even though our intervention is focused on PA, changes in well-being are explained by changes in both depressive symptoms and PA.

This study has some limitations. First, the sample was small, and so the results should be interpreted with caution. Future PP research needs to focus on increasing sample sizes [61]. Second, the predictions of the multiple regression analyses were based on the stepwise method, so the conclusion should be taken as preliminary (i.e., the stepwise method is based on a mathematical criterion and not a theoretical criterion). Third, in our sample, participants had mild or moderate depressive symptoms; thus, it would be important to investigate the effect of PP strategies on patients with more severe depression [22]. Finally, it was not possible to record the number of face-to-face sessions focused on treating depression with the GP (although the available information indicated that they were very scarce and brief) or the medication dose administered to each patient in the iTAU condition. Future studies should consider these variables and analyze whether participants in IBIs receive less medical attention, which could be a cost-effectiveness variable of this treatment. Future research could explore the efficacy of this PP intervention, but in a completely self-guided way, without the support of the GP [59].

Despite the exploratory nature of this work, we consider that this study has several strengths. It may be relevant to the field of PP interventions, as it provides preliminary data on the profile of patients who benefit most of them. It also identifies the mechanisms of change of the intervention showing the improvement in PA, and not only in depression, as a significant predictor of long-term change in well-being. Finally, the study was carried out in a real context in a naturalistic way, which informs us regarding the utility of low-intensity IBIs in PC settings. The findings of the present study suggest that PA promotion can be an effective approach to treat depression by helping to improve both negative symptoms and positive emotions [62]. Furthermore, the PP intervention can be delivered using the Internet and self-guided formats, thus responding to an essential challenge in the field of depression treatments: reaching everyone in need by using new and alternative ways to apply psychological interventions. Therefore, the use of digital interventions helps to fulfill this proposal by contributing to the accessibility and dissemination of evidence-based treatments in the PC context.

5. Conclusions

In conclusion, this was the first study to explore a low-intensity IBI based on PA promotion in the PC setting in Spain. The results suggest that PP strategies might have an impact on clinical symptomatology, but they also contribute to improvements in positive functioning measures. Moreover, income level, education level, mental health, and well-being were significant predictors of the changes in depression severity and positive functioning measures at the end of the treatment and in the follow-up period. In addition, two mechanisms were identified as being responsible for the change in long-term well-being: the improvement in depression severity and the improvement in PA. Nevertheless, these findings should be interpreted with caution given the exploratory nature of the analyses and the small sample size used. Finally, this study highlights the importance of implementing IBIs in PC to produce changes in both negative and positive dimensions of human psychological functioning and promote more comprehensive psychotherapy for depression [63]. Overall, this study provides further support for the application of PP techniques using an IBI [62–64]. Future research should take into account the profile and unique characteristics of each patient to provide reliable tools to guide the choice of effective treatments.

Author Contributions: Conceptualization, A.G.-P., C.B., M.G., J.G.-C., F.M.-C., and R.M.B.; methodology, M.G. and A.G.-P.; software, C.B. and R.M.B.; formal analysis, M.D.V., A.M., M.M., and P.R.-S.; resources, A.G.-P., C.B., and R.M.B.; data curation, M.D.V., A.M., M.M., and P.R.-S.; writing—original draft preparation, M.D.V., A.M., and M.M.; writing—review and editing, all authors; supervision, A.G.-P., C.B., M.G., J.G.-C., F.M.-C., and R.M.B.; funding acquisition, A.G.-P., C.B., M.G., and R.M.B. All authors have read and agreed to the published version of the manuscript.

Funding: This research was funded by the Spanish Ministry of Economy, Industry and Competitiveness, and the Carlos III Health Institute. Health Research Project (grant number PI16/01017).

Acknowledgments: We would like to thank CIBERObn, an initiative of the ISCIII (ISC III CB06 03/0052), and "INTERSABIAS" Project (PROMETEO/2018/110).

Conflicts of Interest: The authors declare no conflict of interest.

References

1. Kessler, R.C. The Costs of Depression. *Psychiatr. Clin. N. Am.* **2012**, *35*, 1–14. [CrossRef]
2. Mrazek, D.A.; Hornberger, J.C.; Altar, C.A.; Degtiar, I. A Review of the Clinical, Economic, and Societal Burden of Treatment-Resistant Depression: 1996–2013. *Psychiatr. Serv.* **2014**, *65*, 977–987. [CrossRef] [PubMed]
3. Roca, M.; Gili, M.; García-García, M.; Salva, J.; Vives, M.; Campayo, J.G.; Comas, A. Prevalence and comorbidity of common mental disorders in primary care. *J. Affect. Disord.* **2009**, *119*, 52–58. [CrossRef] [PubMed]
4. Cuijpers, P.; Van Straten, A.; Andersson, G.; Van Oppen, P. Psychotherapy for depression in adults: A meta-analysis of comparative outcome studies. *J. Consult. Clin. Psychol.* **2008**, *76*, 909–922. [CrossRef] [PubMed]
5. Cuijpers, P.; Beekman, A.T.F.; Reynolds, C.F. Preventing Depression. *JAMA* **2012**, *307*, 1033–1034. [CrossRef] [PubMed]
6. Craven, M.; Bland, R. Depression in Primary Care: Current and Future Challenges. *Can. J. Psychiatry* **2013**, *58*, 442–448. [CrossRef]
7. Al-Harbi, K.S. Treatment-resistant depression: Therapeutic trends, challenges, and future directions. *Patient Prefer Adher* **2012**, *6*, 369–388. [CrossRef] [PubMed]

8. Cuijpers, P.; Karyotaki, E.; Weitz, E.; Andersson, G.; Hollon, S.D.; Van Straten, A. The effects of psychotherapies for major depression in adults on remission, recovery and improvement: A meta-analysis. *J. Affect. Disord.* **2014**, *159*, 118–126. [CrossRef] [PubMed]
9. Linde, K.; Sigterman, K.; Kriston, L.; Rücker, G.; Jamil, S.; Meissner, K.; Schneider, A. Effectiveness of Psychological Treatments for Depressive Disorders in Primary Care: Systematic Review and Meta-Analysis. *Ann. Fam. Med.* **2015**, *13*, 56–68. [CrossRef]
10. Carl, J.R.; Soskin, D.P.; Kerns, C.; Barlow, D.H. Positive emotion regulation in emotional disorders: A theoretical review. *Clin. Psychol. Rev.* **2013**, *33*, 343–360. [CrossRef]
11. Ruini, C. *Positive Psychology in the Clinical Domains*; Springer Science and Business Media LLC: Berlin/Heidelberg, Germany, 2017.
12. Watson, D.; Naragon-Gainey, K. On the specificity of positive emotional dysfunction in psychopathology: Evidence from the mood and anxiety disorders and schizophrenia/schizotypy. *Clin. Psychol. Rev.* **2010**, *30*, 839–848. [CrossRef]
13. Werner-Seidler, A.; Banks, R.; Dunn, B.D.; Moulds, M.L. An investigation of the relationship between positive affect regulation and depression. *Behav. Res. Ther.* **2013**, *51*, 46–56. [CrossRef]
14. Pressman, S.D.; Jenkins, B.N.; Moskowitz, J.T. Positive Affect and Health: What Do We Know and Where Next Should We Go? *Annu. Rev. Psychol.* **2019**, *70*, 627–650. [CrossRef]
15. Dalgleish, T.; Black, M.; Johnston, D.; Bevan, A. Transdiagnostic approaches to mental health problems: Current status and future directions. *J. Consult. Clin. Psychol.* **2020**, *88*, 179–195. [CrossRef]
16. Gray, J.A. Précis of The neuropsychology of anxiety: An enquiry into the functions of the septo-hippocampal system. *Behav. Brain Sci.* **1982**, *5*, 469–484. [CrossRef]
17. Watson, D.; Wiese, D.; Vaidya, J.; Tellegen, A. The two general activation systems of affect: Structural findings, evolutionary considerations, and psychobiological evidence. *J. Pers. Soc. Psychol.* **1999**, *76*, 820–838. [CrossRef]
18. Seligman, M.E.; Csikszentmihalyi, M. Special issue on happiness, excellence, and optimal human functioning. *Am. Psychol.* **2000**, *55*, 5–183. [CrossRef] [PubMed]
19. Sin, N.L.; Lyubomirsky, S. Enhancing well-being and alleviating depressive symptoms with positive psychology interventions: A practice-friendly meta-analysis. *J. Clin. Psychol.* **2009**, *65*, 467–487. [CrossRef]
20. Bolier, L.; Haverman, M.; Westerhof, G.J.; Riper, H.; Smit, F.; Bohlmeijer, E. Positive psychology interventions: A meta-analysis of randomized controlled studies. *BMC Public Health* **2013**, *13*, 119. [CrossRef]
21. Weiss, L.A.; Westerhof, G.J.; Bohlmeijer, E.T. Can We Increase Psychological Well-Being? The Effects of Interventions on Psychological Well-Being: A Meta-Analysis of Randomized Controlled Trials. *PLoS ONE* **2016**, *11*, e0158092. [CrossRef]
22. Chakhssi, F.; Kraiss, J.T.; Sommers-Spijkerman, M.; Bohlmeijer, E.T. The effect of positive psychology interventions on well-being and distress in clinical samples with psychiatric or somatic disorders: A systematic review and meta-analysis. *BMC Psychiatry* **2018**, *18*, 1–17. [CrossRef]
23. Johnson, J.; Wood, A.M. Integrating Positive and Clinical Psychology: Viewing Human Functioning as Continua from Positive to Negative Can Benefit Clinical Assessment, Interventions and Understandings of Resilience. *Cogn. Ther. Res.* **2015**, *41*, 335–349. [CrossRef]
24. Wakida, E.K.; Talib, Z.; Akena, D.; Okello, E.S.; Kinengyere, A.; Mindra, A.; Obua, C. Barriers and facilitators to the integration of mental health services into primary health care: A systematic review. *Syst. Rev.* **2018**, *7*, 211. [CrossRef]
25. Beck, J.S. *Cognitive Therapy: Basics and Beyond*; Guilford Press: New York, NY, USA, 1995.
26. Weissman, M.M.; Markowitz, J.C.; Klerman, G.L. *Comprehensive Guide to Interpersonal Psychotherapy*; Basic Books: New York, NY, USA, 2000.
27. Andrews, G.; Williams, A.D. Up-scaling clinician assisted internet cognitive behavioural therapy (iCBT) for depression: A model for dissemination into primary care. *Clin. Psychol. Rev.* **2015**, *41*, 40–48. [CrossRef]
28. Castro, A.; Garcia-Palacios, A.; Campayo, J.G.; Mayoral, F.; Botella, C.; Garcia-Herrera, J.M.; Pérez-Yus, M.-C.; Vives, M.; Baños, R.; Roca, M.; et al. Efficacy of low-intensity psychological intervention applied by ICTs for the treatment of depression in primary care: A controlled trial. *BMC Psychiatry* **2015**, *15*, 1–10. [CrossRef]
29. Gili, M.; Castro, A.; García-Palacios, A.; García-Campayo, J.; Mayoral-Cleries, F.; Botella, C.; Roca, M.; Barceló-Soler, A.; Hurtado, M.M.; Navarro, M.T.; et al. In primary care: Randomized Controlled Trial. *J. Med. Internet Res.* **2020**, *22*, e15845. [CrossRef]

30. Diez-Quevedo, C.; Rangil, T.; Sanchez-Planell, L.; Kroenke, K.; Spitzer, R.L. Validation and Utility of the Patient Health Questionnaire in Diagnosing Mental Disorders in 1003 General Hospital Spanish Inpatients. *Psychosom. Med.* **2001**, *63*, 679–686. [CrossRef]
31. Sheehan, D.V.; Lecrubier, Y.; Sheehan, K.H.; Amorim, P.; Janavs, J.; Weiller, E.; Hergueta, T.; Baker, R.; Dunbar, G.C. The Mini-International Neuropsychiatric Interview (M.I.N.I.): The development and validation of a structured diagnostic psychiatric interview for DSM-IV and ICD-10. *J. Clin. Psychiatry* **1998**, *59*, 22–33.
32. Bobes, J. A Spanish validation study of the mini international neuropsychiatric interview. *Eur. Psychiatry* **1998**, *13*, 198S–199S. [CrossRef]
33. García-Palacios, A.; Mira, A.; Mayoral, F.; Baños, R.M.; Botella, C. *Psychological Intervention in Primary Care for Mild-Moderate Depression. Protocol for the Promotion of Positive Affect. Therapist's Manual*; Publications of the University Jaume I: Castellón de la Plana, Spain, 2017. (In Spanish)
34. Fernández, A.; Haro, J.M.; Codony, M.; Vilagut, G.; Martinez-Alonso, M.; Autonell, J.; Salvador-Carulla, L.; Ayuso-Mateos, J.L.; Fullana, M.A.; Alonso, J. Treatment adequacy of anxiety and depressive disorders: Primary versus specialised care in Spain. *J. Affect. Disord.* **2006**, *96*, 9–20. [CrossRef]
35. Kroenke, K.; Spitzer, R.L.; Williams, J.B. The PHQ-9: Validity of a brief depression severity measure. *J. Gen. Intern. Med.* **2001**, *16*, 606–613. [CrossRef] [PubMed]
36. American Psychiatric Association. *Diagnostic and Statistical Manual of Mental Disorders, Fourth Edition, Text Revision (DSM-IV-TR)*; Masson: Barcelona, Spain, 1995.
37. Watson, D.; Clark, L.A.; Tellegen, A. Development and Validation of Brief Measures of Positive and Negative Affect: The PANAS Scales. *J. Pers. Soc. Psychol.* **1988**, *54*, 1063–1070. [CrossRef]
38. Sandín, B.; Chorot, P.; Lostao, L.; Joiner, T.E.; Santed, M.A.; Valiente, R.M. Escalas PANAS de afecto positivo y negativo: Validación factorial y convergencia transcultural. *Psicothema* **1999**, *11*, 37–51.
39. Hervás, G.; Vázquez, C. Construction and validation of a measure of integrative well-being in seven languages: The Pemberton Happiness Index. *Heal. Qual. Life Outcomes* **2013**, *11*, 66. [CrossRef]
40. Ware, J.E.; Kosinski, M.; Keller, S.D. A 12-Item Short-Form Health Survey. *Med Care* **1996**, *34*, 220–233. [CrossRef] [PubMed]
41. Vilagut, G.; Valderas, J.M.; Ferrer, M.; Garin, O.; López-García, E.; Alonso, J. Interpretación de los cuestionarios de salud SF-36 y SF-12 en España: Componentes físico y mental. *Medicina Clínica* **2008**, *130*, 726–735. [CrossRef]
42. Badia, X.; Roset, M.; Montserrat, S.; Herdman, M.; Segura, A. [The Spanish version of EuroQol: A description and its applications. European Quality of Life scale]. *Medicina Clínica* **1999**, *112*, 79–85.
43. Azur, M.J.; Stuart, E.A.; Frangakis, C.; Leaf, P.J. Multiple imputation by chained equations: What is it and how does it work? *Int. J. Methods Psychiatr. Res.* **2011**, *20*, 40–49. [CrossRef]
44. Bowerman, B.L.; O'Connell, R.T. *Linear Statistical Models: An. Applied Approach*; Duxbury: Belmont, CA, USA, 1990.
45. Myers, R. *Classical and Modern Regression with Applications*; Duxbury: Boston, MS, USA, 2000.
46. Santos, V.; Paes, F.; Pereira, V.; Arias-Carrión, O.; Silva, A.C.; Carta, M.G.; Nardi, A.E.; Machado, S. The Role of Positive Emotion and Contributions of Positive Psychology in Depression Treatment: Systematic Review. *Clin. Pr. Epidemiology Ment. Heal.* **2013**, *9*, 221–237. [CrossRef]
47. Chaves, C.; Lopez-Gomez, I.; Hervas, G.; Vazquez, C. A Comparative Study on the Efficacy of a Positive Psychology Intervention and a Cognitive Behavioral Therapy for Clinical Depression. *Cogn. Ther. Res.* **2016**, *41*, 417–433. [CrossRef]
48. Geschwind, N.; Arntz, A.; Bannink, F.; Peeters, F. Positive cognitive behavior therapy in the treatment of depression: A randomized order within-subject comparison with traditional cognitive behavior therapy. *Behav. Res. Ther.* **2019**, *116*, 119–130. [CrossRef]
49. Mira, A.; Bretón-López, J.; Enrique, Á.; Castilla, D.; Garcia-Palacios, A.; Baños, R.; Botella, C. Exploring the Incorporation of a Positive Psychology Component in a Cognitive Behavioral Internet-Based Program for Depressive Symptoms. Results Throughout the Intervention Process. *Front. Psychol.* **2018**, *9*, 2360. [CrossRef]
50. Proyer, R.T.; Wellenzohn, S.; Gander, F.; Ruch, W. Toward a better understanding of what makes positive psychology interventions work: Predicting happiness and depression from the person × intervention fit in a follow-up after 3.5 years. *Appl. Psychol. Health Well Being* **2015**, *7*, 108–128. [CrossRef]
51. Bower, J.E.; Moskowitz, J.T.; Epel, E. Is benefit finding good for your health? Pathways linking positive life changes after stress and physical health outcomes. *Curr. Dir. Psychol. Sci.* **2009**, *18*, 337–341. [CrossRef]

52. Craske, M.G.; Meuret, A.E.; Ritz, T.; Treanor, M.; Dour, H.; Rosenfield, D. Positive affect treatment for depression and anxiety: A randomized clinical trial for a core feature of anhedonia. *J. Consult. Clin. Psychol.* **2019**, *87*, 457–471. [CrossRef] [PubMed]
53. Craske, M.G.; Meuret, A.E.; Ritz, T.; Treanor, M.; Dour, H.J. Treatment for Anhedonia: A Neuroscience Driven Approach. *Depress. Anxiety* **2016**, *33*, 927–938. [CrossRef] [PubMed]
54. Gilbert, K.; Nolen-Hoeksema, S.; Gruber, J. Positive emotion dysregulation across mood disorders: How amplifying versus dampening predicts emotional reactivity and illness course. *Behav. Res. Ther.* **2013**, *51*, 736–741. [CrossRef]
55. Fredrickson, B.L. The role of positive emotions in positive psychology: The broaden-and-build theory of positive emotions. *Am. Psychol.* **2001**, *56*, 218–226. [CrossRef]
56. Seligman, M.E.P.; Rashid, T.; Parks, A.C. Positive psychotherapy. *Am. Psychol.* **2006**, *61*, 774–788. [CrossRef]
57. Ryff, C.D. Psychological Well-Being Revisited: Advances in the Science and Practice of Eudaimonia. *Psychother. Psychosom.* **2014**, *83*, 10–28. [CrossRef]
58. Taylor, C.T.; Lyubomirsky, S.; Stein, M.B. Upregulating the positive affect system in anxiety and depression: Outcomes of a positive activity intervention. *Depress. Anxiety* **2017**, *34*, 267–280. [CrossRef]
59. Karyotaki, E.; Riper, H.; Twisk, J.; Hoogendoorn, A.; Kleiboer, A.; Mira, A.; MacKinnon, A.; Meyer, B.; Botella, C.; Littlewood, E.; et al. Efficacy of Self-guided Internet-Based Cognitive Behavioral Therapy in the Treatment of Depressive Symptoms. *JAMA Psychiatry* **2017**, *74*, 351–359. [CrossRef]
60. Bower, P.; Kontopantelis, E.; Sutton, A.; Kendrick, T.; Richards, D.A.; Gilbody, S.; Knowles, S.; Cuijpers, P.; Andersson, G.; Christensen, H.; et al. Influence of initial severity of depression on effectiveness of low intensity interventions: Meta-analysis of individual patient data. *BMJ* **2013**, *346*, f540. [CrossRef]
61. White, C.A.; Uttl, B.; Holder, M.D. Meta-analyses of positive psychology interventions: The effects are much smaller than previously reported. *PLoS ONE* **2019**, *14*, e0216588. [CrossRef]
62. Wood, A.M.; Tarrier, N. Positive Clinical Psychology: A new vision and strategy for integrated research and practice. *Clin. Psychol. Rev.* **2010**, *30*, 819–829. [CrossRef] [PubMed]
63. Rashid, T. Positive interventions in clinical practice. *J. Clin. Psychol.* **2009**, *65*, 461–466. [CrossRef]
64. Fava, G.A.; Ruini, C. Development and characteristics of a well-being enhancing psychotherapeutic strategy: Well-being therapy. *J. Behav. Ther. Exp. Psychiatry* **2003**, *34*, 45–63. [CrossRef]

Publisher's Note: MDPI stays neutral with regard to jurisdictional claims in published maps and institutional affiliations.

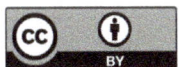

© 2020 by the authors. Licensee MDPI, Basel, Switzerland. This article is an open access article distributed under the terms and conditions of the Creative Commons Attribution (CC BY) license (http://creativecommons.org/licenses/by/4.0/).

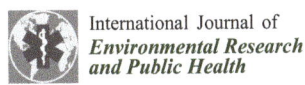

Article

Be a Mom's Efficacy in Enhancing Positive Mental Health among Postpartum Women Presenting Low Risk for Postpartum Depression: Results from a Pilot Randomized Trial

Fabiana Monteiro *, Marco Pereira, Maria Cristina Canavarro and Ana Fonseca

Center for Research in Neuropsychology and Cognitive Behavioral Intervention (CINEICC), Faculty of Psychology and Educational Sciences, the University of Coimbra Rua do Colégio Novo, 3000-315 Coimbra, Portugal; marcopereira@fpce.uc.pt (M.P.); mccanavarro@fpce.uc.pt (M.C.C.); ana.fonseca77@gmail.com (A.F.)
* Correspondence: fgmonteiro.91@gmail.com; Tel.: +351-239-851-450

Received: 18 May 2020; Accepted: 28 June 2020; Published: 29 June 2020

Abstract: In this study, we conducted a preliminary investigation of the efficacy of *Be a Mom*, a web-based self-guided intervention, in enhancing positive mental health among postpartum women at low risk for postpartum depression. Additionally, we examined *Be a Mom*'s efficacy regarding secondary outcomes as well as its acceptability and adherence. A total of 367 participants were randomly assigned to the *Be a Mom* group ($n = 191$) or to the waiting-list control group ($n = 176$) and completed baseline (T1) and postintervention (T2) assessments. The intervention group reported significant increases in positive mental health between T1 and T2 compared to the control group. Additionally, group effects were found for depressive and anxiety symptoms. A significantly higher proportion of participants in the *Be a Mom* group had an improvement trajectory (from not flourishing at T1 to flourishing at T2). A total of 62 (32.5%) women completed *Be a Mom*, and most would use it again if needed ($n = 82/113$; 72.6%). This study provides preliminary evidence of *Be a Mom*'s efficacy in increasing positive mental health among low-risk postpartum women. Our findings support mental health promotion strategies in the postpartum period and highlight the important role of web-based CBT interventions.

Keywords: web-based intervention; be a mom; randomized controlled trial; positive mental health; flourishing; postpartum period

---

1. Introduction

The transition to motherhood is often depicted as a joyful period filled with excitement, but it also involves demanding adjustments to a new role and new responsibilities [1]. Research in this area has suggested that this is a period of increased mental health vulnerability due to the considerable number of stressors that are often experienced, such as increased physical health needs, adjusting to infant care tasks, changes in marital and social relationships, financial strains or transitioning back to work [2–7]. Even under optimal circumstances, the early postpartum period is full of challenging tasks. Although some women may present risk factors that make them more vulnerable to mental illness, such as postpartum depression (PPD; e.g., history of depression, low social support; [8]), this period constitutes a major life transition for all postpartum women, including low-risk women, who can also experience symptoms of depression and anxiety [9,10].

Mental illness during the postpartum period has increasingly been considered a high-priority public health problem due to the long-term negative implications for maternal health, infant health and development [11,12] and economic costs [13,14]. Even the presence of subclinical symptoms of depression has been associated with increased psychosocial difficulties (poorer maternal self-esteem, more negative and less negative positive affect) [15]. Several efforts have targeted the treatment and prevention of psychological disorders during this period, particularly PPD [16,17]. With respect to preventive interventions, there is evidence that cognitive behavioral therapy (CBT) is effective in preventing depression both among women who present risk factors for PPD (selective/indicated prevention) and among all women in the community (universal prevention), although the effects of these preventive interventions may be more robust among groups at a higher risk of perinatal depression [16,18].

In addition to prevention, the promotion of positive mental health has been increasingly recognized as a priority [19,20], with research suggesting the need to address positive mental health directly since interventions that are effective in reducing psychopathological symptoms are not necessarily effective in enhancing levels of positive mental health [21,22]. However, previous research has tended to consider women's psychological adjustment to this period in terms of levels of depression and anxiety, and the promotion of positive mental health has been neglected in favor of a greater focus on the prevention and reduction of mental illness [23]. Positive mental health has received growing attention in recent years as research has shown that it is not simply the absence of mental illness [22,24]. Optimal levels of positive mental health involve the experience of high levels of emotional (positive feelings, e.g., feeling happy, satisfaction with life), psychological (optimal functioning in life, e.g., self-acceptance, purpose in life, personal growth) and social wellbeing (optimal social functioning, e.g., social integration and contribution) [24]. Keyes [24] conceptualized those with high levels of emotional, psychological and social wellbeing as flourishing individuals. Existing studies about the impact of flourishing underline the need for interventions that increase positive mental health. For instance, the presence of flourishing has been associated with better physical health and longevity [25,26], fewer health limitations of activities of daily living and fewer missed days of work [24] and may act as a buffer against future mental illness [27,28]. Although still rarely studied in the postpartum period, higher levels of positive mental health in mothers have been longitudinally associated with better development outcomes in children, specifically cognitive, communication and social development [29]. Thus, proactively addressing and assessing positive mental health in psychological interventions should be a complementary goal of psychological interventions in the postpartum period, including those targeting low-risk women.

Reaching all women in the postpartum period through traditional face-to-face interventions is difficult considering the high amount of human and economic costs involved [30]. Additionally, help-seeking rates for postpartum women with depressive symptoms range from 15% to 40% [31,32]. Suggested barriers that contribute to these low rates include feelings of shame, guilt and stigma and demands associated with infant care [33,34]. eHealth interventions have the potential to effectively address these barriers because they provide an opportunity to enhance the capacity and accessibility of mental health care and can be delivered at a very low cost and with privacy and convenience [35,36]. Moreover, these interventions have been shown to have long-term positive outcomes beyond the reduction of psychopathological symptoms, such as improvements in personal empowerment, self-esteem and quality of life [37]. In a recent review, the role of eHealth in the perinatal period was also highlighted as having the potential to be revolutionary if integrated into standard care [38].

In line with this, *Be a Mom* was developed to be a short-term, fully self-guided web-based intervention for Portuguese postpartum women. It was primarily developed to prevent PPD among at-risk women, and a previous pilot trial demonstrated its efficacy in reducing depressive and anxiety symptoms among a sample at high risk for PPD [39]. Although *Be a Mom* addresses the minimization of psychosocial risk factors for PPD (e.g., lack of social support, poor marital relationship), it does not focus solely on the minimization of such risk factors. Rather, *Be a Mom* specifically targets the development and strengthening of psychological competences and resources, namely, acceptance- and compassion-based skills. *Be a Mom* has already proven its efficacy in promoting self-compassion and emotion regulation skills among a high-risk sample for PPD [40]. Because the enhancement of psychological resources could be useful to all women in the postpartum period, *Be a Mom* may also be effective in the promotion of mental health among postpartum women presenting low risk for PPD. *Be a Mom* is grounded in CBT principles applied to the postpartum context and includes content based on the third wave of CBT, namely, acceptance- and compassion-focused approaches. Third-wave CBT approaches aim not only to reduce psychopathology but also to promote flourishing [41].

There is evidence of web-based CBT interventions as well as acceptance and compassion-based approaches enhancing positive mental health in general population samples [42,43]. However, there is still a lack of studies assessing the efficacy of these interventions in increasing positive mental health in the postpartum period. One study using an eHealth compassion-based intervention found that postpartum women in the intervention group showed an improvement in positive mental health compared to the control group [44], although the effects were small and only significant among participants with lower levels of positive mental health at baseline. Another study using an intervention based on positive psychology and metacognitive therapy only found a significant effect of the intervention with regard to emotional well-being [45]. The majority of web-based intervention studies in the perinatal period focus on the treatment or prevention of psychopathological symptoms using mostly high-risk samples [46]. However, given the characteristics of eHealth interventions and the importance of maternal mental health in influencing lifelong health outcomes, low-risk women may also benefit from these interventions.

Therefore, the present study reports the results of a pilot randomized controlled trial of the *Be a Mom* web-based intervention compared to a waiting-list control (WLC) group. The aims of this study were (1) to explore the efficacy of *Be a Mom* in enhancing positive mental health among low-risk postpartum women; (2) to investigate *Be a Mom*'s efficacy considering secondary outcomes (depressive and anxiety symptoms, maternal self-efficacy, empowerment and relationship satisfaction); and (3) to test *Be a Mom*'s acceptability, adherence and pattern of usage.

2. Materials and Methods

2.1. Study Design

This study was a two-arm, open-label, pilot randomized controlled trial on the efficacy of *Be a Mom* vs. a WLC for postpartum women presenting low risk for PPD. This study is part of a wider research project assessing *Be a Mom*'s efficacy as a web-based program for the promotion of maternal mental health during the postpartum period. The study was conducted in accordance with the Declaration of Helsinki, and the protocol was approved by the Ethics Committee of the Faculty of Psychology and Educational Sciences, University of Coimbra and was registered on ClinicalTrials.gov (NCT04055974). The extensions of the CONSORT 2010 checklist for pilot trials [47] and CONSORT-EHEALTH [48] were used for study reporting.

2.2. Recruitment Procedure and Participants

Participants were recruited online between January 2019 and February 2020. In addition to unpaid cross-posting, paid advertisements were placed on social media websites (Facebook and Instagram) targeting women aged 18–45 years old with interests in maternity topics. The tagline to advertise the study was "Did you have a baby in the last three months? We want to know if *Be a Mom* is effective in promoting postpartum women's mental health, and you can help us! To know if you are eligible to participate in the study fill out the following form and we will contact you". Participants who clicked on the link were then given information about the study's goals and procedures, the participants' and researchers' roles, the voluntary nature of participation, and all aspects related to data protection (anonymity and confidentiality). Participants who gave online informed consent (by clicking the option "I understand and accept the conditions of the study") answered a set of questions to assess eligibility criteria and provided their contact information (email address and telephone number). The inclusion criteria to participate in this study were a) being in the early postpartum period (up to 3 months postpartum); b) being 18 years or older; c) presenting low risk for PPD (having a score lower than 5.5 on the Postpartum Depression Predictors Inventory-Revised; [49]); d) having internet access at home; e) being a resident of Portugal; and f) understanding Portuguese. Exclusion criteria were the presence of a serious medical condition (physical or psychiatric) in the mother or in the infant (self-reported). Participants who did not meet eligibility criteria were sent an email informing them of the reason they could not participate in this study and advising them to seek professional help if needed. Because this study was part of a wider research project, women who presented risk factors for PPD were contacted by the research team to take part in a separate study to assess *Be a Mom*'s efficacy in preventing postpartum depressive symptoms (i.e., the primary outcome was depressive symptoms).

A priori calculations indicated that a sample size of at least 200 participants at postintervention assessment was needed to assess preliminary evidence of efficacy for the primary outcome (detecting a small effect size [$d = 0.10$] with a statistical power of 0.80 in a two-tailed test, $p < 0.05$). Considering the dropout rate of approximately 35% in the pilot study of *Be a Mom* [39], at least 350 participants were needed for randomization.

2.3. Randomization

After completing the baseline assessment, eligible participants were randomly assigned (allocation ratio 1:1) to the intervention group (*Be a Mom*) or to the WLC group. Randomization was performed using a computerized random number generator. After randomization, participants received an email with information about their assigned group. The last author was responsible for randomization, and the first author was responsible for the enrollment and assignment of participants to either the *Be a Mom* group or the WLC group.

2.4. Interventions

Participants in the intervention arm were invited to a password-protected website that contained the *Be a Mom* intervention (beamom.pt). Access to the program was free of cost, and no compensation was given to participants. *Be a Mom* has five sequential modules (Changes and Emotional Reactions; Cognitions; Values and Social Support; Couple's Relationship (only presented to women in a relationship); PPD Alert Signs and Professional Help-seeking) and its contents are presented in an attractive format (simple text, animations, interactive exercises). The modules follow the structured and goal-oriented nature of CBT: first, the module's goals are presented, followed by the thematic content and, finally, a homework activity at the end to guarantee continued therapeutic practice. Each module has an approximate length of 30–45 min, and women can interrupt it whenever they need to and resume when they are available. Asynchronous communication channels (e.g., reminders, email contact for program-related support) are available. The formative evaluation process that informed the design and the intervention components of *Be a Mom* is detailed elsewhere [50].

Participants were given the instructions that they should complete one module per week, but they were allowed to complete the program at their own pace. Those who did not register on *Be a Mom* were sent two email reminders during the course of the eight weeks given to complete *Be a Mom*. Participants who registered on the program and who had a valid telephone number were contacted via telephone by the first author approximately two weeks after registration. This contact aimed to clarify any questions regarding the flow of the program or help with difficulties accessing the website. Email reminders were sent automatically by the *Be a Mom* website to the participants if they went three, seven and 13 days without accessing it. Approximately two days after completing *Be a Mom*, participants were sent an email with the postintervention assessment. Those who did not complete the program were sent an email with the postintervention assessment eight weeks after randomization.

Participants in the WLC arm were offered no intervention but were informed that they would receive access to *Be a Mom* at the end of the study. They were asked to complete the postintervention assessment protocol at the same time as the participants in the *Be a Mom* group (eight weeks after randomization). All participants could access usual care from their health services.

Outcome variables were assessed at baseline (Time 1—T1) and eight weeks after randomization (Time 2—T2) by self-report using the survey platform Limesurvey®. To reduce attrition, email and text message reminders were sent on an alternate basis each week for one month to women in both groups who failed to complete T1 and T2 online questionnaires.

2.5. Measures

Women's sociodemographic (e.g., age, marital status, number of children, employment status, educational level, household monthly income, and residence), clinical (psychopathology history) and infant-related data (e.g., infant's age, infant's sex and infant's gestational weeks at birth) were collected through a self-report questionnaire developed by the researchers.

To identify women presenting low risk for PPD, the Portuguese version of the Postpartum Depression Predictors Inventory-Revised (PDPI-R) was used [51]. This questionnaire comprises 39 items answered on a dichotomous scale (yes vs. no, except for the first two items in which participants report their marital and socioeconomic status). The PDPI-R total score ranges from 0 to 39. Higher scores indicate increased risk for PPD. In Portuguese validation studies, a score of 5 or lower is indicative of lower PPD risk [49].

2.5.1. Primary Outcome-Positive Mental Health

Positive mental health was assessed using the Mental Health Continuum Short Form (MHC-SF; [52]; Portuguese Version [PV]: [53]). The MHC-SF comprises 14 items divided into three dimensions: emotional (3 items; e.g., "During the past month, how often did you feel happy?"), social (five items; e.g., "During the past month, how often did you feel that you had something important to contribute to society?") and psychological wellbeing (six items; e.g., "During the past month, how often did you feel that your life has a sense of direction or meaning to it?"). Each item is rated on a six-point response scale from 0 (*never*) to 5 (*every day*) in reference to the last month. In Portuguese psychometric studies, only the use of the total score was recommended as no adequate support was found for the use of the subscales as measures of distinct dimensions. The MHC-SF can be scored continuously (scores range from 0 to 70, and higher scores indicate better positive mental health) or categorically considering mental health status (flourishing, moderate mental health, languishing). Using Keyes' criteria [52], women who answered *every day* or *almost every day* at least once in the emotional wellbeing subscale and at least six times in the psychological and social wellbeing subscales were categorized as flourishing. Women who answered *never* or *once or twice* for at least one item in the emotional wellbeing subscale and at least six items in the psychological and social wellbeing subscales were categorized as languishing. Finally, women who did not fit the criteria for either flourishing or languishing were considered moderately mentally healthy. In this study, we categorized participants as flourishing and not flourishing (including both languishers and those with moderate mental health). The Cronbach's alpha values in this study ranged from 0.90 (intervention group—T1) to 0.93 (intervention group—T2).

2.5.2. Secondary Outcomes

The Edinburgh Postnatal Depression Scale (EPDS; [54]; PV: [54]) was used to assess postpartum depressive symptoms. EPDS comprises 10 items (e.g., "I have blamed myself unnecessarily when things went wrong") that are rated with an individualized four-point response scale (ranging from 0 to 3). The total score ranges between 0 and 30, and higher scores are indicative of more severe depressive symptoms. In this study, the Cronbach's alpha values ranged from 0.80 (intervention group—T1) to 0.86 (control group—T2).

The Anxiety Subscale of the Hospital Anxiety and Depression Scale (HADS-A; [55]; PV: [56]) was used to assess anxiety symptoms. This widely used seven-item subscale (e.g., "Worrying thoughts go through my mind") employs a four-point response scale (ranging from 0 to 3) that assesses the presence of anxiety symptoms in the week prior to completion. Higher scores denote higher anxiety symptoms. In this study, the Cronbach's alpha values ranged from 0.76 (intervention group—T1) to 0.82 (intervention group—T2).

The Empowerment Scale (ES; [57]; PV: [58]) was used to assess empowerment. The ES is a self-reported questionnaire with 20 items (e.g., "I am usually confident about the decision I make") that are rated with a four-point scale ranging from 1 (*strongly agree*) to 4 (*strongly disagree*). Higher scores indicate higher levels of empowerment. The Cronbach's alpha values in this study ranged from 0.79 (control group—T2) to 0.89 (intervention group—T2).

Women's perception of self-efficacy in the mothering role was assessed using the Perceived Maternal Parenting Self-Efficacy (PMP S-E; [59]). This measure comprises 20 items (e.g., "I am good at understanding what my baby wants") rated with a four-point scale ranging from 1 (*strongly disagree*) to 4 (*strongly agree*). Higher scores indicate higher levels of perceived self-efficacy. In this study, the Cronbach's alpha values ranged from 0.91 (control group—T2) to 0.95 (intervention group—T2).

The Satisfaction subscale of the Investment Model Scale (IMS-S; [60]; PV: [61]) was used to assess satisfaction in the relationship with the woman's partner. This subscale comprises five items (e.g., "Our relationship makes me very happy") answered on nine-point scale ranging from 0 (*do not agree at all*) to 8 (*completely agree*). Higher scores indicate higher satisfaction with the relationship. In this study, the Cronbach's alpha values ranged from 0.81 (intervention group—T1) to 0.83 (control group—T2).

2.5.3. Be a Mom's Web System Data

Data were collected through the *Be a Mom* website regarding the number of completed modules and pages accessed in each module, number of logins, average minutes spent on the website at each login, number of finished exercises and number of times each audio exercise was played.

2.5.4. Be a Mom's Acceptability and Experience

At the postintervention assessment, the intervention group completed an additional set of questions referring to *Be a Mom*'s acceptability. Participants were asked to answer questions with a two-point response scale (1 = *not applicable to me*; 2 = *applicable to me*) regarding their satisfaction with the help provided by the program, their intentions to use it again if needed and to recommend it to a friend, usefulness/relevance of the information learned and demandingness. Additional questions were presented about the participant's experience using *Be a Mom*; these were open-ended questions regarding the presence of others when accessing the program and reasons for not completing all modules of *Be a Mom*, when applicable.

2.6. Data Analysis

Statistical analyses were conducted in accordance with the intention-to-treat principles following the CONSORT statement [62] so that all participants who completed baseline assessment were included even if they did not complete postintervention assessment. Data were analyzed using the Statistical Package for Social Sciences (IBM SPSS, version 23.0 (IBM Corp., Armonk, NY, USA)). Descriptive statistics and comparison tests (t-tests and chi-squared tests) were computed for sample characterization and to examine *Be a Mom*'s usage and acceptability. Comparison analyses were also conducted between completers and dropouts and completers and non-completers. Dropout was defined as not completing the postintervention assessment regardless of the number of modules completed, and non-completers were defined as not completing the intervention.

Linear mixed models (LMMs) were used to determine the effects of the intervention over time on primary and secondary outcomes. LMMs are particularly helpful in longitudinal studies with missing data because they allow incomplete cases to be included in the analysis. All available data are used to obtain parameter estimates with small bias in the presence of data missing completely at random or missing at random [63]. Group, time and time by group interaction and covariates (variables presenting statistically significant differences between intervention and control groups at T1 and between completers and dropouts at T2: previous history of psychopathology, infant's age and category of positive mental health) were fitted as fixed effects. Participants were included as a random intercept. An LMM with an autoregressive covariance matrix was conducted for each outcome with the assumption of data missing completely at random (Little's MCAR test χ^2 = 415.21, p = 0.938). Missing endpoints at posttest ranged from 119/367 (32.4%) on the MHC-SF to 127/367 (34.6%) on the IMS-S.

Additionally, chi-squared tests were used to examine differences in the proportion of patterns of change as a function of group (intervention vs. control group) considering the primary outcome. Based on the cutoff scores of the MHC-SF, participants were categorized as flourishing or not flourishing at both T1 and T2. Participants were then classified in accordance with their pattern of change from T1 to T2: (a) maintenance—flourishing (if they were flourishing at both T1 and T2); (b) maintenance—not flourishing (if they were not flourishing at both T1 and T2); (c) deterioration (if they were flourishing at T1 and not flourishing at T2); and (d) improvement (if they were not flourishing at T1 and flourishing at T2).

3. Results

3.1. Participant Characteristics

Figure 1 shows the flow diagram of the participants throughout the study period. Of the 1657 women who were screened for eligibility, 72.5% (n = 1202) were excluded due to not meeting eligibility criteria (mostly because they presented risk for PPD; n = 1030, 85.7%). Of the 455 eligible participants, 367 completed the baseline assessment and were randomized and allocated to the intervention group (n = 191) or to the WLC group (n = 176).

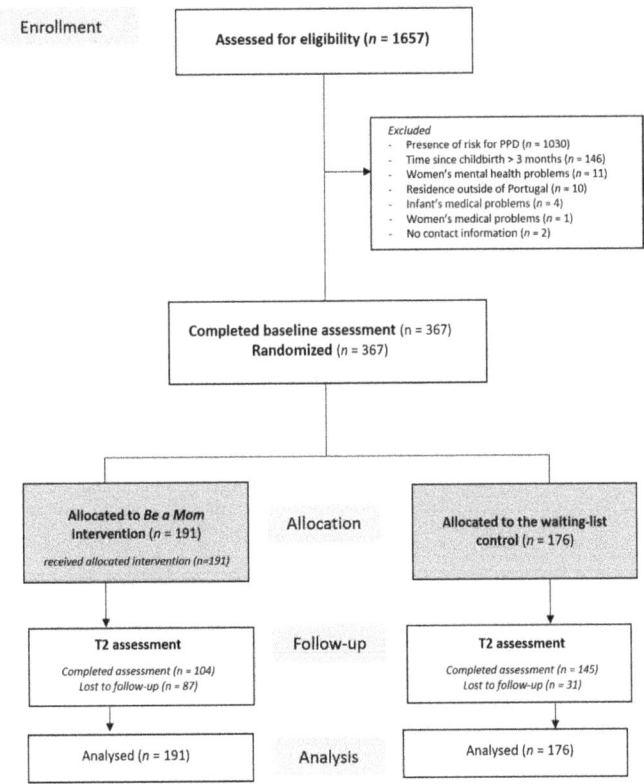

Figure 1. Flowchart of the participants in the study.

Table 1 summarizes the baseline sociodemographic and clinical characteristics of the intervention and control groups. There were no significant differences in most sociodemographic and clinical characteristics. However, a significantly higher proportion of participants in the intervention group had a previous history of psychopathology than in the control group (25.1% vs. 14.2%, $\chi^2 = 6.86$, $p = 0.009$). The control group also had a significantly higher proportion of participants who were flourishing (67% vs. 57.1%, $\chi^2 = 3.86$, $p = 0.049$).

Table 1. Participants' sociodemographic and clinical characteristics at baseline.

Variables	Intervention Group ($n = 191$) M (SD)/n (%)	Control Group ($n = 176$) M (SD)/n (%)	t/χ^2
Age	33 (4.04)	33 (4.43)	−0.14
Marital status			0.53
Married/co-habiting	183 (95.8)	170 (96.6)	
Single	4 (2.1)	2 (1.1)	
In a relationship (without living together)	4 (2.1)	4 (2.3)	
Primiparous	140 (73.3)	122 (69.3)	0.71
Employment status			3.35
Employed	176 (92.1)	170 (96.6)	
Not currently working	15 (7.9)	6 (3.4)	
Educational level			5.66
Up to the 9th grade	2 (1.0)	4 (2.3)	
10th to 12th grade	30 (15.7)	26 (14.8)	
Bachelor's degree	83 (43.5)	58 (33)	
Master's or Doctorate	76 (39.8)	88 (50)	
Household monthly income			4.92
Less than 580€	8 (4.2)	9 (5.1)	
580–1000€	88 (46.1)	80 (45.5)	
1000–2000€	87 (45.5)	70 (39.8)	
More than 2000€	8 (4.2)	17 (9.7)	
Residence			1.06
Urban	141 (73.8)	138 (78.4)	
Rural	50 (26.2)	38 (21.6)	
Psychopathology history			6.86 *
Yes	48 (25.1)	25 (14.2)	
No	143 (74.9)	151 (85.8)	
Positive mental health			3.86 *
Flourishing	109 (57.1)	118 (67)	
Not flourishing	82 (42.9)	58 (33)	
Infant's age (in months)	1.89 (0.94)	1.87 (1.32)	0.16
Infant's sex			0.43
Male	98 (51.3)	93 (53.1)	
Infant's gestational weeks (at birth)	38.89 (1.64)	38.95 (1.77)	−0.33

Note. * $p < 0.05$.

The overall retention rate at the postintervention assessment was 67.8%. The intervention arm had significantly higher loss to follow-up than the control arm (intervention group: $n = 87$, 45.5% vs. control group: $n = 31$, 17.6%, $\chi^2 = 32.77$, $p < 0.001$). Potential differences between completers and dropouts on baseline sociodemographic and clinical characteristics were explored but did not reveal any significant differences. The only exception was infant age, with infants of the participants who dropped out of the study being older than the infants of those who completed the postintervention assessment ($M = 2.11$ months, $SD = 0.97$ vs. $M = 1.77$ months, $SD = 1.20$, $t = -2.68$, $p = 0.008$). The proportion of women who had psychological/psychiatric treatment after the baseline assessment was also similar in both groups (intervention group: $n = 8$, 7.7% vs. control group: $n = 7$, 4.9%, $\chi^2 = 0.85$, $p = 0.356$).

3.2. Be a Mom's Preliminary Evidence of Efficacy: Comparison with the Control Group

Table 2 presents the estimated marginal means of all outcome measures and fixed effects for time, group and time × group interaction as well as for covariates (psychopathology history, infant's age and category of positive mental health at baseline).

Table 2. Estimated marginal means and fixed effects for primary and secondary outcome measures.

Variables	Group	Time 1 M (SE)	Time 2 M (SE)	Effect	B (SE)	95% CI	p
MHC-SF	Intervention	51.17 (0.54)	53.94 (0.69)	Time	−2.77 (0.69)	[−4.13, −1.40]	<0.001
	Control	50.47 (0.57)	51.19 (0.61)	Group	−2.74 (0.93)	[−4.56, −0.92]	0.003
				Time × Group	2.05 (0.93)	[0.22, 3.87]	0.028
				Psychopathology history	0.43 (0.88)	[−1.31, 2.16]	0.630
				MHC-SF baseline category	13.75 (0.73)	[12.31, 15.18]	<0.001
				Infant's age	−0.10 (0.31)	[−0.70, 0.50]	0.748
EPDS	Intervention	6.38 (0.26)	5.26 (0.33)	Time	1.12 (0.34)	[0.45, 1.80]	0.001
	Control	6.72 (0.27)	6.19 (0.29)	Group	0.93 (0.45)	[−0.06, 1.81]	0.036
				Time × Group	−0.60 (0.46)	[−1.50, 0.31]	0.194
				Psychopathology history	−1.43 (0.42)	[−2.25, −0.61]	0.001
				MHC-SF baseline category	−2.75 (0.34)	[−3.42, −2.08]	<0.001
				Infant's age	−0.05 (0.14)	[−0.33, 0.23]	0.739
HADS-A	Intervention	4.40 (0.22)	3.88 (0.28)	Time	0.53 (0.29)	[−0.04, 1.09]	0.069
	Control	4.54 (0.23)	4.72 (0.25)	Group	0.84 (0.38)	[0.09, 1.59]	0.028
				Time × Group	−0.71 (0.38)	[−1.46, 0.05]	0.067
				Psychopathology history	−2.02 (0.36)	[−2.73, −1.31]	<0.001
				MHC-SF baseline category	−1.62 (0.30)	[−2.20, −1.04]	<0.001
				Infant's age	0.05 (0.12)	[−0.20, 0.29]	0.710
PMPS-E	Intervention	69.06 (0.48)	73.09 (0.59)	Time	−4.11 (0.58)	[−5.14, −2.92]	<0.001
	Control	67.87 (0.50)	72.57 (0.53)	Group	−0.56 (0.81)	[−2.09, 1.05]	0.517
				Time × Group	−0.63 (0.77)	[−2.15, 0.81]	0.375
				Psychopathology history	−0.80 (0.79)	[−2.41, 0.72]	0.285
				MHC-SF baseline category	3.84 (0.65)	[2.54, 5.10]	<0.001
				Infant's age	0.94 (0.27)	[0.40, 1.47]	0.001
ES	Intervention	61.05 (0.38)	61.52 (0.46)	Time	−0.47 (0.40)	[−1.27, 0.32]	0.244
	Control	61.32 (0.40)	61.05 (0.42)	Group	−0.47 (0.63)	[−1.70, 0.76]	0.454
				Time × Group	0.74 (0.54)	[−0.32, 1.79]	0.170
				Psychopathology history	0.73 (0.65)	[−0.55, 2.01]	0.264
				MHC-SF baseline category	4.29 (0.53)	[3.24, 5.34]	<0.001
				Infant's age	−0.22 (0.22)	[−0.66, 0.22]	0.331
IMS-S	Intervention	6.54 (0.09)	6.36 (0.11)	Time	0.19 (0.09)	[0.00, 0.37]	0.046
	Control	6.48 (0.09)	6.30 (0.10)	Group	−0.05 (0.14)	[−0.33, 0.23]	0.718
				Time × Group	−0.02 (0.12)	[−0.26, 0.23]	0.901
				Psychopathology history	0.20 (0.15)	[−0.08, 0.49]	0.166
				MHC-SF baseline category	0.57 (0.12)	[0.33, 0.81]	<0.001
				Infant's age	−0.11 (0.05)	[−0.21, −0.02]	0.024

Note. MHC-SF—Mental Health Continuum-Short Form; EPDS—Edinburgh Postnatal Depression Scale; HADS-A—Hospital Anxiety and Depression Scale-Anxiety; ES—Empowerment Scale; PMPSE—Perceived Maternal Parenting Self-Efficacy; IMS-S—Investment Model Scale-Satisfaction.

Regarding the primary outcome, the LMM revealed a significant effect of time × group interaction, with women in the intervention group reporting a greater increase in positive mental health levels than participants in the control group (see Figure 2).

Regarding the secondary outcomes, significant effects of group were found for depressive and anxiety symptoms. Specifically, we found that these symptoms were higher overall in the control group. Although no significant time × group interactions were found, Figure 2 shows that a greater decrease in depressive and anxiety symptoms was found from T1 to T2 in the intervention group.

Regarding the remaining secondary outcomes, no interaction effects of time × group were found. For maternal self-efficacy and relationship satisfaction, significant effects of time were found. In both the intervention and control groups, there was a decrease in satisfaction in the relationship with the partner and an increase in maternal self-efficacy from T1 to T2, but there were no significant differences between the *Be a Mom* group and the WLC group.

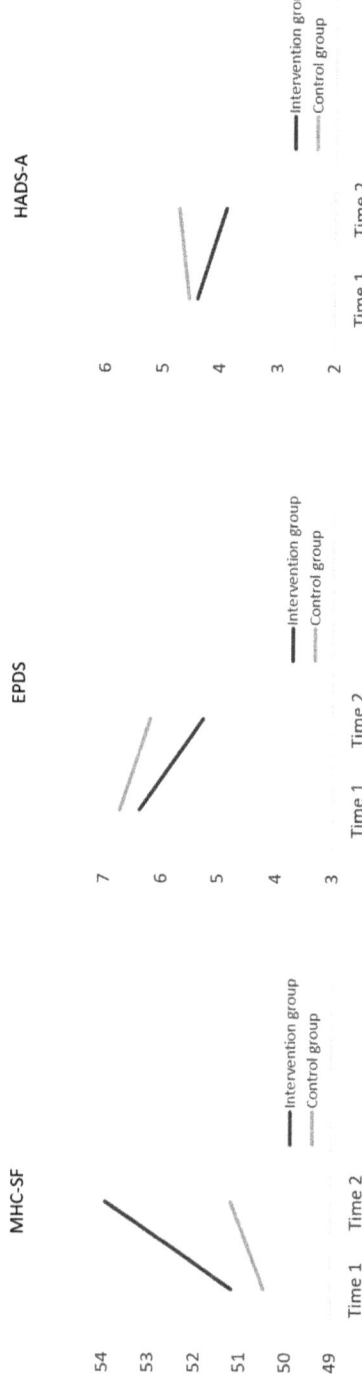

Figure 2. Intervention and control group trajectories for the Mental Health Continuum-Short Form, the Edinburgh Postnatal Depression Scale and the Anxiety subscale of the Hospital Anxiety and Depression Scale from T1 to T2 (based on mean estimates from linear mixed models).

Figure 3 shows that a significantly higher proportion of women in the intervention group had an improvement trajectory (from not flourishing at T1 to flourishing at T2) compared to women in the control group ($n = 21$, 20.2% vs. $n = 14$, 9.7%, $\chi^2 = 10.59$, $p = 0.014$). Additionally, a higher proportion of women in the control group had a deterioration trajectory (from flourishing at T1 to not flourishing at T2) compared to women in the intervention group ($n = 18$, 12.4% vs. $n = 4$, 3.8%).

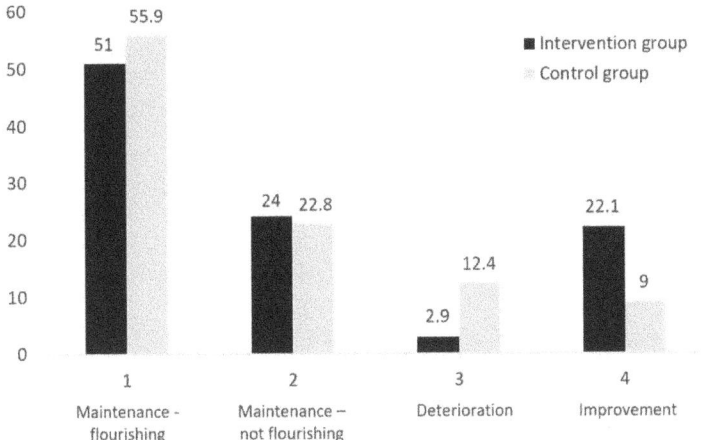

Figure 3. Trajectory of participants in the intervention and control groups from Time 1 to Time 2 regarding category of positive mental health. Maintenance—flourishing: flourishing at both T1 and T2; Maintenance—not flourishing: not flourishing at both T1 and T2; Deterioration: flourishing at T1 and not flourishing at T2; Improvement: not flourishing at T1 and flourishing at T2.

3.3. Adherence to the Intervention, Be a Mom's Usage and Acceptability

A total of 191 participants received an email invite to access the *Be a Mom* website. Of these, 62 (32.5%) completed the intervention, 23 (12%) completed half of the program, and 20 (10.5%) did not register on the website and initiate the intervention. Of the participants who registered on the *Be a Mom* website, 29 (17%) participants did not complete any module.

Considering all 171 participants who registered on the *Be a Mom* website, the average number of logins was 6 ($SD = 3.78$, range: 1–20) and the average number of minutes spent on the website in each login was 16 ($SD = 11.80$, range: 0–73). The majority of participants finished all four exercises of module 1 ($n = 128$, 74.9%) and the two exercises of module 2 ($n = 103$; 60.2%). Considering the participants who completed modules three, four and five, most of them finished all exercises proposed (four in module three, two in modules four and five; $n = 73/80$, 91.3%; $n = 58/60$, 96.7%; $n = 30/59$, 50.8%, respectively). Most of the participants who completed module 2 listened to the two audio exercises provided (observing thoughts and distancing of thoughts) ($n = 78/103$, 75.7% and $n = 48/103$, 46.6%, respectively).

Moreover, 113 participants in the intervention group answered a questionnaire about their experience using *Be a Mom* and its acceptability. Of these, 55 (48.7%) did not complete the intervention. Regarding the reasons for not completing *Be a Mom*, 53 (96.4%) participants highlighted lack of time, one (1.8%) participant answered that it was due to personal issues and one (1.8%) answered that *Be a Mom* was not useful in her case. Most women accessed *Be a Mom* on their own ($n = 102$; 90.3%). The remaining 11 participants accessed *Be a Mom* with their partners ($n = 10$; 90.9%) and other family members ($n = 1$; 9.1%), and all considered it beneficial for them and for the other person.

Of the 113 participants who answered the acceptability questionnaire, 65.5% ($n = 74$) were satisfied with the help provided by *Be a Mom*, 85% ($n = 96$) would recommend it to a friend, and 72.6% ($n = 82$) would use it again if needed. Moreover, 92% ($n = 104$) of participants rated the quality of *Be a Mom* as good/excellent. Additionally, 74.3% ($n = 84$) felt that they had learned relevant information with *Be a Mom*. Finally, 21 women (5.7%) considered participating in *Be a Mom* to be too demanding.

When comparing completers and non-completers of *Be a Mom*, a higher proportion of completers was satisfied with the help provided by *Be a Mom* ($n = 43$, 74.1% vs. $n = 31$, 56.4%, $\chi^2 = 3.95$, $p = 0.047$). Moreover, when compared to non-completers, a higher proportion of completers would recommend *Be a Mom* to a friend ($n = 54$, 93.1% vs. $n = 42$, 76.4%, $\chi^2 = 6.19$, $p = 0.013$), would use it again if they needed ($n = 48$, 82.8% vs. $n = 34$, 61.8%, $\chi^2 = 6.22$, $p = .013$) and felt that they learned relevant information with the program ($n = 49$, 84.5% vs. $n = 35$, 63.6%, $\chi^2 = 6.43$, $p = 0.011$). A higher proportion of non-completers considered participating in the *Be a Mom* program to be too demanding compared to completers ($n = 17$, 30.9% vs. $n = 4$, 6.9%, $\chi^2 = 10.76$, $p = 0.001$).

4. Discussion

The current study examined the efficacy of a web-based intervention, *Be a Mom*, in increasing positive mental health among postpartum women presenting low risk for PPD compared to a waiting-list condition. The efficacy of *Be a Mom* on secondary outcomes (depressive and anxiety symptoms, maternal self-efficacy, empowerment and relationship satisfaction) was also examined. The results of our study suggest that *Be a Mom* was superior to the WLC in increasing positive mental health. Additionally, there was a decreasing trend over time in depressive and anxiety symptoms in the *Be a Mom* group. *Be a Mom* was also shown to be an acceptable web-based intervention among low-risk postpartum women with satisfactory adherence and usage.

The significant improvement of positive mental health in the *Be a Mom* group is in line with previous evidence supporting the efficacy of web-based CBT interventions to promote positive mental health [42,43]. However, this is one of the first trials to successfully demonstrate this in the postpartum period. Additionally, our results showed that *Be a Mom* increased the proportion of flourishers over time. Conversely, a higher proportion of women in the control group had a deterioration trajectory (from flourishing at baseline to not flourishing at postintervention assessment). This is an important finding given the demonstrated importance of flourishing in protecting against future adversities and mental disorders, such as anxiety and depression [27,28], as well as its association with several health and psychosocial outcomes [24,64]. Thus, *Be a Mom* could have an important impact on mental health outcomes in the long term and, as such, enhance public mental health. Future studies using long-term assessments could test this hypothesis.

Regarding the secondary outcomes, the interaction effects of time and group failed to reach statistical significance. However, regarding depressive and anxiety symptoms, we found significant group effects (these symptoms were higher in the control group) as well as a trend of a greater decrease in the intervention group, particularly for anxiety symptoms. When looking at mean estimates, we found that from T1 to T2, there was an increase in anxiety symptoms in the control group contrasting with a reduction in the intervention group. This suggests that participants who received the *Be a Mom* program had greater benefits than those in the control group. However, although the efficacy of *Be a Mom* in reducing depressive and anxiety symptoms was previously demonstrated [39], it is important to note that *Be a Mom* seems to not have a substantial impact on such symptoms among low-risk postpartum women. A possible explanation may be the relatively low levels of depressive and anxiety symptoms at baseline, which leaves limited space for improvement.

Moreover, we found an increase over time in maternal self-efficacy in both study groups. This is consistent with the existing literature [65,66]: infants' demands become more predictable as they grow older, providing the opportunity to increase the mother's ability to successfully perform childcare tasks. However, we found that *Be a Mom* did not have a significant impact on the maternal self-efficacy of low-risk women. Although *Be a Mom* does not target caregiving behaviors, we expected that the emotional state of participants would influence the assessment of their self-efficacy, in line with Bandura's self-efficacy theory [67] and previous studies associating depressive symptoms with lower maternal self-efficacy [68]. This result is consistent with those previously found on the efficacy of *Be a*

Mom among a high-risk sample [39] and provides further evidence that *Be a Mom* may not be a suitable intervention to contribute to maternal confidence and self-efficacy, at least in the short term.

With respect to the results on empowerment, small, nonsignificant differences were found between the groups over time. Looking at mean estimates, the results suggest an increase in empowerment in the *Be a Mom* group compared with a decrease in the control group. A previous trial in the general population highlighted the significant impact of a web-based intervention on empowerment levels [37], suggesting that individuals who access the intervention may feel that they are more informed and involved in managing their own health outcomes. However, this was not found for *Be a Mom*. Future trials with follow-up assessments could provide more information on the pattern of this finding.

Finally, we found that both groups presented a decline in relationship satisfaction over time. Previous studies have emphasized that the arrival of an infant can strain the romantic relationship and produce changes in the couple, with a decline in satisfaction [69]. Although *Be a Mom* has a module that focuses on the changes that can happen within the couple during this period, most participants (90.3%) accessed *Be a Mom* on their own. The strategies that are presented (e.g., acknowledging the difficulties experienced by the other member of the couple, assertive and open communication skills, accepting differences in backgrounds and parental values) should ideally be implemented in a joint effort by the two members of the couple. In the future, further efforts and instructions to involve partners when accessing *Be a Mom* could help clarify its impact on relationship satisfaction.

In addition to the results on the efficacy of *Be a Mom*, our study provided results on *Be a Mom*'s acceptability as well as its usage and adherence. Extending on previous acceptability results among postpartum women presenting risk factors for PPD [39], *Be a Mom* appears to also be an acceptable option for low-risk postpartum women. However, adherence to the intervention was relatively low (only 32.5% women completed *Be a Mom*). This result is congruent with those found by previous research with web-based interventions applied to universal samples during the perinatal period [44,45] and could be explained by the hectic and challenging period women are experiencing, which leaves them with limited time for themselves. Additionally, *Be a Mom* is a fully self-guided intervention that was delivered to a low-risk sample with relatively good levels of overall mental health at baseline. It is possible that participants perceived that they did not need to complete the intervention and prioritized their limited time with other tasks. Nevertheless, those who completed the intervention or accessed half of the modules adhered to most of the exercises that were proposed.

Overall, the results of our study are very encouraging: they support mental health promotion strategies in the postpartum period and highlight the important role of web-based CBT interventions in achieving this. First, the postpartum represents an appropriate period to implement mental health promotion strategies given the pervasive consequences of mental health problems during this period and how they might shape children's development and health outcomes in the long term [11]. Second, the finding that low-risk women may significantly benefit from *Be a Mom* gives strength to the argument that mental health promotion strategies at a population level are needed. Growing research has emphasized that it is not sufficient to target only groups suffering from mental disorders or at-risk groups as new cases of mental illness will emerge [70,71]. A small change in the average level of positive mental health per individual could lead to significant benefits in population terms and shift the population distribution of positive mental health [70], with a possible impact on the prevalence and burden of mental disorders. Finally, *Be a Mom*'s brief and unguided format provides the opportunity to be delivered with low costs and to be easily disseminated at a population level. If implemented in healthcare, *Be a Mom* could be used as an early intervention of a stepped-care model, which is highly recommended by international guidelines [72], and could consequently provide a more efficient use of resources.

Although the results of our study are innovative and may add important input to public health policies, some limitations should be considered when interpreting our findings. First, the generalizability of the results is limited because the participants in the current study were self-selected, and it is possible that women with an interest in the topic were more likely to participate.

Moreover, one criterion to be included in this study was having internet access and this could also represent a selection bias. Additionally, our sample was mainly composed of highly educated and employed women. Future studies could build on current findings by investigating the efficacy of *Be a Mom* in more heterogeneous and representative samples. Second, there was a high attrition rate and low adherence in the intervention group. This is in line with previous intervention studies in the perinatal period [46] and, as previously mentioned, could be explained by the demanding nature of the early postpartum period. The lower attrition rate in the control group could be explained by the added incentive of gaining access to *Be a Mom* by continuing participation in the study. Future intervention studies during the postpartum period need to take into account the challenging and time-restricted period women are experiencing when designing research. Brief assessment protocols could help improve attrition rates. Additionally, future studies using the *Be a Mom* program must be mindful of this study's low adherence. Although a great proportion of participants answered that they did not complete the program due to lack of time, it is important to understand the reasons underlying this low rate and how much does it reflect the demandingness of the early postpartum period or the intervention's structure, length and contents. Third, the lack of an active control group does not allow us to rule out the possibility that the effects found were due to social desirability or placebo effects. Fourth, while the present study found evidence of the efficacy of *Be a Mom* in enhancing positive mental health, the observed effect was only a short-term improvement. Thus, the results presented are best interpreted as providing promising evidence. Future RCTs with follow-up assessments are needed to test *Be a Mom*'s efficacy in producing enduring positive effects. Examining the long-term impact of this approach with added input from a cost-effectiveness analysis could meaningfully inform public health policies. Finally, the mechanisms that explain the participants' response to treatment were not directly explored in this study. Because *Be a Mom* was developed to mainly target psychological resources such as self-compassion and emotion regulation, further studies exploring whether these mechanisms are involved in explaining the increase in levels of positive mental health are needed.

5. Conclusions

The promotion of positive mental health in the perinatal period has received very little attention to date. This is one of the first trials to test a web-based CBT intervention for this purpose among postpartum women presenting low risk for PPD. Given our findings, *Be a Mom* could be considered a new mental health promotion strategy among Portuguese postpartum women. The results of this pilot trial support its preliminary efficacy in increasing positive mental health to a flourishing mental health status with the potential to reduce depressive and anxiety symptoms among a nonclinical population. As an unguided web-based intervention, *Be a Mom* offers an accessible intervention option that could easily be disseminated among all postpartum women. Further research with a larger sample and long-term follow-up assessments is required to consolidate our findings and significantly inform public health policies.

Author Contributions: Conceptualization, F.M. and A.F.; Formal analysis, F.M. and A.F.; Investigation, F.M.; Methodology, F.M., M.P. and A.F.; Supervision, M.P., M.C.C. and A.F.; Writing—original draft, F.M.; Writing—review & editing, M.P., M.C.C. and A.F. All authors have read and agreed to the published version of the manuscript.

Funding: This project was co-funded by the European Regional Development Fund (FEDER), through the Portugal-2020 program (PT2020), under the Centre's Regional Operational Program (CENTRO-01-0145-FEDER-028699), and by the Portuguese Foundation for Science and Technology/MCTES through national funds (PIDDAC). Fabiana Monteiro was supported by a doctoral grant from the Portuguese Foundation for Science and Technology (SFRH/BD/115585/2016).

Acknowledgments: This study is part of the research project "Promoting maternal mental health: Applicability and effectiveness of an eHealth intervention for Portuguese postpartum women", integrated in the research group Relationships, Development & Health of the R&D Unit Center for Research in Neuropsychology and Cognitive Behavioral Center Intervention (CINEICC) of the Faculty of Psychology and Educational Sciences, University of Coimbra.

Conflicts of Interest: The authors declare no conflict of interest.

References

1. Winson, N. Transition to motherhood. In *The Social Context of Birth*, 3rd ed.; Squire, C., Ed.; Routledge: London, UK, 2017. [CrossRef]
2. Kanotra, S.; D'Angelo, D.; Phares, T.M.; Morrow, B.; Barfield, W.D.; Lansky, A. Challenges faced by new mothers in the early postpartum period: An analysis of comment data from the 2000 Pregnancy Risk Assessment Monitoring System (PRAMS) survey. *Matern. Child Health J.* **2007**, *11*, 549–558. [CrossRef] [PubMed]
3. Woolhouse, H.; Gartland, D.; Perlen, S.; Donath, S.; Brown, S.J. Physical health after childbirth and maternal depression in the first 12 months post partum: Results of an Australian nulliparous pregnancy cohort study. *Midwifery* **2014**, *30*, 378–384. [CrossRef] [PubMed]
4. Woolhouse, H.; McDonald, E.; Brown, S. Women's experiences of sex and intimacy after childbirth: Making the adjustment to motherhood. *J. Psychosom. Obstet. Gynaecol.* **2012**, *33*, 185–190. [CrossRef] [PubMed]
5. Grice, M.M.; Feda, D.; McGovern, P.; Alexander, B.H.; McCaffrey, D.; Ukestad, L. Giving birth and returning to work: The impact of work-family conflict on women's health after childbirth. *Ann. Epidemiol.* **2007**, *17*, 791–798. [CrossRef] [PubMed]
6. Nowak, M.J.; Naude, M.; Thomas, G. Returning to work after maternity leave: Childcare and workplace flexibility. *J. Ind. Relat.* **2013**, *55*, 118–135. [CrossRef]
7. Jevitt, C.M.; Groer, M.W.; Crist, N.F.; Gonzalez, L.; Wagner, V.D. Postpartum stressors: A content analysis. *Issues Ment. Health Nurs.* **2012**, *33*, 309–318. [CrossRef]
8. Norhayati, M.N.; Hazlina, N.H.; Asrenee, A.R.; Emilin, W.M. Magnitude and risk factors for postpartum symptoms: A literature review. *J. Affect. Disord.* **2015**, *175*, 34–52. [CrossRef]
9. Murphey, C.; Carter, P.; Price, L.R.; Champion, J.D.; Nichols, F. Psychological distress in healthy low-risk first-time mothers during the postpartum period: An exploratory study. *Nurs. Res. Pract.* **2017**, *2017*, 8415083. [CrossRef]
10. Weisman, O.; Granat, A.; Gilboa-Schechtman, E.; Singer, M.; Gordon, I.; Azulay, H.; Kuint, J.; Feldman, R. The experience of labor, maternal perception of the infant, and the mother's postpartum mood in a low-risk community cohort. *Arch. Womens Ment. Health* **2010**, *13*, 505–513. [CrossRef]
11. Slomian, J.; Honvo, G.; Emonts, P.; Reginster, J.Y.; Bruyere, O. Consequences of maternal postpartum depression: A systematic review of maternal and infant outcomes. *Womens Health (Lond.)* **2019**, *15*, 1745506519844044. [CrossRef]
12. Wen, D.J.; Poh, J.S.; Ni, S.N.; Chong, Y.S.; Chen, H.; Kwek, K.; Shek, L.P.; Gluckman, P.D.; Fortier, M.V.; Meaney, M.J.; et al. Influences of prenatal and postnatal maternal depression on amygdala volume and microstructure in young children. *Transl. Psychiatry* **2017**, *7*, e1103. [CrossRef] [PubMed]
13. Bauer, A.; Knapp, M.; Parsonage, M. Lifetime costs of perinatal anxiety and depression. *J. Affect. Disord.* **2016**, *192*, 83–90. [CrossRef] [PubMed]
14. Ladd, C.; Rodriguez McCullough, N.; Carmaciu, C. Perinatal mental illness. *InnovAiT* **2017**, *10*, 653–658. [CrossRef]
15. Weinberg, M.K.; Tronick, E.Z.; Beeghly, M.; Olson, K.L.; Kernan, H.; Riley, J.M. Subsyndromal depressive symptoms and major depression in postpartum women. *Am. J. Orthopsychiatry* **2001**, *71*, 87–97. [CrossRef]
16. Sockol, L.E. A systematic review of the efficacy of cognitive behavioral therapy for treating and preventing perinatal depression. *J. Affect. Disord.* **2015**, *177*, 7–21. [CrossRef]
17. Lin, P.Z.; Xue, J.M.; Yang, B.; Li, M.; Cao, F.L. Effectiveness of self-help psychological interventions for treating and preventing postpartum depression: A meta-analysis. *Arch. Womens Ment. Health* **2018**, *21*, 491–503. [CrossRef]
18. Dennis, C.L.; Creedy, D. Psychosocial and psychological interventions for preventing postpartum depression. *Cochrane Database Syst. Rev.* **2004**. [CrossRef]
19. Barry, M.M.; Clarke, A.M.; Petersen, I.; Jenkins, R. *Implementing Mental Health Promotion*; SpringerNature Switzerland: Cham, Switzerland, 2019.
20. Forsman, A.K.; Wahlbeck, K.; Aaro, L.E.; Alonso, J.; Barry, M.M.; Brunn, M.; Cardoso, G.; Cattan, M.; de Girolamo, G.; Eberhard-Gran, M.; et al. Research priorities for public mental health in Europe: Recommendations of the ROAMER project. *Eur. J. Public Health* **2015**, *25*, 249–254. [CrossRef]

21. Newnham, E.A.; Hooke, G.R.; Page, A.C. Progress monitoring and feedback in psychiatric care reduces depressive symptoms. *J. Affect. Disord.* **2010**, *127*, 139–146. [CrossRef]
22. Trompetter, H.R.; Lamers, S.M.A.; Westerhof, G.J.; Fledderus, M.; Bohlmeijer, E.T. Both positive mental health and psychopathology should be monitored in psychotherapy: Confirmation for the dual-factor model in acceptance and commitment therapy. *Behav. Res. Ther.* **2017**, *91*, 58–63. [CrossRef]
23. Smith, V.; Daly, D.; Lundgren, I.; Eri, T.; Benstoem, C.; Devane, D. Salutogenically focused outcomes in systematic reviews of intrapartum interventions: A systematic review of systematic reviews. *Midwifery* **2014**, *30*, e151–e156. [CrossRef] [PubMed]
24. Keyes, C.L. Mental illness and/or mental health? Investigating axioms of the complete state model of health. *J. Consult. Clin. Psychol.* **2005**, *73*, 539–548. [CrossRef] [PubMed]
25. Howell, R.T.; Kern, M.L.; Lyubomirsky, S. Health benefits: Meta-analytically determining the impact of well-being on objective health outcomes. *Health Psychol. Rev.* **2007**, *1*, 83–136. [CrossRef]
26. Keyes, C.L.; Simoes, E.J. To flourish or not: Positive mental health and all-cause mortality. *Am. J. Public Health* **2012**, *102*, 2164–2172. [CrossRef] [PubMed]
27. Schotanus-Dijkstra, M.; Keyes, C.L.M.; de Graaf, R.; Ten Have, M. Recovery from mood and anxiety disorders: The influence of positive mental health. *J. Affect. Disord.* **2019**, *252*, 107–113. [CrossRef]
28. Keyes, C.L.; Dhingra, S.S.; Simoes, E.J. Change in level of positive mental health as a predictor of future risk of mental illness. *Am. J. Public Health* **2010**, *100*, 2366–2371. [CrossRef]
29. Phua, D.Y.; Kee, M.; Koh, D.X.P.; Rifkin-Graboi, A.; Daniels, M.; Chen, H.; Chong, Y.S.; Broekman, B.F.P.; Magiati, I.; Karnani, N.; et al. Positive maternal mental health during pregnancy associated with specific forms of adaptive development in early childhood: Evidence from a longitudinal study. *Dev. Psychopathol.* **2017**, *29*, 1573–1587. [CrossRef]
30. Kazdin, A.E.; Blase, S.L. Rebooting Psychotherapy Research and Practice to Reduce the Burden of Mental Illness. *Perspect. Psychol. Sci.* **2011**, *6*, 21–37. [CrossRef]
31. McGarry, J.; Kim, H.; Sheng, X.; Egger, M.; Baksh, L. Postpartum depression and help-seeking behavior. *J. Midwifery Womens Health* **2009**, *54*, 50–56. [CrossRef]
32. Fonseca, A.; Gorayeb, R.; Canavarro, M.C. Womens help-seeking behaviours for depressive symptoms during the perinatal period: Socio-demographic and clinical correlates and perceived barriers to seeking professional help. *Midwifery* **2015**, *31*, 1177–1185. [CrossRef]
33. Moore, D.; Ayers, S.; Drey, N. A Thematic Analysis of Stigma and Disclosure for Perinatal Depression on an Online Forum. *JMIR Ment. Health* **2016**, *3*, e18. [CrossRef] [PubMed]
34. Dennis, C.L.; Chung-Lee, L. Postpartum depression help-seeking barriers and maternal treatment preferences: A qualitative systematic review. *Birth* **2006**, *33*, 323–331. [CrossRef] [PubMed]
35. Lal, S.; Adair, C.E. E-mental health: A rapid review of the literature. *Psychiatr. Serv.* **2014**, *65*, 24–32. [CrossRef] [PubMed]
36. Andersson, G.; Titov, N. Advantages and limitations of Internet-based interventions for common mental disorders. *World Psychiatry* **2014**, *13*, 4–11. [CrossRef] [PubMed]
37. Crisp, D.; Griffiths, K.; Mackinnon, A.; Bennett, K.; Christensen, H. An online intervention for reducing depressive symptoms: Secondary benefits for self-esteem, empowerment and quality of life. *Psychiatry Res.* **2014**, *216*, 60–66. [CrossRef] [PubMed]
38. van den Heuvel, J.F.; Groenhof, T.K.; Veerbeek, J.H.; van Solinge, W.W.; Lely, A.T.; Franx, A.; Bekker, M.N. eHealth as the Next-Generation Perinatal Care: An Overview of the Literature. *J. Med. Internet Res.* **2018**, *20*, e202. [CrossRef]
39. Fonseca, A.; Alves, S.; Monteiro, F.; Gorayeb, R.; Canavarro, M.C. Be a Mom, a Web-Based Intervention to Prevent Postpartum Depression: Results From a Pilot Randomized Controlled Trial. *Behav. Ther.* **2019**. [CrossRef]
40. Fonseca, A.; Monteiro, F.; Alves, S.; Gorayeb, R.; Canavarro, M.C. Be a Mom, a web-based intervention to prevent postpartum depression: The enhancement of self-regulatory skills and its association with postpartum depressive symptoms. *Front. Psychol.* **2019**, *10*, 265. [CrossRef]
41. Ciarrochi, J.; Kashdan, T.B. (Eds.) The foundations of flourishing. In *Mindfulness, Acceptance and Positive Psychology*; New Harbinger Press: Oakland, CA, USA, 2013; pp. 1–29.

42. Powell, J.; Hamborg, T.; Stallard, N.; Burls, A.; McSorley, J.; Bennett, K.; Griffiths, K.M.; Christensen, H. Effectiveness of a web-based cognitive-behavioral tool to improve mental well-being in the general population: Randomized controlled trial. *J. Med. Internet Res.* **2012**, *15*, e2. [CrossRef]
43. Rasanen, P.; Lappalainen, P.; Muotka, J.; Tolvanen, A.; Lappalainen, R. An online guided ACT intervention for enhancing the psychological wellbeing of university students: A randomized controlled clinical trial. *Behav. Res. Ther.* **2016**, *78*, 30–42. [CrossRef]
44. Gammer, I.; Hartley-Jones, C.; Jones, F.W. A Randomized Controlled Trial of an Online, Compassion-Based Intervention for Maternal Psychological Well-Being in the First Year Postpartum. *Mindfulness* **2020**, *11*, 928–939. [CrossRef]
45. Haga, S.M.; Kinser, P.; Wentzel-Larsen, T.; Lisøy, C.; Garthus-Niegel, S.; Slinning, K.; Drozd, F. Mamma Mia—A randomized controlled trial of an internet intervention to enhance subjective well-being in perinatal women. *J. Posit. Psychol.* **2020**. [CrossRef]
46. Lee, E.W.; Denison, F.C.; Hor, K.; Reynolds, R.M. Web-based interventions for prevention and treatment of perinatal mood disorders: A systematic review. *BMC Pregnancy Childbirth* **2016**, *16*, 38. [CrossRef] [PubMed]
47. Eldridge, S.M.; Chan, C.L.; Campbell, M.J.; Bond, C.M.; Hopewell, S.; Thabane, L.; Lancaster, G.A. PAFS consensus group (2016) CONSORT 2010 statement: Extension to randomised pilot and feasibility trials. *BMJ* **2016**, *355*, i5239. [CrossRef] [PubMed]
48. Eysenbach, G.; Group, C.-E. CONSORT-EHEALTH: Improving and standardizing evaluation reports of Web-based and mobile health interventions. *J. Med. Internet Res.* **2011**, *13*, e126. [CrossRef]
49. Alves, S.; Fonseca, A.; Canavarro, M.C.; Pereira, M. Predictive validity of the Postpartum Depression Predictors Inventory-Revised (PDPI-R): A longitudinal study with Portuguese women. *Midwifery* **2019**, *69*, 113–120. [CrossRef]
50. Fonseca, A.; Pereira, M.; Araújo-Pedrosa, A.; Gorayeb, R.; Ramos, M.M.; Canavarro, M.C. Be a Mom: Formative evaluation of a web-based psychological intervention to prevent postpartum depression. *Cogn. Behav. Pract.* **2018**, *25*, 473–495. [CrossRef]
51. Alves, S.; Fonseca, A.; Canavarro, M.C.; Pereira, M. Preliminary Psychometric Testing of the Postpartum Depression Predictors Inventory-Revised (PDPI-R) in Portuguese Women. *Matern. Child Health J.* **2018**, *22*, 571–578. [CrossRef]
52. Keyes, C.L.; Wissing, M.; Potgieter, J.P.; Temane, M.; Kruger, A.; van Rooy, S. Evaluation of the Mental Health Continuum-Short Form (MHC-SF) in Setswana-speaking South Africans. *Clin. Psychol. Psychother.* **2008**, *15*, 181–192. [CrossRef]
53. Monteiro, F.; Fonseca, A.; Pereira, M.; Canavarro, M.C. Measuring positive mental health in the postpartum period: The bifactor structure of the Mental Health Continuum-Short Form in Portuguese women. *Assessment* **2020**. [CrossRef]
54. Areias, M.E.; Kumar, R.; Barros, H.; Figueiredo, E. Comparative incidence of depression in women and men, during pregnancy and after childbirth. Validation of the Edinburgh Postnatal Depression Scale in Portuguese mothers. *Br. J. Psychiatry* **1996**, *169*, 30–35. [CrossRef] [PubMed]
55. Zigmond, A.S.; Snaith, R.P. The hospital anxiety and depression scale. *Acta Psychiatr. Scand.* **1983**, *67*, 361–370. [CrossRef] [PubMed]
56. Pais-Ribeiro, J.; Silva, I.; Ferreira, T.; Martins, A.; Meneses, R.; Baltar, M. Validation study of a Portuguese version of the Hospital Anxiety and Depression Scale. *Psychol. Health Med.* **2007**, *12*, 225–235. [CrossRef] [PubMed]
57. Rogers, E.S.; Chamberlin, J.; Ellison, M.L.; Crean, T. A consumer-constructed scale to measure empowerment among users of mental health services. *Psychiatr. Serv.* **1997**, *48*, 1042–1047. [CrossRef] [PubMed]
58. Jorge-Monteiro, M.F.; Ornelas, J.H. Properties of the Portuguese version of the empowerment scale with mental health organization users. *Int. J. Ment. Health Syst.* **2014**, *8*, 48. [CrossRef]
59. Barnes, C.R.; Adamson-Macedo, E.N. Perceived Maternal Parenting Self-Efficacy (PMP S-E) tool: Development and validation with mothers of hospitalized preterm neonates. *J. Adv. Nurs* **2007**, *60*, 550–560. [CrossRef]
60. Rusbult, C.E.; Martz, J.M.; Agnew, C.R. The Investment Model Scale: Measuring commitment level, satisfaction level, quality of alternatives, and investment size. *Pers. Relatsh.* **1998**, *5*, 357–387. [CrossRef]
61. Rodrigues, D.; Lopes, D. The Investment Model Scale (IMS): Further studies on construct validation and development of a shorter version (IMS-S). *J. Gen. Psychol.* **2013**, *140*, 16–28. [CrossRef]

62. Schulz, K.F.; Altman, D.G.; Moher, D.; Group, C. CONSORT 2010 statement: Updated guidelines for reporting parallel group randomised trials. *BMJ* **2010**, *340*, c332. [CrossRef]
63. Siddiqui, O.; Hung, H.M.; O'Neill, R. MMRM vs. LOCF: A comprehensive comparison based on simulation study and 25 NDA datasets. *J. Biopharm. Stat.* **2009**, *19*, 227–246. [CrossRef]
64. Dyrbye, L.N.; Harper, W.; Moutier, C.; Durning, S.J.; Power, D.V.; Massie, F.S.; Eacker, A.; Thomas, M.R.; Satele, D.; Sloan, J.A.; et al. A multi-institutional study exploring the impact of positive mental health on medical students' professionalism in an era of high burnout. *Acad. Med.* **2012**, *87*, 1024–1031. [CrossRef] [PubMed]
65. Zheng, X.; Morrell, J.; Watts, K. Changes in maternal self-efficacy, postnatal depression symptoms and social support among Chinese primiparous women during the initial postpartum period: A longitudinal study. *Midwifery* **2018**, *62*, 151–160. [CrossRef]
66. Law, K.H.; Dimmock, J.; Guelfi, K.J.; Nguyen, T.; Gucciardi, D.; Jackson, B. Stress, Depressive Symptoms, and Maternal Self-Efficacy in First-Time Mothers: Modelling and Predicting Change across the First Six Months of Motherhood. *Appl. Psychol. Health Well Being* **2019**, *11*, 126–147. [CrossRef] [PubMed]
67. Bandura, A. Regulation of cognitive processes through perceived self-efficacy. *Dev. Psychol.* **1989**, *25*, 729–735. [CrossRef]
68. Bornstein, M.H.; Hendricks, C.; Hahn, C.-S.; Haynes, O.M.; Painter, K.M.; Tamis-LeMonda, C.S. Contributors to Self-Perceived Competence, Satisfaction, Investment, and Role Balance in Maternal Parenting: A Multivariate Ecological Analysis. *Parent. Sci. Pract.* **2003**, *3*, 285–326. [CrossRef]
69. Dyrdal, G.M.; Roysamb, E.; Nes, R.B.; Vitterso, J. Can a Happy Relationship Predict a Happy Life? A Population-Based Study of Maternal Well-Being During the Life Transition of Pregnancy, Infancy, and Toddlerhood. *J. Happiness Stud.* **2011**, *12*, 947–962. [CrossRef] [PubMed]
70. Huppert, F.A. A New Approach to Reducing Disorder and Improving Well-Being. *Perspect. Psychol. Sci.* **2009**, *4*, 108–111. [CrossRef]
71. Herrman, H.; Saxena, S.; Moodie, R. *Promoting Mental Health: Concepts, Emerging Evidence, Practice. A WHO Report in Collaboration with the Victoria Health Promotion Foundation and the University of Melbourne*; World Health Organization: Geneva, Switzerland, 2005.
72. National Institute for Health and Excellence. *Antenatal and Postnatal Mental Health: Clinical Management and Service Guidance.* Updated February 2020. 2014. Available online: https://www.nice.org.uk/guidance/cg192/resources/antenatal-and-postnatal-mental-health-clinical-management-and-service-guidance-pdf-35109869806789 (accessed on 8 May 2020).

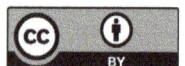

© 2020 by the authors. Licensee MDPI, Basel, Switzerland. This article is an open access article distributed under the terms and conditions of the Creative Commons Attribution (CC BY) license (http://creativecommons.org/licenses/by/4.0/).

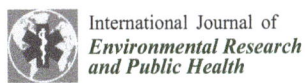

Article

Effectiveness of Psychological Capital Intervention and Its Influence on Work-Related Attitudes: Daily Online Self-Learning Method and Randomized Controlled Trial Design

Shu Da, Yue He and Xichao Zhang *

Beijing Key Laboratory of Applied Experimental Psychology, National Demonstration Center for Experimental Psychology Education (Beijing Normal University), Faculty of Psychology, Beijing Normal University, Beijing 100875, China; zhuriyinv@163.com (S.D.); hyue0917@163.com (Y.H.)
* Correspondence: xchzhang@bnu.edu.cn

Received: 29 September 2020; Accepted: 22 November 2020; Published: 25 November 2020

Abstract: Research on positive psychology intervention is in its infancy; only a few empirical studies have proved the effectiveness and benefits of psychological capital interventions in workplaces. From a practical perspective, a more convenient intervention approach is needed for when organizations have difficulties in finding qualified trainers. This study aims to extend the psychological capital intervention (PCI) model and examine its influence on work-related attitudes. A daily online self-learning approach and a randomized controlled trial design are utilized. A final sample of 104 full-time employees, recruited online, is randomly divided into three groups to fill in self-report questionnaires immediately before (T1), immediately after (T2), and one week after (T3) the intervention. The results indicate that the intervention is effective at improving psychological capital (PsyCap), increasing job satisfaction, and reducing turnover intention. The practical implications for human resource managers conducting a flexible and low-cost PsyCap intervention in organizations are discussed. Limitations related to sample characteristics, short duration effect, small sample size, and small effect size are also emphasized. Due to these non-negligible drawbacks of the study design, this study should only be considered as a pilot study of daily online self-learning PsyCap intervention research.

Keywords: psychological capital intervention; online self-learning; job satisfaction; turnover intention; job embeddedness; cost-effectiveness

1. Introduction

In the wake of the influential positive psychology movement, Luthans and Church [1] (p. 59) defined positive organizational behavior (POB) as "the study and application of positively oriented human resource strengths and psychological capacities that can be measured, developed, and effectively managed for performance improvement in today's workplace". Instead of emphasizing relatively stable individual differences such as positive personality traits, POB tries to pay more attention to state-like factors that can be developed through well-designed workplace interventions and targeted managerial policies [2].

It is widely assumed that POB can result in highly valued outcomes that benefit employees and organizations [3]. However, compared to the large number of studies that focus on cross-sectional or longitudinal relationships between POB and outcome variables, empirical research focusing on organizational positive psychology interventions is still in its early stages [4]. In the current situation, we do not have enough evidence to support the supposed benefits of positive psychology interventions in organizations, so it will be difficult for human resource (HR) managers to implement positive psychology practices [5], which reveals the huge gap between the requirements from organizations to promote employees' POB and the tough reality that HR managers do not know how to do so. Therefore, more research on POB interventions is required to not only prove the real value of POBs but also show HR managers how to conduct POB interventions.

Psychological capital (PsyCap), which goes beyond human and social capital, might be one of the most popular POB in both academic and practical fields, and includes four elements: self-efficacy, optimism, hope, and resilience. Many studies have focused on what influences PsyCap and what it leads to [6] but not on PsyCap interventions. Luthans et al. [7] put forward an intervention model, the psychological capital intervention (PCI) model, to operationalize and implement PsyCap interventions. Several intervention studies explore the effectiveness of the PCI model [8–11]. These interventions are typically conducted by training facilitators using face-to-face or online training, lasting one to three consecutive hours, and utilizing a series of group activities, discussions, or individual exercises [7,9,10]. To sum up, previous PsyCap intervention studies have something in common. First, they are mainly based on the PCI model. Second, they provide one to three hours' centralized training and do not clarify trainers' qualifications and styles. Third, they mainly focus on the effectiveness of PsyCap intervention but ignore its influence on other work-related outcomes, except for one study that tests the effect of the intervention on on-the-job performance [9]. Fourth, the participants are all from Western countries.

However, in workplaces, it might be difficult to implement interventions in this way, especially in China. For instance, it is difficult to find a training time suitable for all employees. If employees have emergency work but must attend intervention workshops due to pressure from HR managers, they may be absent-minded or participate halfheartedly, which would counteract the intervention's effect. In addition, if HR managers make employee participation voluntary, it will cost more money for organizations to make all employees get access to the training. Furthermore, small or middle-sized organizations in small or middle-sized cities in China might face difficulties in finding qualified trainers, as the development of psychological talent is uneven in different regions of mainland China.

Therefore, this study aims to extend the PsyCap intervention literature from both a theoretical and a practical perspective in the cultural context of mainland China. First, we add a goal-as-journey metaphor [12] in the hope of supplementing the PCI model. Second, we utilize a daily online self-learning approach to conduct the intervention. Third, based on the conservation of resources (COR) [13,14] theory, we examine the intervention effect on PsyCap and also other work-related attitudes: job satisfaction, turnover intention, and job embeddedness.

1.1. Psychological Capital Development

PsyCap is defined as "an individual's positive psychological state of development and is characterized by: (1) having confidence (self-efficacy) to take on and put in the necessary effort to succeed at challenging tasks; (2) making a positive attribution (optimism) about succeeding now and in the future; (3) persevering toward goals, and when necessary, redirecting paths to goals (hope) in order to succeed; and (4) when beset by problems and adversity, sustaining and bouncing back and even beyond (resiliency) to attain success" [15] (p. 3). It has been argued that these four elements have a synergistic effect and have more influence when combined than separate [7], which indicates that PsyCap, as a core construct, is better than any of its individual components at predicting outcome variables [16].

Moreover, as the concept of PsyCap is derived from the USA and European countries, it is important to illustrate how we can directly apply the PCI model to non-Western countries. From a theoretical perspective, Lomas [17] introduces the idea of positive cross-cultural psychology and argues that most research actually offers a synthesizing perspective on positive psychology, which recognizes universals in the way well-being is sought, constructed, and experienced, but it also allows for extensive variation in the ways these universals are shaped by culture. However, to the best of our knowledge, the literature on cultural differences in PsyCap interventions is still deficient.

From an empirical perspective, although the concept of PsyCap originates from Western countries, it also attracts wide research interest from many other different countries, such as South Africa [18], Ethiopia [19], Russia [20], Korea [21], Malaysia [22], Pakistan [23], China [24–27], and so on, which all support the positive effect of PsyCap. A recent meta-analysis [28] suggests that positive psychology interventions that are conducted in non-Western countries have larger effects than those in Western countries. However, research in the field of positive psychology interventions in non-Western countries is still in its infancy, and researchers urge articles from non-Western countries, even when there is a finding of no effect, as this is likely to reduce the publication bias in positive psychology intervention research [28,29].

Therefore, our study aims to generalize the effectiveness of the PCI model in mainland China in order to enrich the literature on positive psychology interventions in non-Western countries. The theory of the development of the four core constructs of PsyCap has been illustrated in detail in the literature [1,7]. Here, we summarize it briefly.

1.1.1. Developing Efficacy

Bandura's [30] social cognitive theory, especially the content related to efficacy, has been widely accepted. He classified sources of efficacy into four categories: task mastery, modeling or vicarious learning, social persuasion and positive feedback, and physiological or psychological arousal. This became the basic foundation of the PCI model [31]. In the PCI model [7], employees who participate in the intervention will be encouraged to experience and model success through social persuasion and arousal, which will give them a positive emotional experience and confidence to generate plans to achieve their goals. Additionally, combined with hope development, participants can create an imaginary task mastery experience by generating pathways, inventorying resources, and identifying subgoals to enhance and develop their efficacy.

1.1.2. Developing Hope

Positive psychologist Rick Snyder's work [32] is also the foundation of PsyCap development. He identified the basic components of hope as agency, pathways, and goals. In the PCI model, Luthans and colleagues [7] use a three-pronged strategy, embedded in a goal-oriented framework, which included goal design, pathway generation, and overcoming obstacles. First, employees who participate in the intervention will be guided to form personal goals. Then, they will be asked to divide their goals into several steps. After that, they will be encouraged to think about as many different pathways to the goal as possible. They will also consider the obstacles they might face and figure out alternative solutions to overcome them.

In this study, we add a goal-as-journey metaphor as a prime picture to stimulate participants' motivation to put their goals into action. Combining the conceptual metaphor theory [33] and identity-based motivation theory [34], researchers have shown that the journey metaphor implies a feeling of knowing how to achieve a goal and promote identity connection [12].

1.1.3. Developing Resilience

The resilience component in the PCI model [7,35,36] mainly comes from Masten [37], who considered asset factors, risks factors, and influence processes as three major components of resiliency. The most effective strategies to build resilience are based on enhancing assets (e.g., becoming more employable) and proactively avoiding risky, potentially adverse events (e.g., meeting critical deadlines) [37]. In the PCI model, employees who participate in the intervention will be encouraged to write down their reactions to recent feedback at work. Then, they will be guided to form a view of reality and how to react with resilience.

1.1.4. Developing Optimism

Luthans and his colleagues [7] developed the optimism dimension of PsyCap from both an expectancy-value orientation and a positive attributional, explanatory style [38], with realistic optimism being the ideal. They proposed that self-efficacy and hope training can both be used to build optimism [7]. Specifically, employees who participate in PCI will be guided to consider "bad events" as potential challenges or obstacles and then use the methods to develop hope to create alternative pathways to overcome problems.

1.2. Daily Online Self-Learning Method

In order to widely promote PsyCap interventions in China, HR managers should consider more flexible methods of conducting PsyCap interventions. With the development of the Internet, distance education has gradually become more popular. Increasingly, employees have arranged their spare time to allow for self-learning through distance education. Therefore, online self-learning might replace centralized workshops to implement PsyCap intervention in organizations, and intervention time could be divided into several days to allow employees to autonomously choose an appropriate schedule.

In the literature, self-learning modules are defined as self-contained instructional tools that guide learners through a step-by-step process for achieving educational objectives [39]. It contains some basic elements, including clear objectives and directions, materials needed for accomplishing objectives, and post-tests to examine the effectiveness. The instructional materials usually contain text and images that explain what is to be learnt and include examinations for self-assessment after self-learning. Compared with traditional learning methods with teachers, self-learning is a low-cost, nontechnical, and easily and widely disseminated strategy, which is commonly used by students, nurses, and other groups [40–42].

Moreover, traditionally, educators have focused on lecture/discussion teaching methods [43], in which learners are dependent upon instructors and are assumed to have a passive role in learning activities. Lectures assume that all participants are at the same level and learning at the same pace. By contrast, self-learning shows some distinct characteristics. It fosters learners' personal autonomy, allows them to realize self-management, and lets them control the learning process and utilize an independent approach to learning [44].

To conclude, an online-based self-learning intervention approach enjoys the benefits of speed, convenience, cost, and effectiveness, which can be applied to interventions in workplaces to promote employees' PsyCap and further human resource development [8]. Additionally, there have been a number of studies examining the effectiveness of online methods to deliver education, training, and interventions [45]. Therefore, we decided to adopt a daily online self-learning method to implement PsyCap intervention and proposed the following hypothesis:

Hypothesis 1. *The daily online self-learning PsyCap intervention will effectively improve the PsyCap level of employees.*

1.3. Work-Related Attitudes

In this study, we not only pay attention to the effectiveness of an online self-learning method for promoting PsyCap but also assess the influence of PsyCap interventions on work-related attitudes.

According to psychological resource theories such as the conservation of resources (COR) theory [13,14], individuals are motivated to acquire, maintain, and foster the necessary resources, as found in PsyCap, to attain successful performance outcomes. If an individual builds abundant resources including personal, social, economic, etc., he or she will be more capable of overcoming obstacles, enduring severe stress, and seeing accomplishments [46]. PsyCap, as an underlying capacity consisting of four positive psychological resources, is supposed to be beneficial to employees' attitudes and performance [47], both in the workplace and in their personal lives, through the mechanism of improving motivation and cognitive processing.

In addition, plenty of empirical studies have already demonstrated the influence of PsyCap on work-related outcomes, such as satisfaction or commitment [48,49], absenteeism [50], and performance [16]. However, except for Luthans et al. [9], who provided evidence that short training interventions can develop participants' PsyCap and improve on-the-job performance, few intervention studies have attempted to determine whether PsyCap development has a positive influence on employees' work-related attitudes. In this study, we choose job satisfaction, turnover intention, and job embeddedness as outcome indicators of PsyCap intervention, as they are the most common and fundamental work-related attitudes.

1.3.1. Job Satisfaction

Job satisfaction is a multidimensional construct including cognitive and affective perspectives [51]. From the perspective of cognition, job satisfaction is decided by how much an employee's physical and psychological needs are fulfilled by his or her work [52]. From the perspective of affect, job satisfaction is the overall feeling toward different aspects of one's job, including payments, leaders, colleagues, subordinates, environment, content, and so on [53].

With the general expectation of success derived from optimism and the belief in personal abilities derived from efficacy, employees with higher PsyCap show a higher level of job satisfaction, which was also supported by a meta-analysis [54].

1.3.2. Turnover Intention

Employee turnover—employees' voluntary severance of employment ties [55]—has long attracted the attention of scholars and practitioners [56]. March [57] identifies two main factors that affect employees' decision to relinquish their job: movement desirability (or job satisfaction) and ease (or perceived job opportunities). Before actual turnover behavior, employees usually generate initial behavior intentions [58] to indicate their possible choices. Avey, Luthans, and Youssef [59] prove that employees' level of PsyCap has a positive effect on reducing turnover intention as employees with high efficacy are prone to have confidence when facing obstacles (such as high job demands) during work and have higher motivation to overcome difficulties in order to better perform in the organizations; thus, they are more likely to stay within the organization [60].

1.3.3. Job Embeddedness

Mitchell et al. [61] introduce the notion of job embeddedness to elucidate why people stay at an organization or leave. It has been gradually recognized that the motives for leaving and staying are not necessarily opposite to each other [56]. That is, what triggers someone to quit the job (e.g., interpersonal conflicts or low pay) may differ from what makes people want to stay (e.g., opportunities for development or supervisor guidance). Sun et al. [62] prove that, in nurses, high levels of PsyCap are related to higher levels of job embeddedness and performance.

Therefore, we propose the following hypotheses:

Hypothesis 2. *The daily online self-learning PsyCap intervention will effectively promote the job satisfaction of employees.*

Hypothesis 3. *The daily online self-learning PsyCap intervention will effectively reduce the turnover intention of employees.*

Hypothesis 4. *The daily online self-learning PsyCap intervention will effectively promote the job embeddedness of employees.*

2. Materials and Methods

2.1. Participants

Both the recruitment and the intervention in this study were conducted through WeChat, the most popular online social and work connection application in mainland China. The study was open to all who met the following inclusion criteria: 20–60 years old; full-time employees in mainland China; working for five consecutive workdays every week; and ability to access WeChat on a daily basis. Participants were excluded from the study if they had a psychology degree, just in case they were familiar with the procedures of psychology interventions and responded to the surveys in accordance with the purpose of the intervention. We utilized a convenience sampling method, posting the recruitment advertisement on researchers' WeChat. Due to the snowball effect, we recruited 171 participants at time 1 (T1). Due to dropout, 118 participants completed the questionnaire at time 2 (T2), and 110 participants finished the questionnaire at time 3 (T3). After data cleaning, the final sample consisted of 104 participants (Figure 1). The rate of valid data was 60.82%.

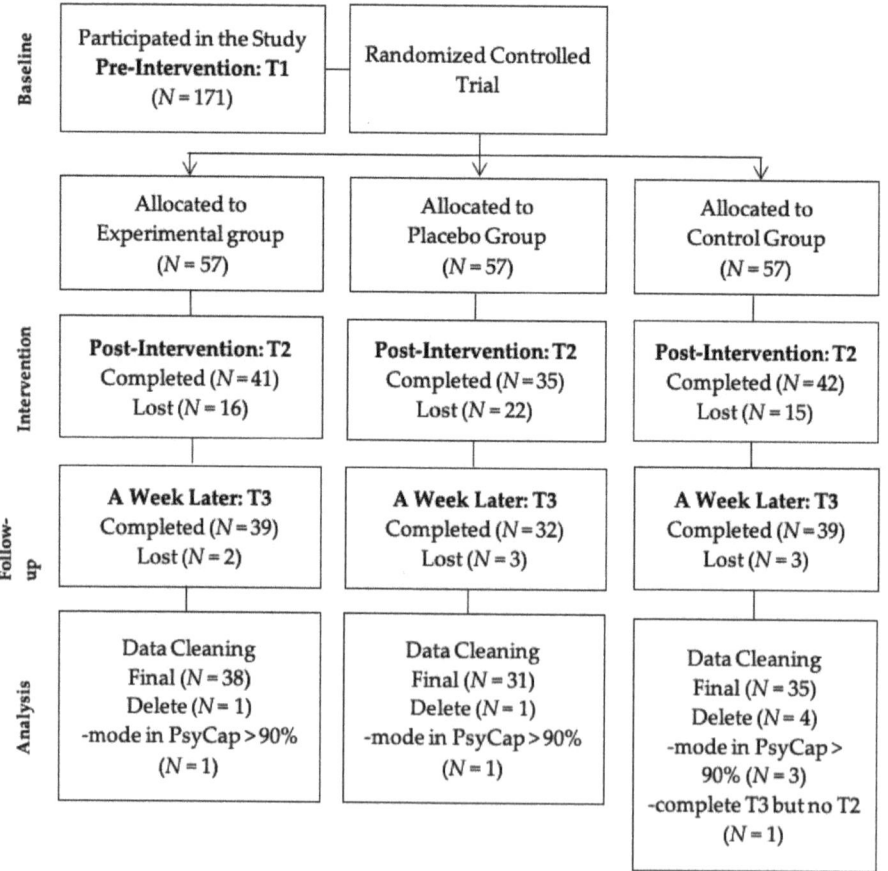

Figure 1. Participants' flowchart.

To check for potential selection bias due to dropout, independent-samples *t* tests and chi-square tests were calculated for the study variables and demographic variables. The results showed that the dropouts—those who did not complete post-intervention and follow-up questionnaires—differed with regard to gender, $\chi^2(1, N = 104) = 7.497$, $p < 0.01$: more men dropped out of the study than women. The means of the study variables (PsyCap, job satisfaction, turnover intention, and job embeddedness) and other demographic variables (age, job tenure, education, and marital status) did not differ significantly.

The final sample included 38 participants in the experimental group, 31 participants in the placebo group, and 35 participants in the control group; 27 of the total participants were men and 77 were women. Most participants (61.5%) were aged between 26 and 35 years, with 31.7% between 36 and 45, 3.8% between 46 and 55, and 2.9% under 25. As for work experience, 47.1% of the participants had five to 10 years of work experience, 38.5% had more than 10 years, and 14.4% had under five years. Regarding education, 57.7% of the participants had a bachelor's degree, 33.7% had a Master's degree, and 8.7% had a high school or associate's degree. Most participants were married (60.6%), while 34.6% were unmarried, 3.8% were divorced, and 1% were remarried. The sample represented a broad range of industries: the three most common were healthcare (20.0%), education (19.0%), and information technology (9.5%). In addition, the three most common job positions in this sample were consultants (12.4%), human resources personnel (11.4%), and managers (11.4%). The complicated composition of the final sample, the small sample size, and the short follow-up appeared to be limitations of our study and are discussed in detail at the end of the study.

2.2. Procedure

All subjects gave their informed consent for inclusion before they participated in the study. The study was conducted in accordance with the Declaration of Helsinki, and the protocol was approved by Institutional Review Board of the Faculty of Psychology, BNU on 19th, December 2019 (201912190084). This study was conducted using a randomized controlled trial (RCT) intervention method.

First, participants voluntarily filled out the informed consent form, baseline questionnaire (T1), and contact information (e-mail address and nickname) online after they viewed the study's advertisement and decided to participate. We made the study purpose, inclusion and exclusion criteria, and rewards very clear in our online recruitment advertisement. It was stated that this was a three-fold survey on occupational psychological health and the lucky participants could get access to a five-day online activity to promote mental health.

Then, after finishing a pretest questionnaire, participants were randomly assigned to one of three WeChat online groups (assigned by e-mail) according to the sequence in which they finished the pretest: experimental group, placebo group, and control group. After creating three WeChat online groups, the researcher again explained the study purpose and procedures to the different groups. Participants in the control group were thanked for participating in a survey on occupational psychological health and told when and how to complete the online questionnaires three times. As to the experimental and placebo groups, the researcher thanked them for their participation in a survey on occupational psychological health and told them that they were the lucky ones, getting an opportunity for a five-day activity to promote mental health. Therefore, it was a single-blind design, as the participants in the placebo group had the same study guidance but a different intervention from the experimental group to ensure that the results were due to the experimental design instead of the organizational process or instruction. Next, interventions were conducted by sending daily online links to reading materials and practice activities to the experimental group and online links to write down self-reflections to the placebo group for five consecutive workdays. The links were sent in the morning, and participants could choose a convenient time to read and complete the content before the next day. Nothing was sent to the control group. On day six, participants in all three groups were sent a posttest questionnaire (T2). One week later, they were sent a follow-up questionnaire (T3). Participants were asked to complete the intervention in a quiet setting, free from interference. It took approximately 20 min to finish the intervention each day. Each participant won 10-yuan rewards every time they completed a survey.

For PsyCap intervention according to the PCI model and journal metaphor, in the links sent to experimental group, participants were asked to read materials or engage in related activities and record their answers to questions (Figure 2).

In order to balance the Hawthorne effect that may exist in an experimental group, we utilized an expressive writing [63] and a self-reflection [64] intervention method for participants in the placebo group. A growing number of studies have found that expressive writing improves a variety of outcomes, ranging from improved immunity and reduced stress [65]. A meta-analysis [66] reveals that emotional disclosure confers lots of benefits, including increased physical and psychological well-being. Therefore, in the links sent to the placebo group, participants were guided to engage in self-reflection and record anything impressive from the work in at least 50 Chinese characters every day.

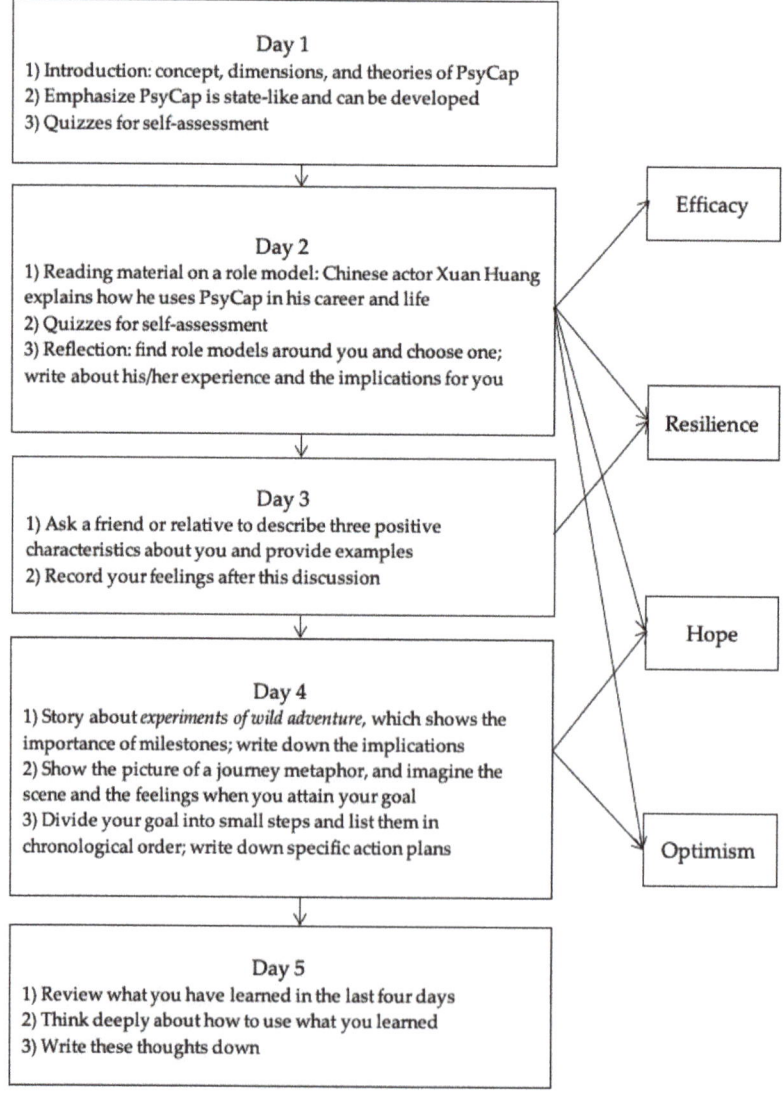

Figure 2. The intervention process.

2.3. Measures

All four study variables (psychological capital, job satisfaction, turnover intention, and job embeddedness) were assessed at all three measurement points (T1, T2, and T3) using the scales outlined below with the exception of demographic variables, which were collected only at T1. All participants created unique nicknames for themselves, which were used to match the three questionnaires. Given that the nicknames might reveal a participant's identity, we stored them in a separate file. All scales showed good internal consistency at all measurement times (see Table 1).

Psychological capital. Psychological capital was measured by the Psychological Capital Questionnaire-24 developed by Luthans, Avolio, and Norman [16], which included four dimensions: efficacy, optimism, hope, and resilience. All 24 items were rated on a six-point Likert scale, ranging from 1 (*completely disagree*) to 6 (*completely agree*).

Job satisfaction was measured by the six-item Overall Job Satisfaction short form developed by Agho, Price, and Mueller [67]. Items such as "I find real enjoyment in my job" and "I am seldom bored with my job" were rated on a five-point Likert scale, ranging from 1 (*completely disagree*) to 5 (*completely agree*).

Turnover intention was measured with a five-item scale used in previous research by Bluedom [68], including items such as "I intend to quit my present job." Respondents indicated their answers on a seven-point Likert scale, ranging from 1 (*completely disagree*) to 7 (*completely agree*).

We used the seven-item version of a global measure of job embeddedness [69]. Items such as "I feel attached to this organization" and "It would be easy for me to leave this organization" were accompanied by responses on a five-point Likert scale, ranging from 1 (*completely disagree*) to 5 (*completely agree*).

Table 1. Correlations and reliability of all study variables.

	1	2	3	4	5	6	7	8	9	10	11	12
1. PC T1	(0.89)											
2. PC T2	0.77 **	(0.91)										
3. PC T3	0.75 **	0.89 **	(0.93)									
4. JS T1	0.61 **	0.51 **	0.53 **	(0.83)								
5. JS T2	0.48 **	0.55 **	0.58 **	0.80 **	(0.89)							
6. JS T3	0.49 **	0.57 **	0.63 **	0.77 **	0.89 **	(0.90)						
7. TI T1	−0.30 **	−0.27 **	−0.31 **	−0.60 **	−0.53 **	−0.57 **	(0.94)					
8. TI T2	−0.30 **	−0.29 **	−0.36 **	−0.59 **	−0.61 **	−0.63 **	0.90 **	(0.93)				
9. TI T3	−0.27 **	−0.28 **	−0.34 **	−0.57 **	−0.59 **	−0.62 **	0.90 **	0.95 **	(0.96)			
10. JE T1	0.21 *	0.20 *	0.26 **	0.51 **	0.58 **	0.55 **	−0.62 **	−0.65 **	−0.64 **	(0.81)		
11. JE T2	0.19	0.24 *	0.27 **	0.49 **	0.60 **	0.59 **	−0.58 **	−0.65 **	−0.66 **	0.87 **	(0.87)	
12. JE T3	0.21 *	0.28 **	0.34 **	0.47 **	0.57 **	0.64 **	−0.62 **	−0.68 **	−0.70 **	0.83 **	0.88 **	(0.83)

Note. T1 = Time 1; T2 = Time 2; T3 = Time 3. PC = Psychological capital; JS = Job Satisfaction; TI = Turnover Intention; JE = Job Embeddedness. Coefficient alphas appear in parentheses along the diagonal. * $p < 0.05$. ** $p < 0.01$.

2.4. Data Analysis

SPSS 18.0 and MPLUS 7.0 were used to analyze the data. Descriptive analyses and tests of baseline homogeneity of three groups were conducted using analysis of variance (ANOVA) and chi-square analysis. Data are available from the corresponding author.

To test the hypotheses, we conducted a mixed between-within ANOVA. The interaction of Group (experimental, placebo, control) × Time (T1, T2, T3) was analyzed to test whether three groups showed different development over time. Moreover, we conducted post hoc analyses to test mean differences between three groups at T1, T2, and T3 with three multivariate analyses of variance (MANOVAs). In addition, analysis of covariance (ANCOVA) was used to support the differences between the groups. Then, pairwise comparisons were conducted to test within-group differences, that is, whether the experimental group showed a significant difference in the study variables at different time points. Partial eta-squared (η_p^2), Cohen's *d*, and 95% confidence intervals were calculated to examine the effect size. Cohen's *d* was considered to be a small effect if $d \geq 0.2$, a medium effect if $d \geq 0.5$, and a large effect if $d \geq 0.8$ [70]. Partial eta-squared was interpreted as a small effect if $\eta_p^2 \geq 0.01$, a medium effect if $\eta_p^2 \geq 0.06$, and a large effect if $\eta_p^2 \geq 0.14$ [70].

3. Results

3.1. Preliminary Analysis

The ANOVA indicated that random assignment was truly effective at establishing an initial equivalence between the three groups, as no significant differences were found between their levels of PsyCap ($p = 0.981$). Furthermore, at the baseline, no significant differences were found between groups for job satisfaction ($p = 0.952$); turnover intention ($p = 0.731$); job embeddedness ($p = 0.514$) (Table 2); gender, χ^2 (1, $N = 104$) = 0.98, $p = 0.612$; age, χ^2 (3, $N = 104$) = 4.51, $p = 0.608$; job tenure, χ^2 (4, $N = 104$) = 12.81, $p = 0.118$; education, χ^2 (3, $N = 104$) = 4.24, $p = 0.644$; or marriage, χ^2 (3, $N = 104$) = 3.35, $p = 0.764$.

Table 2. Means, standard deviations, and results of the multivariate analyses of variance (MANOVAs) for study variables at pretest (time 1), posttest (time 2), and follow-up (time 3), comparing experimental, placebo, and control groups.

Variable	Group	M (SD)			Results of MANOVA					
		Pre (T1)	Post (T2)	Follow-up (T3)	Pre (T1)		Post (T2)		Follow-up (T3)	
					Univariate F, p-Value	η_p^2	Univariate F, p-Value	η_p^2	Univariate F, p-Value	η_p^2
PsyCap	E	4.47 (0.559)	4.66 (0.503)	4.69 (0.513)	0.020, 0.981	0.000	1.673, 0.193	0.032	1.705, 0.187	0.033
	P	4.48 (0.434)	4.52 (0.489)	4.51 (0.473)						
	C	4.49 (0.514)	4.44 (0.554)	4.49 (0.532)						
Job Satisfaction	E	3.29 (0.651)	3.52 (0.632)	3.57 (0.636)	0.048, 0.952	0.001	0.438, 0.646	0.009	0.852, 0.430	0.017
	P	3.34 (0.689)	3.38 (0.812)	3.41 (0.785)						
	C	3.33 (0.795)	3.38 (0.774)	3.35 (0.782)						
Turnover Intention	E	3.65 (1.64)	3.45 (1.51)	3.48 (1.59)	0.314, 0.731	0.006	0.725, 0.487	0.014	0.308, 0.736	0.006
	P	3.69 (1.80)	3.90 (1.63)	3.77 (1.59)						
	C	3.39 (1.69)	3.62 (1.58)	3.52 (1.59)						
Job Embeddedness	E	3.12 (0.471)	3.16 (0.618)	3.15 (0.535)	0.671, 0.514	0.013	0.051, 0.950	0.001	0.172, 0.842	0.003
	P	2.99 (0.899)	3.14 (0.904)	3.15 (0.861)						
	C	3.18 (0.671)	3.20 (0.763)	3.07 (0.609)						

Note. Group: E = Experimental; P = Placebo; C = Control. N (experimental group) = 38; N (placebo group) = 31; N (control group) = 35. $df = 2$; η_p^2 = partial eta-squared.

3.2. Intervention Effects on PsyCap

To test the first hypothesis, which proposed that the intervention would effectively improve the PsyCap level, we performed a mixed between-within ANOVA. The results revealed a significant interaction effect for groups by time for PsyCap, $F = 3.77$, $df = 3.439$, $p = 0.009$, $\eta_p^2 = 0.069$. As a post hoc analysis, we conducted MANOVA to test whether the three groups differed significantly regarding their means at T1, T2, and T3 for PsyCap. The results indicated no significant differences between the groups (Table 2).

In addition, we conducted ANCOVA for a more rigorous test for mean differences. Specifically, PsyCap data at T2 and T3 were compared among the experimental, placebo, and control groups, controlling for PsyCap at T1. In addition to controlling for the effect of PsyCap at T1, we also included the covariates of age, gender, job tenure, education, and marriage. The results (Table 3) suggested that the group variable was a significant predictor of PsyCap at T2 and T3 ($p < 0.05$), whereas age, gender, job tenure, education, and marriage were not ($p > 0.05$).

Table 3. Analysis of covariance (ANCOVA) controlling for study variables at T1, demographic, and job variables.

Dependent Variable	Variables	F Value	p-Value	Dependent Variable	Variables	F Value	p-Value
PsyCap at T2	PsyCap at T1	159.629	<0.001	JS at T2	JS at T1	176.522	<0.001
	Age	0.855	0.357		Age	0.001	0.979
	Gender	0.131	0.719		Gender	0.170	0.681
	Job Tenure	0.144	0.705		Job Tenure	0.221	0.639
	Education	0.589	0.455		Education	0.072	0.790
	Marriage	0.534	0.467		Marriage	0.221	0.639
	Group	4.546	0.013		Group	1.688	0.190
PsyCap at T3	PsyCap at T1	129.698	<0.001	JS at T3	JS T1	140.703	<0.001
	Age	0.028	0.867		Age	0.822	0.367
	Gender	2.132	0.148		Gender	0.018	0.893
	Job Tenure	0.092	0.762		Job Tenure	0.813	0.370
	Education	0.663	0.417		Education	0.298	0.587
	Marriage	0.102	0.750		Marriage	0.095	0.758
	Group	5.018	0.008		Group	3.089	0.050
TI at T2	TI at T1	433.628	<0.001	JE at T2	JE at T1	314.839	<0.001
	Age	0.265	0.608		Age	0.013	0.908
	Gender	2.175	0.144		Gender	0.483	0.489
	Job Tenure	0.125	0.724		Job Tenure	0.398	0.530
	Education	2.470	0.119		Education	0.499	0.482
	Marriage	0.616	0.434		Marriage	0.929	0.338
	Group	5.017	0.008		Group	1.044	0.356
TI at T3	TI at T1	419.907	<0.001	JE at T3	JE at T1	230.827	<0.001
	Age	0.182	0.670		Age	0.037	0.848
	Gender	0.397	0.530		Gender	0.701	0.405
	Job Tenure	0.005	0.943		Job Tenure	0.923	0.339
	Education	1.416	0.237		Education	5.835	0.018
	Marriage	0.044	0.835		Marriage	0.405	0.526
	Group	1.544	0.219		Group	3.028	0.053

Note. T1 = Time 1; T2 = Time 2; T3 = Time 3. JS = Job Satisfaction; TI = Turnover Intention; JE = Job Embeddedness.

We also analyzed whether the means in the experimental group were significantly distinct from T1 to T2 and from T1 to T3, expecting an increase across this time frame. Pairwise comparison showed a significant promotion in PsyCap over time in the experimental group (Figure 3): the means changed significantly from T1 to T2 (Δ(T2−T1) = 0.198, $p = 0.001$, $d = 0.501$, 95% CI [0.044, 0.958]) and from T1 to T3 (Δ(T3−T1) = 0.224, $p = 0.000$, $d = 0.557$, 95% CI [0.098, 1.015]). For the placebo group, pairwise comparison showed no significant distinctions from T1 to T2 (Δ(T2−T1) = 0.043, $p = 1.000$, $d = 0.136$, 95% CI [−0.363, 0.634]) or from T1 to T3 (Δ(T3−T1) = 0.03, $p = 1.000$, $d = 0.098$, 95% CI [−0.4, 0.596]). For the control group, pairwise comparison also showed no significant differences from T1 to T2 (Δ(T2−T1) = −0.043, $p = 1.000$, $d = −0.143$, 95% CI [−0.613, 0.326]) or from T1 to T3 (Δ(T3−T1) = 0, $p = 1.000$, $d = 0$, 95% CI [−0.469, 0.469]). Thus, only the experimental group saw a significant promotion in PsyCap level, which supported Hypothesis 1.

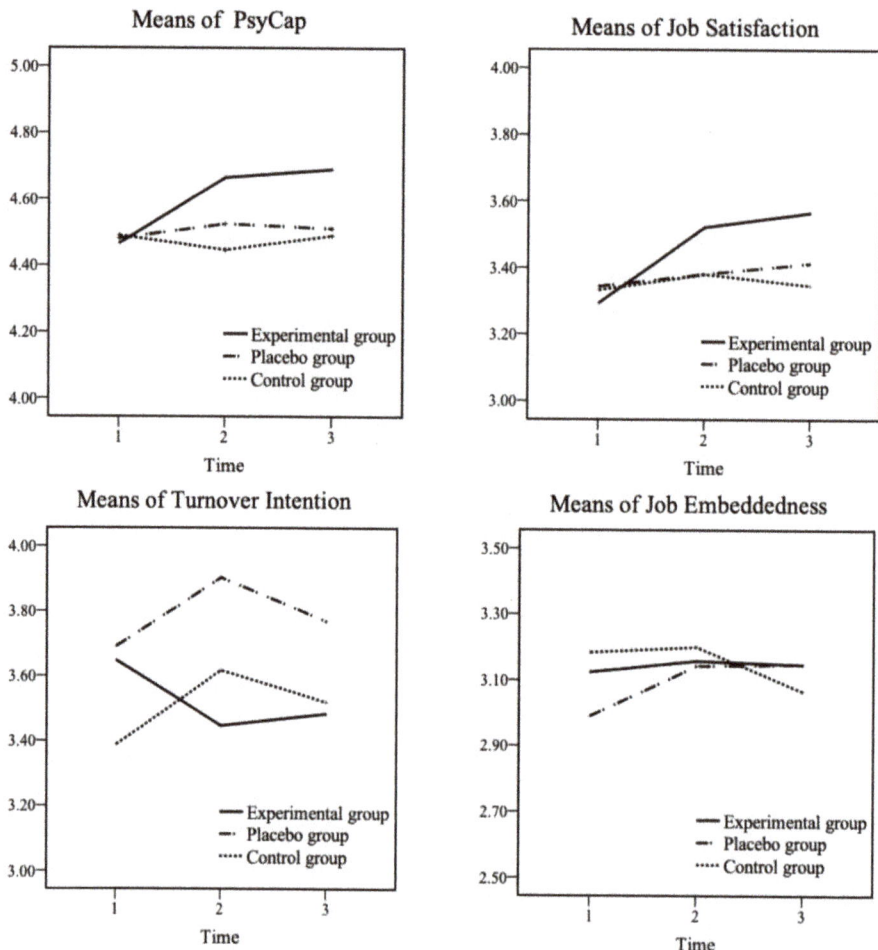

Figure 3. Development of PsyCap and work-related attitudes for the three groups over time.

3.3. Intervention Effects on Work-Related Attitudes

For job satisfaction, the mixed between-within ANOVA showed no significant interaction effect of group by time, $F = 2.015$, $df = 3.643$, $p = 0.101$, $\eta_p^2 = 0.038$. However, the main effect of time was significant, $F = 4.571$, $df = 1.821$, $p = 0.014$, $\eta_p^2 = 0.043$, whereas the main effect of group was not significant, $F = 0.242$, $df = 2$, $p = 0.786$, $\eta_p^2 = 0.005$.

Furthermore, we conducted ANCOVA for a more rigorous test for mean differences of job satisfaction. The results (Table 3) suggested that the group variable was not a significant predictor of job satisfaction at T2 ($p > 0.05$) but was a marginally significant one at T3 ($p = 0.050$), whereas age, gender, job tenure, education, and marriage were not significant at either interval ($p > 0.05$).

In addition, pairwise comparison showed a significant promotion in job satisfaction over time in the experimental group (Figure 3): the means changed significantly from T1 to T2 (Δ(T2–T1) = 0.228, $p = 0.002$, $d = 0.559$, 95% CI (0.1, 1.017)) and from T1 to T3 (Δ(T3–T1) = 0.272, $p = 0.001$, $d = 0.634$, 95% CI (0.173, 1.095)). For the placebo group, pairwise comparison showed no significant differences from T1 to T2 (Δ(T2–T1) = 0.038, $p = 0.642$, $d = 0.092$, 95% CI (−0.406, 0.59)) or between T1 and T3 (Δ(T3–T1) = 0.070, $p = 0.424$, $d = 0.15$, 95% CI (−0.349, 0.648)). For the control group, pairwise comparison showed no significant differences from T1 to T2 (Δ(T2–T1) = 0.048, p = 0.531, d = 0.099, 95% CI (−0.369, 0.568)) or from T1 to T3 (Δ(T3–T1) = 0.014, p = 0.082, d = 0.037, 95% CI (−0.431, 0.506)). Thus, the experimental group saw a significant promotion of job satisfaction level, which supported Hypothesis 2.

For turnover intention, the mixed between-within ANOVA showed a marginally significant interaction effect of group by time, F = 2.476, df = 3.607, p = 0.052, η_p^2 = 0.047. However, neither the main effect of time, F = 0.842, df = 1.804, p = 0.422, η_p^2 = 0.008, nor the main effect of group, F = 0.318, df = 2, p = 0.728, η_p^2 = 0.006, was significant.

Nevertheless, the mixed between-within ANOVA revealed a significant interaction effect of group at two time points (T1 and T2), F = 4.022, df = 2, p = 0.021, η_p^2 = 0.074, which indicated that the effect of the PsyCap intervention on turnover was significant at T2, but the significant effect did not persist to T3. We conducted ANCOVA for a more rigorous test for mean differences of turnover intention; the results shown in Table 3 suggested that the group variable was a significant indicator of turnover intention at T2 (p < 0.05) but not at T3 (p > 0.05), whereas age, gender, job tenure, education levels, and marriage status were not significant at either interval (p > 0.05).

We also analyzed whether the means of turnover intention in the experimental group were significantly changed from T1 to T2, indicating a decrease across this time frame. However, pairwise comparison showed no significant reduction in turnover intention in any of the groups between T1 and T2: the experimental group, Δ(T2–T1) = 0.200, p = 0.094, d = −0.273, 95% CI (−0.724, 0.179) (Figure 3); the placebo group, Δ(T2–T1) = −0.213, p = 0.107, d = 0.261, 95% CI (−0.239, 0.761); or control group, Δ(T2–T1) = −0.229, p = 0.067, d = 0.304, 95% CI (−0.167, 0.776). Although the experimental group did not exhibit a significant reduction in turnover intention level, it appeared that the intervention did prevent participants from increasing turnover intention, which was observed in both the placebo and control groups. Thus, Hypothesis 3 was partially supported.

For job embeddedness, the mixed between-within ANOVA showed a marginally significant interaction effect of group by time, F = 2.422, df = 4, p = 0.050, η_p^2 = 0.046. However, neither the main effect of time, F = 1.794, df = 2, p = 0.169, η_p^2 = 0.017, nor main effect of group, F = 0.067, df = 2, p = 0.936, η_p^2 = 0.001, was significant. Additionally, the ANCOVA results (Table 3) suggested that the group variable was not a significant predictor of job embeddedness at T2 (p > 0.05) but was a marginally significant one at T3 (p = 0.053), whereas age, gender, job tenure, education, and marriage were not significant at either interval (p > 0.05).

In addition, despite expecting an increase over time, pairwise comparison of the means of job embeddedness from T1 to T2 and from T1 to T3 showed no significant promotion in job embeddedness over time in the experimental group (Figure 3): the means did not differ significantly from T1 to T2 (Δ(T2–T1) = 0.034, p = 0.572, d = 0.167, 95% CI (−0.284, 0.617)) or from T1 to T3 (Δ(T3–T1) = 00.023, p = 0.712, d = 0.109, 95% CI (−0.341, 0.559)). However, for the placebo group, the pairwise comparison showed significant changes from T1 to T2 (Δ(T2–T1) = 0.152, p = 0.023, d = 0.327, 95% CI (−0.174, 0.828)) and from T1 to T3 (Δ(T3–T1) = 00.157, p = 0.027, d = 0.305, 95% CI (−0.196, 0.806)). For the control group, the pairwise comparison showed no significant differences from T1 to T2 (Δ(T2–T1) = 0.016, p = 0.794, d = 0.058, 95% CI (−0.41, 0.527)) or from T1 to T3 (Δ(T3–T1) = −0.118, p = 0.075, d = −0.281, 95% CI (−0.752, 0.19)). Thus, the experimental group did not see a significant improvement in job embeddedness. Thus, Hypothesis 4 was not supported.

4. Discussion

The purpose of this study was to extend PsyCap intervention studies from both theoretical and practical perspectives in the cultural context of mainland China, which creatively contributes to the academic literature and, to some degree, organizational practice on PsyCap intervention. Theoretically, we added a goal-as-journey metaphor [12] in the development of the hope dimension. To the best of our knowledge, this is the first attempt to extend the existing content of the PCI model. We believe that it is crucial to generalize the effectiveness of PsyCap interventions [7–10] and at the same time continuously develop previous theories and models. However, it is regrettable that we could not evaluate the effect of adding the journal metaphor into the PCI model. It has been argued by many researchers that the effectiveness of workplace interventions cannot look only at final outcomes [71]. The combination of an outcome evaluation and an evaluation of the process of the intervention is encouraged by researchers [72–74].

Moreover, based on the conservation of resources (COR) theory [13,14], we examined not only the effectiveness of this PsyCap intervention but also its influence on other work-related attitudes: job satisfaction, turnover intention, and job embeddedness. Consistent with both our hypothesis and the results of other studies [8–10], we found that our intervention based on the PCI model significantly enhanced PsyCap. In addition, we found that our intervention significantly improved the job satisfaction level in the experimental group over time, despite the group difference at the three time points not being significant. Moreover, we found that our intervention significantly reduced the turnover intention at time 2, whereas the intervention effect at time 3 was not significant. Specifically, the group difference was significant at time 2, despite the fact that the time difference was not significant. Even though the effect size of PsyCap intervention's influence on job satisfaction and turnover intention was not strong, it still showed a positive tendency in the experimental group, which is worth further exploration.

Contrary to our expectations, we found no significant intervention effects for job embeddedness. However, it is surprising that the time effect for the placebo group was significant, which means that job embeddedness significantly improved in the placebo group from T1 to T3. Although we did not verify our hypothesis on job embeddedness, we proved that job embeddedness and turnover intention are not opposite to each other and may be influenced by different factors in workplaces [56]. The adverse effects of job embeddedness have also been found by other researchers. For example, Ng and Feldman [75] note that employees with high levels of embeddedness are associated with declining social capital development, which is presumably because they have already amassed contacts and felt less need to cultivate new ones. The reason why the intervention effect of PsyCap on job embeddedness was not significant may be related to the different emphases of PsyCap and job embeddedness. Specifically, PsyCap may pay more attention to the difficulties of work and help people to deal with or overcome them, while job embeddedness may pay more attention to the positive sides of work. We consider this a very interesting finding and encourage future studies that examine the relationships between PsyCap and job embeddedness, as well as the influence of PsyCap intervention on this variable and also on some other work-related outcomes.

Practically, a daily online self-learning approach was utilized to conduct the intervention, which provides more possible methods for implementing PsyCap interventions in workplaces. As discussed, ascertaining that a proposed training intervention is effective per se, regardless of the person or method delivering it, is meaningful to the intervention itself and also to practice [10]. A self-learning perspective also challenges the traditional mindset of interventions with trainers. With the development of technology, the Internet can be quite a useful and convenient medium for psychological interventions; it is able to reach a broad audience, flexible and time-efficient, cost-effective, and anonymous [76], which can help organizations and employees overcome different kinds of difficulties, such as getting access to professional trainers, gathering employees together at the same time, increasing more active participation, and so on. Our study encourages future researchers and managers to be creative and flexible when designing targeted and suitable interventions for organizations and employees.

Furthermore, our study enriches the literature of PsyCap interventions in non-Western countries. To the best of our knowledge, this study is one of very few PsyCap intervention studies in Asia or China. According to a previous meta-analysis [29], 78% of the randomized controlled trials on the effectiveness of positive psychology interventions are conducted in Western countries. A systematic review [28] also reveals that research in the field of positive psychology intervention in non-Western countries is still in its infancy, and the low quality of the studies from non-Western countries may explain the larger difference in effect sizes. Therefore, our study utilized a rigid randomized controlled trial design to practice PsyCap intervention in China and may contribute to the field of positive psychology interventions by better comparing the cultural differences between Western and non-Western countries.

4.1. Limitations and Implications for Future Research

Meanwhile, we admit the following limitations of our study. First, our study sample was not confined to one organization. Participants from various occupations were recruited online using a convenience sampling method and then randomly allocated into three groups. Although this makes the sample more representative, this diversity may have produced differences during the intervention, despite no significant difference being found between three groups at T1. Due to differences in organizational culture, the intervention effect may have been contaminated, and the effect of the PsyCap intervention may have been underestimated. This might explain why Hypotheses 2 and 3 were partially supported: employees' job attitudes and behaviors may have been influenced by some organizational elements. Future research should consider conducting the interventions in the same organizations to further test the effect of the PsyCap intervention. In addition, conducting interventions in the same organizations would allow for the addition of some group-level or organization-level outcome variables to verify the intervention effect on both groups and organizations. Furthermore, our use of self-report methods to measure all variables may have led to common method bias; an intervention study confined to one organization could include other measurements, such as objective data, peer assessment, and leader assessment, to reduce such bias.

Second, our study tested all four variables just before (T1), just after (T2), and one week after (T3) the intervention. A one-week follow-up is definitely not strong enough to verify the duration effect of the intervention. When designing the study, as participants are all recruited online, it is difficult to maintain connections with participants for a month or several months, which may lead to a higher rate of dropout. Therefore, we chose a one-week follow-up. However, there is no doubt that one-week follow-up is not sufficient to prove the duration effect of the intervention. Therefore, future research on PsyCap intervention should consider test the duration effect through a longer follow-up, such as one month or three months.

Third, the final sample size was quite small, with about 30 to 40 participants in each group. Based on the limited sample size, it should be stressed that this is at best a pilot study and no valid conclusions can be reached. In addition, more men dropped out of our study than women, which produced a final sample composed mostly of women (68.4%), suggesting gender bias. Future research should attempt to enlarge the sample size and balance the gender distribution. Last but not least, the effect size of some of our significant findings is also small, and it may have resulted from the short duration of the intervention, the small sample size, and so on. Future research could extend the intervention duration to several weeks, as researchers have found that long-term training can lead to a higher effect than short-term training [77].

To conclude, this study has some non-negligible drawbacks to the study design, such as the short follow-up and small sample size, which makes the conclusions of this study unconvincing. Therefore, this study should only be considered as a pilot study [78] of PsyCap intervention, and future research is required to further verify the effectiveness of a daily online self-learning PsyCap intervention and its influence on other work-related variables.

4.2. Practical Implications

Our results are promising for human resources development and management because we demonstrate that a daily self-learning PsyCap intervention over five working days can promote employees' PsyCap level, increase their job satisfaction, and decrease their turnover intention to some degree. Our findings encourage managers to flexibly apply the PCI model to meet the needs of their organizations and employees. Our study also indicates that PsyCap intervention can be provided through daily self-learning materials without professional trainers, which allows employees to receive a PsyCap intervention more conveniently and at lower cost.

5. Conclusions

This study reveals that a daily online self-learning PsyCap intervention is effective at improving PsyCap levels and has positive influences, increasing job satisfaction and decreasing turnover intention. This is another replication and extension of the PCI model and proves the effectiveness of the model on PsyCap and several work-related attitudes.

Author Contributions: Conceptualization, S.D., Y.H., and X.Z.; methodology, S.D., Y.H., and X.Z.; software, S.D.; validation, S.D., Y.H., and X.Z.; formal analysis, Y.H. and X.Z.; investigation, Y.H. and X.Z.; resources, Y.H. and X.Z.; data curation, S.D. and Y.H.; writing—original draft preparation, S.D.; writing—review and editing, S.D., Y.H., and X.Z.; visualization, S.D.; supervision, X.Z.; project administration, X.Z.; funding acquisition, X.Z. All authors have read and agreed to the published version of the manuscript.

Funding: This research was funded by the Research on National Key R&D Program of China, grant number 2018YFC0810600.

Acknowledgments: The authors thank Liuqin Yang for insightful comments on a previous version of this article, Siw Tone Innstrand for the help on manuscript revision, and the two anonymous reviewers and the action editor for their constructive comments during the review process.

Conflicts of Interest: The authors declare no conflict of interest.

References

1. Luthans, F.; Church, A.H. Positive Organizational Behavior: Developing and Managing Psychological Strengths. *Acad. Manag. Exec.* **2002**, *16*, 57–75. [CrossRef]
2. Luthans, F.; Youssef, C.M. Human, Social, and Now Positive Psychological Capital Management: Investing in People for Competitive Advantage. *Organ. Dyn.* **2004**, *33*, 143–160. [CrossRef]
3. Cameron, K.S.; Caza, A. Contributions to the Discipline of Positive Organizational Scholarship. *Am. Behav. Sci.* **2004**, *47*, 731–739. [CrossRef]
4. Meyers, M.C.; Woerkom, M.V.; Bakker, A.B. The Added Value of the Positive: A Literature Review of Positive Psychology Interventions in Organizations. *Eur. J. Work Organ. Psychol.* **2013**, *22*, 618–632. [CrossRef]
5. Cameron, K.S.; Mora, C.; Leutscher, T.; Calarco, M. Effects of Positive Practices on Organizational Effectiveness. *J. Appl. Behav. Sci.* **2011**, *47*, 266–308. [CrossRef]
6. Nolzen, N. The concept of psychological capital: A comprehensive review. *Manag. Rev. Q.* **2018**, *68*, 237–277. [CrossRef]
7. Luthans, F.; Avey, J.B.; Avolio, B.J.; Norman, S.M.; Combs, G.M. Psychological capital development: Toward a micro-intervention. *J. Organ. Behav.* **2006**, *27*, 387–393. [CrossRef]
8. Luthans, F.; Avey, J.B.; Patera, J.L. Experimental Analysis of a Web-Based Training Intervention to Develop Positive Psychological Capital. *Acad. Manag. Learn. Educ.* **2008**, *7*, 209–221. [CrossRef]
9. Luthans, F.; Avey, J.B.; Avolio, B.J.; Peterson, S.J. The Development and Resulting Performance Impact of Positive Psychological Capital. *Hum. Resour. Dev. Q.* **2010**, *21*, 41–67. [CrossRef]
10. Dello Russo, S.; Stoykova, P. Psychological Capital Intervention (PCI): A Replication and Extension. *Hum. Resour. Dev. Q.* **2015**, *26*, 329–347. [CrossRef]
11. Demerouti, E.; van Eeuwijk, E.; Snelder, M.; Wild, U. Assessing the effects of a "personal effectiveness" training on psychological capital, assertiveness and self-awareness using self-other agreement. *Career Dev. Int.* **2011**, *16*, 60–81. [CrossRef]
12. Landau, M.J.; Oyserman, D.; Keefer, L.A.; Smith, G.C. The College Journey and Academic Engagement: How Metaphor Use Enhances Identity-Based Motivation. *J. Personal. Soc. Psychol.* **2014**, *106*, 679–698. [CrossRef] [PubMed]
13. Hobfoll, S.E. Social and psychological resources and adaptation. *Rev. Gen. Psychol.* **2002**, *6*, 307. [CrossRef]
14. Wright, T.A.; Hobfoll, S.E. Commitment, psychological well-being and job performance: An examination of conservation of resources (COR) theory and job burnout. *J. Bus. Manag.* **2004**, *9*, 389–406.
15. Luthans, F.; Youssef, C.M.; Avolio, B.J. *Psychological Capital: Developing the Human Competitive Edge*; Oxford University Press: Oxford, UK, 2007.
16. Luthans, F.; Avolio, B.J.; Avey, J.B.; Norman, S.M. Positive Psychological Capital: Measurement and Relationship with Performance and Satisfaction. *Pers. Psychol.* **2007**, *60*, 541–572. [CrossRef]

17. Lomas, T. Positive cross-cultural psychology: Exploring similarityand difference in constructions and experiences of wellbeing. *Int. J. Wellbeing* **2015**, *5*, 60–77. [CrossRef]
18. Reichard, R.J.; Dollwet, M.; Louw-Potgieter, J. Development of Cross-Cultural Psychological Capital and Its Relationship with Cultural Intelligence and Ethnocentrism. *J. Leadersh. Org. Stud.* **2014**, *21*, 150–164. [CrossRef]
19. Tsegaye, W.K.; Su, Q.; Ouyang, Z. Cognitive adjustment and psychological capital influences on expatriate workers' job performance: An Ethiopian study. *J. Psychol. Afr.* **2019**, *29*, 1–6. [CrossRef]
20. Tatarko, A. Are Individual Value Orientations Related to Socio-Psychological Capital? A Comparative Analysis Data from Three Ethnic Groups in Russia. *Glob. Bus. Issues Ejournal* **2012**. [CrossRef]
21. Jin, C.-H. The effect of psychological capital on start-up intention among young start-up entrepreneurs: A cross-cultural comparison. *Chin. Manag. Stud.* **2017**, *11*, 707–729. [CrossRef]
22. Chua, R.; Ng, Y.L.; Park, M. Mitigating Academic Distress: The Role of Psychological Capital in a Collectivistic Malaysian University Student Sample. *Open Psychol. J.* **2018**, *11*, 171–183. [CrossRef]
23. Nawaz, M.; Bhatti, G.; Ahmad, S.; Ahmed, Z. How Can the Organizational Commitment of Pakistan Railways' Employees Be Improved? The Moderating Role of Psychological Capital. *J. Entrep. Manag. Innov.* **2018**, *14*, 123–142. [CrossRef]
24. Shen, X.; Yang, Y.; Wang, Y.; Liu, L.; Wang, S.; Wang, L. The association between occupational stress and depressive symptoms and the mediating role of psychological capital among Chinese university teachers: A cross-sectional study. *BMC Psychiatry* **2014**, *14*. [CrossRef]
25. Li, X.; Kan, D.; Liu, L.; Shi, M.; Wang, Y.; Yang, X.; Wang, J.; Wang, L.; Wu, H. The mediating role of psychological capital on the association between occupational stress and job burnout among bank employees in China. *Int. J. Environ. Res. Public Health* **2015**, *12*, 2984–3001. [CrossRef] [PubMed]
26. Chen, Q.; Kong, Y.; Niu, J.; Gao, W.; Li, J.; Li, M. How Leaders' Psychological Capital Influence Their Followers' Psychological Capital: Social Exchange or Emotional Contagion. *Front. Psychol.* **2019**, *10*. [CrossRef] [PubMed]
27. Tian, F.; Shu, Q.; Cui, Q.; Wang, L.-l.; Liu, C.; Wu, H. The Mediating Role of Psychological Capital in the Relationship between Occupational Stress and Fatigue: A Cross-Sectional Study among 1104 Chinese Physicians. *Front. Public Health* **2020**, *8*. [CrossRef]
28. Hendriks, T.; Schotanus-Dijkstra, M.; Hassankhan, A.; Graafsma, T.; Bohlmeijer, E.; Jong, J.D. The efficacy of positive psychology interventions from non-Western countries: A systematic review and meta-analysis. *Int. J. Wellbeing* **2018**, *8*, 71–98. [CrossRef]
29. Hendriks, T.; Warren, M.A.; Schotanus-Dijkstra, M.; Hassankhan, A.; Graafsma, T.; Bohlmeijer, E.; Jong, J.D. How WEIRD are positive psychology interventions? A bibliometric analysis of randomized controlled trials on the science of well-being. *J. Posit. Psychol.* **2019**, *14*, 489–501. [CrossRef]
30. Bandura, A. *Self-Efficacy: The Exercise of Control*; W.H. Freeman and Company: New York, NY, USA, 1997.
31. Stajkovic, A.D.; Luthans, F. Social Cognitive Theory and Self Efficacy: Goin beyond Traditional Motivational and Behavioral Approaches. *Organ. Dyn.* **1998**, *26*, 62–74. [CrossRef]
32. Snyder, C.R. *Handbook of Hope*; Academic Press: San Diego, CA, USA, 2000.
33. Lakoff, G.; Johnson, M. *Metaphors We Live By*; University of Chicago Press: Chicago, IL, USA, 1980.
34. Oyserman, D. Not just any path: Implications of identity-based motivation for disparities in school outcomes. *Econ. Educ. Rev.* **2013**, *33*, 179–190. [CrossRef]
35. Luthans, F.; Vogelgesang, G.R.; Lester, P.B. Developing the Psychological Capital of Resiliency. *Hum. Resour. Dev. Rev.* **2006**, *5*, 25–44. [CrossRef]
36. Luthans, F. The Need for and Meaning of Positive Organizational Behavior. *J. Organ. Behav.* **2002**, *23*, 695–706. [CrossRef]
37. Masten, A.S. Ordinary Magic: Resilience Processes in Development. *Am. Psychol.* **2001**, *56*, 227–238. [CrossRef] [PubMed]
38. Seligman, M.E.P. *Learned Optimism*; Pocket Books: New York, NY, USA, 1998.
39. De Tornyay, R.T.M. *Strategies for Teaching Nursing*, 3rd ed.; Delmar Publishers: Albany, NY, USA, 1987.
40. Khalil, M.K.; Nelson, L.D.; Kibble, J.D. The Use of Self-learning Modules to Facilitate Learning of Basic Science Concepts in an Integrated Medical Curriculum. *Anat. Sci. Educ.* **2010**, *3*, 219–226. [CrossRef]
41. Feldman, M.A.; Case, L. Teaching Child-Care and Safety Skills to Parents with Intellectual Disabilities through Self-learning. *J. Intellect. Dev. Disabil.* **1999**, *24*, 27–44. [CrossRef]

42. Kalbfeld, K. *Evaluating the Effect of a Self-Learning Packet on Change in Nursing Practice*; Southern Connecticut State University: New Haven, CT, USA, 2006.
43. Dougal, J.; Gonterman, R. A Comparison of Three Teaching Methods on Learning and Retention. *J. Nurses Staff Dev.* **1999**, *15*, 205–209. [CrossRef]
44. Candy, P.C. *Self-Direction for Lifelong Learning: A Comprehensive Guide to Theory and Practice*; Jossey-Bass: San Francisco, CA, USA, 1991.
45. Sitzmann, T.; Kraiger, K.; Stewart, D.; Wisher, R. The Comparative Effectiveness of Web-based and Classroom Instruction: A Meta-Analysis. *Pers. Psychol.* **2006**, *59*, 623–664. [CrossRef]
46. Updegraff, J.A.; Taylor, S.E. From Vulnerability to Growth: Positive and Negative Effects of Stressful Life Events. In *Loss and Trauma: General and Close Relationship Perspectives*; Harvey, J., Miller, E., Eds.; Brunner-Routledge: Philadelphia, PA, USA, 2000; pp. 3–28.
47. Peterson, S.J.; Luthans, F.; Avolio, B.J.; Walumbwa, F.O.; Zhang, Z. Psychological Capital and Employee Performance: A Latent Growth Modeling Approach. *Pers. Psychol.* **2011**, *64*, 427–450. [CrossRef]
48. Luthans, F.; Norman, S.M.; Avolio, B.J.; Avey, J.B. The Mediating Role of Psychological Capital in the Supportive Organizational Climate-Employee Performance Relationship. *J. Organ. Behav.* **2008**, *29*, 219–238. [CrossRef]
49. Youssef, C.M.; Luthans, F. Positive Organizational Behavior in the Workplace: The Impact of Hope, Optimism, and Resilience. *J. Manag.* **2007**, *33*, 774–800. [CrossRef]
50. Avey, J.B.; Patera, J.L.; West, B.J. The Implications of Positive Psychological Capital on Employee Absenteeism. *J. Leadersh. Organ. Stud.* **2006**, *13*, 42–60. [CrossRef]
51. Locke, E.A. What is Job Satisfaction? *Organ. Behav. Hum. Perform.* **1969**, *4*, 309–336. [CrossRef]
52. Wolf, M.G. Nedd Gratification Theory: A Theoretical Reformulation of Job Satisfaction/Dissatisfaction and Job Motivation. *J. Appl. Psychol.* **1970**, *54*, 87–94. [CrossRef]
53. Spector, P.E. *Job Satisfaction*; Sage Publications Inc.: New York, NY, USA, 1997.
54. Avey, J.B.; Reichard, R.J.; Luthans, F.; Mhatre, K.H. Meta-Analysis of the Impact of Positive Psychological Capital on Employee Attitudes, Behaviors, and Performance. *Hum. Resour. Dev. Q.* **2011**, *22*, 127–152. [CrossRef]
55. Hom, P.W.; Griffeth, R.W. *Employee Turnover*; South-Western College Publishing: Cincinnati, OH, USA, 1995.
56. Hom, P.W.; Lee, T.W.; Shaw, J.D.; Hausknecht, J.P. One Hundred Years of Employee Turnover Theory and Research. *J. Appl. Psychol.* **2017**, *102*, 530–545. [CrossRef]
57. March, J.G.; Simon, H.A. *Organizations*; Wiley: New York, NY, USA, 1958.
58. Ajzen, I. The Theory of Planned Behavior. *Organ. Behav. Hum. Decis. Process.* **1991**, *50*, 179–211. [CrossRef]
59. Avey, J.B.; Luthans, F.; Youssef, C.M. The Additive Value of Positive Psychological Capital in Predicting Work Attitudes and Behaviors. *J. Manag.* **2010**, *36*, 430–452. [CrossRef]
60. Siu, O.L.; Cheung, F.; Lui, S. Linking Positive Emotions to Work Well-Being and Turnover Intention among Hong Kong Police Officers: The Role of Psychological Capital. *J. Happiness Stud.* **2015**, *16*, 367–380. [CrossRef]
61. Mitchell, T.R.; Holtom, B.C.; Wee, T.W.; Sablyskyi, C.J.; Erez, M. Why People Stay: Using Job Embeddedness to Predict Voluntary Turnonver. *Acad. Manag. J.* **2001**, *44*, 1102–1121. [CrossRef]
62. Sun, T.; Zhao, X.W.; Yang, L.B.; Fan, L.H. The Impact of Psychological Capital on Job Embeddedness and Job Performance among Nurses: A Structural Equation Approach. *J. Adv. Nurs.* **2012**, *68*, 69–79. [CrossRef]
63. Lu, Q.; Dong, L.; Wu, I.H.C.; You, J.; Huang, J.; Hu, Y. The impact of an expressive writing intervention on quality of life among Chinese breast cancer patients undergoing chemotherapy. *Supportive Care Cancer* **2018**, *27*, 165–173. [CrossRef] [PubMed]
64. Dolev-Amit, T.; Rubin, A.; Zilcha-Mano, S. Is Awareness of Strengths Intervention Sufficient to Cultivate Wellbeing and Other Positive Outcomes? *J. Happiness Stud.* **2020**, 1–22. [CrossRef]
65. Smyth, J.M. Written Emotional Expression: Effect Sizes, Outcome Types, and Moderating Variables. *J. Consult. Clin. Psych.* **1998**, *66*, 174–184. [CrossRef]
66. Frattaroli, J. Experimental Disclosure and Its Moderators: A Meta-Analysis. *Psychol. Bull.* **2006**, *132*, 823–865. [CrossRef] [PubMed]
67. Agho, A.O.; Price, J.L.; Mueller, C.W. Discriminant Validity of Measures of Job Satisfaction, Positive Affectivity and Negative Affectivity. *J. Occup. Organ. Psychol.* **1992**, *65*, 185–195. [CrossRef]
68. Bluedom, A.C. A Unified Model of Turnover from Organizations. *Hum. Relat.* **1982**, *35*, 135–153. [CrossRef]

69. Crossley, C.D.; Bennett, R.J.; Jex, S.M.; Burnfield, J.L. Development of a Global Measure of Job Embeddedness and Integration into a Traditional Model of Voluntary Turnover. *J. Appl. Psychol.* **2007**, *92*, 1031–1042. [CrossRef]
70. Cohen, J. *Statistical Power Analysis for the Behavioral Sciences*, 2nd ed.; Erlbaum: Hillsdale, NJ, USA, 1988.
71. Innstrand, S.T.; Christensen, M. Healthy Universities. The development and implementation of a holistic health promotion intervention programme especially adapted for staff working in the higher educational sector: The ARK study. *Promot. Educ.* **2018**, *27*, 68–76. [CrossRef]
72. Nielsen, K.; Randall, R. The importance of employee participation and perceptions of changes in procedures in a teamworking intervention. *Work Stress* **2012**, *26*, 91–111. [CrossRef]
73. Abildgaard, J.S.; Saksvik, P.Ø.; Nielsen, K. How to measure the intervention process? An assessment of qualitative and quantitative approaches to data collection in the process evaluation of organizational interventions. *Front. Psychol.* **2016**, *7*, 1380. [CrossRef]
74. Nielsen, K. Organizational occupational health interventions: What works for whom in which circumstances? *Occup. Med. Oxf.* **2017**, *67*, 410–412. [CrossRef] [PubMed]
75. Ng, T.W.H.; Feldman, D.C. The Effects of Organizational Embeddedness on Development of Social Capital and Human Capital. *J. Appl. Psychol.* **2010**, *95*, 696–712. [CrossRef] [PubMed]
76. Leykin, Y.; Thekdi, S.M.; Shumay, D.; MuÒoz, R.; Riba, M.; Dunn, L. Internet interventions for improving psychological welå being in psycho oncology: Review and recommendations. *Psychè Oncol.* **2012**, *21*. [CrossRef]
77. Walter, N.; Nikoleizig, L.; Alfermann, D. Effects of Self-Talk Training on Competitive Anxiety, Self-Efficacy, Volitional Skills, and Performance: An Intervention Study with Junior Sub-Elite Athletes. *Sports* **2019**, *7*. [CrossRef] [PubMed]
78. Hertzog, M.A. Considerations in determining sample size for pilot studies. *Res. Nurse Health* **2008**, *31*, 180–191. [CrossRef]

Publisher's Note: MDPI stays neutral with regard to jurisdictional claims in published maps and institutional affiliations.

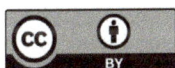

© 2020 by the authors. Licensee MDPI, Basel, Switzerland. This article is an open access article distributed under the terms and conditions of the Creative Commons Attribution (CC BY) license (http://creativecommons.org/licenses/by/4.0/).

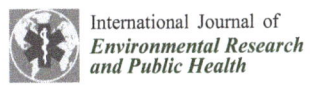

Article

A Blended Cognitive–Behavioral Intervention for the Treatment of Postpartum Depression: Study Protocol for a Randomized Controlled Trial

Mariana Branquinho *, Maria Cristina Canavarro and Ana Fonseca

Center for Research in Neuropsychology and Cognitive Behavioral Intervention, Faculty of Psychology and Educational Sciences, University of Coimbra, Rua do Colégio Novo, 3000-115 Coimbra, Portugal; mccanavarro@fpce.uc.pt (M.C.C.); ana.fonseca77@gmail.com (A.F.)
* Correspondence: marianacjbranquinho@hotmail.com; Tel.: +351-239-851-450

Received: 11 September 2020; Accepted: 18 November 2020; Published: 20 November 2020

Abstract: Despite the existence of effective treatment for postpartum depression, few women seek professional help, indicating the need for a new and innovative format of treatment that can overcome help-seeking barriers. This article presents the study protocol for a blended cognitive–behavioral intervention for the treatment of postpartum depression, by integrating face-to-face sessions with a web-based program (Be a Mom) into one treatment protocol. This study will be a two-arm, noninferiority randomized controlled trial comparing blended intervention to usual treatment for postpartum depression provided in healthcare centers. Portuguese postpartum adult women diagnosed with postpartum depression (according to the DSM-5 diagnostic criteria for major depressive disorder) will be recruited during routine care appointments in local healthcare centers and will be eligible to participate. Measures will be completed at baseline, postintervention, and at three- and six-month follow-ups. The primary outcome will be depressive symptoms. Secondary outcomes will include anxiety symptoms, fatigue, quality of life, marital satisfaction, maternal self-efficacy, and mother–child bonding. Cost-effectiveness analysis and mediator and moderator analysis will be conducted. This study will provide insight into the efficacy and cost-effectiveness of a blended psychological intervention in the Portuguese context and increase the empirically validated treatment options for postpartum depression.

Keywords: postpartum depression; cognitive–behavioral therapy; blended treatment; Be a Mom; study protocol

1. Introduction

Postpartum depression (PPD) is a serious clinical condition affecting approximately 13% of Portuguese women after childbirth [1]. When left untreated, PPD poses adverse and persistent consequences for the entire family system. It affects the woman's health (e.g., increased tiredness [2], decreased quality of life [3]) and mother–child interaction (e.g., mother-child bonding, lower parenting self-efficacy) [3,4]. Moreover, it can have consequences for the infant's development (e.g., infant sleep patterns, emotional development) [3] and for the entire family environment, including the couple's relationship [5].

Despite the existence of effective treatments (e.g., cognitive–behavioral therapy [CBT]) [6], few women with PPD seek professional help [7]. A Portuguese study revealed that only 13.6% of women with depressive symptoms during the perinatal period sought professional help to address their emotional difficulties [8]. Time and financial constraints and struggles with transportation and childcare issues are some of the structural barriers to seeking professional help reported by postpartum women [9,10], suggesting the need for new delivery formats to improve women's access to evidence-based PPD interventions.

E-mental health tools are an innovative form of treatment delivery that use digital technology, including web-based technology, in the mental health field [11]. These tools can overcome PPD treatment uptake barriers given their reduced costs, flexibility, and improved accessibility [12]. Women in the postpartum period already use the internet frequently to search for information about PPD [10]. Moreover, e-mental health tools have been perceived as acceptable and useful among Portuguese women in the perinatal period, particularly among those women presenting clinically relevant depressive symptoms [13].

Existing web-based interventions for PPD treatment based on CBT have proven to be effective in the reduction of postpartum depressive symptoms [14–16]. Interventions such as MomMoodBooster [17], NetMums [18], and Mom-Net [19] have shown promising results not only in reducing postpartum depressive symptoms but also in improving self-efficacy, marital relationship, and mother–child bonding.

However, there is also evidence that web-based interventions suffer from important limitations related to the accuracy of diagnosis, which is based only on online assessments [20], and with low engagement and high attrition rates [15,16] due to the absence of therapist support during the intervention [15,20]. Web-based interventions also lack nonverbal communication as well as the opportunity to discuss specific problems and to deal with crises [21,22]. Instead of replacing traditional psychological interventions, e-mental health tools can be an important complement to them [23].

Blended treatment is the combination of face-to-face treatment with web-based interventions that are integrated and used sequentially in one treatment protocol [24]. Therefore, delivering PPD treatment using a blended format could benefit from the potential of both treatment modalities (face-to-face and online) [23]. Blended treatment presents the advantages of the utilization of e-mental health tools, namely, flexibility in application, good accessibility, and travel time savings [21,25]. Additionally, online sessions can improve patient self-management and help patients better prepare for a session with a therapist [21,22]. Blended treatment allows professional guidance in the therapeutic process, which increases adherence, prevents dropout, facilitates increased treatment intensity, and leads to better results compared to unguided treatments [20]. CBT therapists recognize that blended intervention formats support the patient's motivation, can be adjusted to the patient's specific needs, and reduce the treatment gap between sessions [23,26]. Online sessions can also replace some face-to-face sessions with the therapist, allowing for time savings in healthcare systems as well as decreased treatment costs [24,27].

There is growing evidence of the efficacy of blended treatments for several psychological disorders [24], including depression [21,28,29]. Existing studies have indicated that blended treatment for depression is perceived positively by patients [22,28]. Despite its advantages and considering the aforementioned barriers to professional help-seeking in the postpartum period [9,10], to our knowledge, there is no blended treatment format targeting PPD.

This article presents the study protocol for a blended CBT intervention combining face-to-face sessions with the online program Be a Mom for the treatment of PPD in the Portuguese context. In Portugal, the Be a Mom program was developed as a culturally sensitive web-based CBT intervention that is designed as a self-guided tool for the prevention of PPD. Preliminary evidence of Be a Mom's pilot trial suggests its effectiveness in reducing depressive symptoms among women presenting early-onset PPD symptoms [30], thus supporting its potential as a PPD treatment tool integrated into a blended treatment protocol.

Therefore, we herein outline the protocol for a randomized controlled trial to examine the acceptability and efficacy of a blended CBT intervention for PPD treatment, considering postintervention and follow-up improvements in primary and secondary outcomes. It is expected that the blended CBT intervention will be as effective as treatment usually provided for PPD in decreasing depressive symptoms. In this study, we will evaluate the mediating role of psychological competences (self-compassion, emotion regulation, psychological flexibility) in treatment response. These mechanisms have been core psychological processes underlying the development of the Be a Mom program [31]. Moreover, previous studies have found that these psychological mechanisms were associated with improvements in depressive symptoms in the perinatal period [30,32,33]. We will also examine the moderator effect of characteristics of the patient (e.g., sociodemographic characteristics, motivation for therapy) and of the therapeutic process (e.g., therapeutic relationship, user's satisfaction) in the efficacy of the blended intervention for PPD.

2. Materials and Methods

2.1. Study Design

This study will be a two-arm, noninferiority randomized controlled trial (RCT) comparing blended CBT intervention for PPD (Blended Be a Mom) to the usual treatment that women receive to treat PPD in primary healthcare centers (treatment as usual; TAU). Participants in both the Blended Be a Mom and TAU conditions will complete baseline, postintervention, and follow-up (three and six months postintervention) assessments through a link sent by email that gives access to the survey.

2.2. Ethical Issues

This study was approved by the Ethics Committee of the Faculty of Psychology and Educational Sciences, University of Coimbra, and it will follow the ethical standards and procedures for research with human beings [34,35]. This study protocol was registered with ClinicalTrial.gov (Protocol Record NCT04441879). Participants will be informed about the study goals and procedures and the researcher and participants' roles. An informed consent form to participate in the study will be signed by participants. Participation in the study will be free of cost to women, and no compensation will be given. Women can withdraw at any time, and dropout will not compromise medical care. All collected data will be stored in a secure server in accordance with the General Data Protection Regulation (GDPR) and will only be used for the purposes of the present study. Participants' information will be confidential and anonymized (i.e., no personal data that allow the participant's identification) and will only be treated at a collective level. Trial results will be shared with both the scientific community and health professionals, through publications in scientific peer-reviewed journals and presentations at national and international conferences.

2.3. Participants (Inclusion and Exclusion Criteria)

Adult women during the postpartum period (up to 12 months postpartum) with a confirmed diagnosis of PPD (according to the Structured Clinical Interview for DSM-5 [SCID-5] disorders criteria) will be eligible to participate in this study. Additionally, participants must be residents of Portugal, be able to write and read Portuguese, and have regular access to computers and the internet.

Exclusion criteria will include the presence of psychiatric comorbidity requiring alternative treatment primary to depression treatment, the presence of suicidal ideation, a serious medical condition of either the mother or the baby, and current treatment for depression (e.g., other psychological interventions). Participants who are not eligible to participate in the study will be referred to intervention by local providers.

2.4. Recruitment and Eligibility Assessment

Participants will be recruited in primary healthcare units of the region in routine care appointments during the postpartum period. Alternative recruitment methods (e.g., other institutions, online advertisement) will be considered if sample recruitment difficulties arise (e.g., if the sample size is not achieved, or if the current COVID-19 pandemic disrupts the contact with patients within healthcare institutions). Local healthcare providers (e.g., primary care nurses) will be informed about the study and will ask women if they are interested in participating. Women will be informed in detail about the study, both verbally and through a written flyer. If they are willing to participate, they will be asked to sign an informed consent form and to complete a questionnaire including sociodemographic information, a questionnaire to screen for the presence of depressive symptoms (Edinburgh Postnatal Depression Scale), and other eligibility criteria questions (e.g., technology access, not currently undergoing treatment for PPD). Assessment of depressive symptoms will be conducted every two weeks during the period of the study. When women have a positive screen (indicating the presence of clinically relevant depressive symptoms) and meet the remaining eligibility criteria, they will be further contacted by the researchers through telephone or email to inform them that they will proceed to the second phase of the study. In the second phase, an interview (SCID-5) will be conducted by the researcher (licensed psychologist) to assess the presence of the diagnosis of PPD. Women with a clinical diagnosis of PPD will be eligible to participate in the study and will be included in the third phase of the study. In the third phase of the study, eligible women will receive an email containing a link to complete an online self-report questionnaire (baseline assessment). The flowchart of the study is presented in Figure 1, demonstrating the recruitment and eligibility assessment.

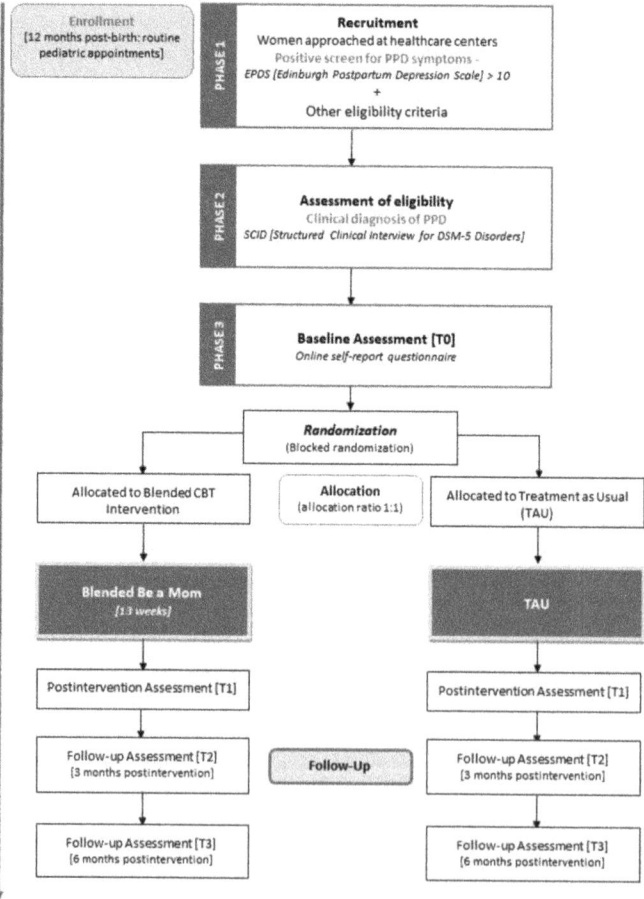

Figure 1. Flowchart of the study.

2.5. Randomization

After completing the baseline assessment, participants will be randomly assigned (blocked randomization, allocation 1:1) to the intervention (Blended Be a Mom) or the TAU conditions (see Figure 1). Randomization will be conducted by a researcher blind to the assessment procedure and will be performed using a computerized random number generator. Women in both conditions will be informed about their assigned treatment condition. Blinding for treatment conditions will not be possible.

2.6. Interventions

2.6.1. Blended Intervention

The blended protocol will be developed based on existing evidence-based CBT interventions for PPD delivered both face-to-face (e.g., [36]) and online (e.g., [37]). The final blended CBT intervention protocol for PPD (Blended Be a Mom) will be developed by the research team and reviewed and approved by a panel of researchers with clinical expertise in the area of PPD. A pilot study with women with a clinical diagnosis of PPD will be conducted prior to the RCT, to assess the acceptability and feasibility of the structure and content of the blended intervention, and to gather preliminary evidence of its clinical efficacy (noncontrolled). Appropriate adjustments to the blended intervention protocol will be done accordingly.

The Blended Be a Mom intervention will integrate 7 face-to-face CBT sessions that are weekly alternated with 6 online sessions over a period of 13 weeks. The online part of the blended intervention will be adapted from the Be a Mom program. Both face-to-face and online sessions will be designed according to CBT principles: problem-oriented, structured, time-limited, educative, and promoting the active participation of the patient [38]. The content of sessions will include psychoeducation, cognitive strategies for negative thoughts, behavioral activation, and relapse prevention (more detailed information is presented in Figure 2). The intervention will also include the utilization of a mobile phone application to conduct ecological momentary assessment, a method to collect information in real time and in the natural environment of participants, over a period of time [39].

Each face-to-face session (with an approximate length of 45–60 min) begins with mood checking and discussion of women's symptoms. The therapist then reviews the experience with the online program and each module's content (i.e., to discuss homework assignments and to practice the strategies learned in the online session), provides feedback, and discusses any doubts. The session ends with the presentation of the upcoming online program module's objectives. The face-to-face sessions will be delivered by a predoctoral-level licensed psychologist, with the supervision of an experienced postdoctoral-level psychologist. To ensure fidelity to treatment protocol, a detailed therapist manual will be available and weekly supervision will be provided by a senior psychologist. At the end of each session, the therapist will fill a checklist to confirm that the topics of the session were covered.

The Be a Mom program was originally designed for the prevention of PPD among Portuguese women. It contains five modules addressing several thematic contents (e.g., Changes and Emotional Reactions, Managing Negative Thoughts, Values and Social Support) and incorporates the recent contributions of third-wave CBT approaches (e.g., self-compassion and acceptance and commitment therapy). Adaptation will be made to the modules to address the specific needs of PPD intervention. Each online session (with an approximate length of 30–45 min) opens with an introduction to the session goals and content, followed by specific information and strategies. Exercises and activities are included to practice the session's specific content, and information is presented through different formats, such as text, interactions, animation, and videos.

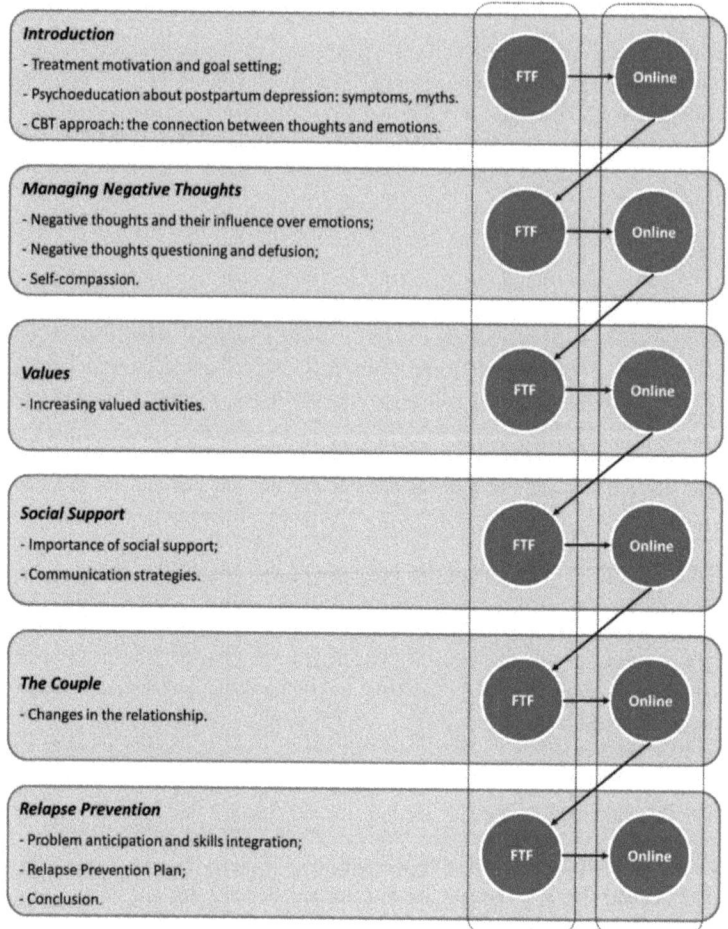

Note. FTF: Face-to-face sessions; Online: Online sessions (Be a Mom).

Figure 2. Blended Be a Mom—structure and content of sessions.

After participants access the program, all modules will be available. Participants will be instructed to complete one module at a time (one session per week) alternating with face-to-face sessions. Online sessions (Be a Mom modules) will be self-guided and an asynchronous communication channel with the therapist through the program will be available. Before entering a new module, participants must confirm that it is in accordance with the therapist. Participants can pause the module at any time and resume the last page visited during subsequent access. Email reminders will be sent to participants to motivate and encourage engagement in online sessions.

The blended intervention will be discontinued if there is a high risk for suicide, possibility to harm others, or the development of severe depressive symptoms. Risk assessment during the intervention, postintervention, and at follow-up assessments will be conducted, through both self-reported and EPDS scores and specific suicidal intention item on the questionnaires that will be administered. These participants will be immediately referred to other mental health services (psychological or psychiatric services) and their participation in the blended intervention will end.

2.6.2. Treatment as Usual

TAU involves the treatment provided in routine healthcare for PPD. It can include different types of traditional face-to-face treatment (e.g., CBT, interpersonal psychotherapy). TAU will be conducted by healthcare center providers (e.g., psychologists), and information concerning the type and duration of therapy (e.g., number of sessions) will be obtained.

2.7. Measures

Table 1 presents the study variables and assessment times.

Table 1. Study variables and assessment points.

Variables	Baseline [T0]	Postintervention [T1]	Follow-Up [T2]	Follow-Up [T3]
Sociodemographic, clinical and obstetric information	x			
Depressive symptoms	x	x	x	x
Anxiety symptoms	x	x	x	x
Fatigue	x	x	x	x
Quality of life	x	x	x	x
Marital satisfaction	x	x	x	x
Maternal self-efficacy	x	x	x	x
Mother–child bonding	x	x	x	x
Self-compassion	x	x		
Emotion regulation	x	x		
Psychological flexibility	x	x		
Motivation for therapy	x	x		
Therapeutic relationship		x		
Acceptability, satisfaction, and usability		x		
Economic evaluation	x	x		

2.7.1. Sociodemographic, Clinical, and Obstetric Information

Women's sociodemographic (e.g., age, marital status, number of children, educational level, professional status, average monthly income, socioeconomic status and residence) and obstetric (e.g., parity, pregnancy complications, type of labor, postpartum data) information will be collected through a questionnaire developed by the researchers. It will also include self-reported clinical information concerning history of psychological/psychiatric problems ("Have you had psychological or psychiatric problems [e.g., depression, anxiety]?", Yes or No) and history of psychological/psychiatric treatment ("Have you had psychological or psychiatric treatment?", Yes or No). Infant-related information (e.g., infant age, infant sex, infant gestational weeks at birth, infant feeding patterns) will also be collected.

2.7.2. Primary Outcome

Changes in depressive symptoms, the primary outcome, will be measured with the Portuguese version of the Edinburgh Postnatal Depression Scale (EPDS) [40]. The EPDS is a 10-item scale (e.g., "I have felt sad or miserable") that assesses how women felt over the last seven days concerning several symptoms using an individualized four-point Likert scale (from 0 to 3). The total score can range between 0 and 30, and higher scores are indicative of more severe depressive symptoms. In Portuguese validation studies, a score of 10 or higher suggests the presence of clinically relevant depressive symptoms. The Portuguese version of EPDS showed good levels of internal consistency (Cronbach's alpha = 0.85) and adequate validity [40].

2.7.3. Secondary Outcomes

Anxiety symptoms will be measured with the Anxiety Subscale of the Portuguese version of the Hospital Anxiety and Depression Scale (HADS-A) [41]. This subscale comprises seven items (e.g., "Worrying thoughts go through my mind") answered on a four-point response scale (ranging from 0 to 3). Higher scores indicate more symptomatology. A score of 11 or higher is indicative of the presence of clinically relevant anxiety symptoms. The Portuguese version of HADS [41] is a reliable scale, with an adequate internal consistency (Cronbach's alpha = 0.76 for the Anxiety Subscale).

Fatigue will be measured with the Portuguese version of the Fatigue Severity Scale (FSS) [42]. The FSS is composed of nine items (e.g., "Fatigue interferes with my work, family, or social life") answered on a seven-point scale ranging from 1 (strongly disagree) to 7 (strongly agree). Higher scores suggest more severe fatigue. The Portuguese version of FSS proved to be a reliable and valid instrument, with a good internal consistency (Cronbach's alpha = 0.87) [42].

Quality of life will be assessed with the Portuguese version of the Euroqol Five-Dimension Scale (EQ-5D) [43]. It is composed of five items (mobility, self-care, usual activities, pain/discomfort, and anxiety/depression), and each item is rated on a scale ranging from 1 (no problems) to 3 (extreme problems). Additionally, participants are asked to rate their own health through visual analogue on a scale ranging from 0 (worst imaginable health state) to 100 (best imaginable health state). The total score is obtained through an algorithm (the digits of the answers to five dimensions) and describes the health state. The Portuguese version of EQ-5D has adequate levels of internal consistency (Cronbach's alpha = 0.72) and was found to be a valid and reliable measure [43].

Marital satisfaction will be assessed with the Portuguese version of the Investment Model Scale—Satisfaction subscale (IMS) [44]. This subscale comprises five items (e.g., "My relationship is close to ideal") rated on a nine-point scale ranging from 0 (do not agree at all) to 8 (completely agree). Higher scores suggest higher satisfaction with the relationship. The Portuguese version of IMS presented good reliability and validity, and found a Cronbach's alpha of 0.91 for the Satisfaction subscale [44].

Maternal self-efficacy will be assessed with the Portuguese version of the Perceived Maternal Parenting Self-Efficacy Questionnaire (PMPS-E; psychometric studies ongoing) [45]. This instrument comprises 20 items (e.g., "I can read my baby's cues") answered on a four-point scale ranging from 1 (strongly disagree) to 4 (strongly agree). Higher scores are indicative of higher perceived maternal self-efficacy.

Mother–child bonding will be measured with the Portuguese version of the Postpartum Bonding Questionnaire (PBQ) [46]. The PBQ is a 12-item instrument (e.g., "I feel close to my baby") with a six-point Likert answer scale ranging from 0 (never) to 5 (always). Higher scores are indicative of a more impaired mother–child bond. The Portuguese version of PBQ found good levels of internal consistency (Cronbach's alpha = 0.71) and validity [46].

Ecological momentary assessments of mood (rated on a scale from "very low" to "very good"), self-esteem, motivation, ability to feel pleasure, depressed mood, and insomnia (Yes or No) will be conducted on a daily basis.

2.7.4. Psychological Competences

Emotion regulation difficulties will be assessed with the Portuguese version of the Difficulties in Emotion Regulation Scale—Short Form (DERS-SF; psychometric studies ongoing) [47]. The DERS-SF is a self-report instrument composed of 18 items (e.g., "When I'm upset, I believe there is nothing I can do to make myself feel better") answered on a five-point scale ranging from 1 (almost never) to 5 (almost always). Higher scores indicate more difficulties in emotion regulation.

Self-compassion will be measured with the Portuguese version of the Self-Compassion Scale—Short Form (SCS-SF) [48]. This is a 12-item instrument (e.g., "I try to see my failings as part of the human condition") with a five-point response scale ranging from 1 (almost never) to 5 (almost always).

Higher scores suggest higher levels of self-compassion. The Portuguese version of SCS-SF is a valid and reliable instrument, with good internal consistency (Cronbach's alpha = 0.86) [48].

Psychological flexibility will be assessed with the Portuguese version of the Acceptance and Action Questionnaire-II (AAQ-II) [49]. The AAQ-II comprises seven items (e.g., "I'm afraid of my feelings") rated on a seven-point scale ranging from 1 (never true) to 7 (always true). Higher scores are indicative of lower psychological flexibility (i.e., higher psychological inflexibility). The Portuguese version of AAQ-II showed good internal consistency (Cronbach's alpha = 0.90) and adequate validity [49].

2.7.5. Intervention-Related Outcomes

Motivation for therapy will be measured with the Portuguese version of the Client Motivation for Therapy Scale (CMTS; psychometric studies ongoing) [50]. The CMTS comprises 24 items (e.g., "Because I would like to make changes to my current situation") rated on a seven-point response scale ranging from 1 (not true at all) to 7 (totally true). Higher scores suggest higher motivation for therapy.

The therapeutic relationship will be assessed with the Portuguese version of the Working Alliance Inventory—Short revised (WAI-SR) [51], a 12-item instrument with a five-point response scale ranging from 1 (rarely or never) to 5 (always). Higher scores indicate better therapeutic alliance. The Portuguese version of WAI-SR is a reliable measure and has good levels of internal consistency (Cronbach's alpha = 0.85).

Acceptability, satisfaction, and usability of the blended treatment will be measured through specific questions developed by the researchers (e.g., satisfaction with the program, usefulness, acceptability, demandingness, recruitment rate, dropout rate, web system data).

The feasibility of the program will be assessed through website utilization (e.g., number of logins, average visit length, total time spent on the website, number of exercises completed) and dropout rate.

2.7.6. Economic Evaluation

Cost-effectiveness will be assessed with an adapted version of the Treatment Inventory Cost in Psychiatric Patients (TiC-P) [52]. This instrument measures medical costs and indirect nonmedical costs, through the assessment of the participant's healthcare use in the last three months (i.e., the number of contacts with healthcare providers), productivity losses (i.e., the number of days of absence from work due to illness), and efficiency at work in the last four weeks.

2.8. Sample Size and Statistical Analyses

The sample size for this study was determined based on power analysis (G*Power). A sample of 45 women per condition is required to detect medium effects in comparison analyses, considering the primary outcome. Considering an expected dropout rate of 20%, we plan to recruit a sample of at least 110 participants (55 per condition) to account for attrition effects.

Statistical analyses to examine the efficacy of the program will be conducted following the intention-to-treat (ITT) and per-protocol (PP) principles in accordance with the CONSORT recommendations [53]. ITT analyses allow us to examine data from all randomized participants, even those with missing values on outcome measures. In contrast, PP analysis includes only participants who followed the assigned treatment protocol. Statistical analyses will be performed using the Statistical Package for the Social Sciences (SPSS, Version 25.0; IBM SPSS) and the Mplus program (Version 7). Linear mixed models will be conducted to determine the effects of the intervention over time (time × group interaction effects) on primary and secondary outcomes and changes in psychological competences. Other appropriate statistical analyses such as two-wave latent change score models, reliable change index, Chi-square tests, and within-group effect sizes will be performed, as well as mediator and moderator analysis. Preliminary cost-effectiveness analysis will be conducted from a healthcare cost perspective and a societal perspective, comparing the differences between

3. Discussion

Despite the existence of effective treatment, few women seek professional help to deal with their depressive symptoms in the postpartum period [7,8], indicating the need for a new and innovative format of treatment that can overcome help-seeking barriers. This study aims to evaluate the acceptability and effectiveness of a blended CBT intervention for the treatment of PPD in the Portuguese context by integrating face-to-face sessions with the web-based program Be a Mom.

To our knowledge, this will be the first study to develop a blended CBT treatment protocol for PPD. Blended Be a Mom benefits from both treatment formats, offering the flexibility, accessibility, and self-management of e-health tools as well as clinical support, increased motivation, and higher treatment intensity [21]. Moreover, it can potentially decrease the number of face-to-face sessions and reduce costs in healthcare systems. A blended CBT intervention can therefore increase help-seeking behaviors among women in the postpartum period by providing treatment that mitigates the impact of the identified barriers in professional help-seeking.

Existing studies have revealed that blended treatment for depression can be effective in reducing depressive symptoms and maintaining these gains over a period of six months [28]. Additionally, previous findings have shown that blended interventions are more effective compared to control groups without intervention (i.e., waiting lists) [24] and that it can be as effective as standard CBT treatments [29]. We expect that Blended Be a Mom will be as effective as TAU with regard to long-term effects on primary and secondary outcomes. The feasibility, acceptability, and usability of the blended intervention will be considered in addition to its cost-effectiveness.

Despite its advantages, there is still limited knowledge about the suitability of blended treatment for every patient [20]. Characteristics such as age, severity of symptoms, or the ability to use technology should be considered and further studied to optimize the effectiveness of blended interventions. The results of our study will provide insights into the processes underlying the treatment effects of blended intervention and the characteristics that moderate the effectiveness of blended intervention.

Our study will also be innovative due to the inclusion of daily ecological momentary assessments during the intervention. This approach allows the collection of information in women's natural environment in real time and therefore prevents retrospective biases [39]. This will provide important information about intraindividual variations over the treatment, the dynamic evolution of PPD symptoms over time, and temporal relationships between mood and other experiences. The inclusion of ecological momentary assessment is recommended in RCTs because it can optimize statistical power effects, improve measurements precision, and potentially increase treatment's adherence [54]. This data collection method has previously been used both in the postpartum period and in depression disorders, and it was considered feasible and acceptable by the users [55,56].

4. Conclusions

This will be the first study to develop and test the effectiveness of a blended CBT intervention for the treatment of PPD in the Portuguese context. This innovative format of treatment delivery can potentially reduce costs in healthcare systems, increase its efficiency, and promote help-seeking behaviors among women in the postpartum period.

We will contribute to the existing research on the topic of e-health technologies applied to mental health. This study is in line with the current directions from the Portuguese e-health Strategy [57] and the European e-Health Action Plan 2012–2020 [58] that encourage the integration of web-based technologies into clinical practice and the use of these tools to enhance patient-centered care and to increase health systems' sustainability and efficiency. We will provide the Portuguese population with access to an evidence-based blended psychological intervention for PPD treatment while contributing to the more effective management of resources in healthcare services.

Author Contributions: Conceptualization, M.B. and A.F.; methodology, M.B. and A.F.; formal analysis, M.B. and A.F.; investigation, M.B.; writing—original draft preparation, M.B.; writing—review and editing, M.C.C. and A.F.; supervision, M.C.C. and A.F. All authors have read and agreed to the published version of the manuscript.

Funding: Mariana Branquinho was supported by a doctoral grant from the Portuguese Foundation for Science and Technology (SFRH/BD/145563/2019).

Acknowledgments: This study is part of the research project "bBeaMom Trial: A randomized controlled trial to test the effectiveness of a cognitive-behavioral blended intervention for postpartum depression in Portuguese women", integrated in the research group Relationships, Development & Health of the R&D Unit Center for Research in Neuropsychology and Cognitive Behavioral Intervention (CINEICC) of the Faculty of Psychology and Educational Sciences, University of Coimbra.

Conflicts of Interest: The authors declare no conflict of interest.

References

1. Maia, B.R.; Marques, M.; Bos, S.; Pereira, A.T.; Soares, M.J.; Valente, J.; Macedo, A.; Azevedo, M.H. Epidemiology of perinatal depression in Portugal: Categorical and dimensional approach. *Acta Med. Port.* **2011**, *24*, 443–448.
2. Woolhouse, H.; Gartland, D.; Perlen, S.; Donath, S.; Brown, S.J. Physical health after childbirth and maternal depression in the first 12 months post partum: Results of an Australian nulliparous pregnancy cohort study. *Midwifery* **2014**, *30*, 378–384. [CrossRef] [PubMed]
3. Slomian, J.; Honvo, G.; Emonts, P.; Reginster, J.Y.; Bruyère, O. Consequences of maternal postpartum depression: A systematic review of maternal and infant outcomes. *Women's Health* **2019**, *15*, 1–55. [CrossRef] [PubMed]
4. Field, T. Postpartum depression effects on early interactions, parenting, and safety practices: A review. *Infant Behav. Dev.* **2010**, *33*, 1–6. [CrossRef] [PubMed]
5. Barnes, D.L. Postpartum depression: Its impact on couples and marital satisfaction. *J. Syst. Ther.* **2006**, *25*, 25–42. [CrossRef]
6. Sockol, L.E. A systematic review of the efficacy of cognitive behavioral therapy for treating and preventing perinatal depression. *J. Affect. Disord.* **2015**, *177*, 7–21. [CrossRef]
7. Henshaw, E.; Sabourin, B.; Warning, M. Treatment-seeking behaviors and attitudes survey among women at risk for perinatal depression or anxiety. *J. Obs. Gynecol. Neonatal Nurs.* **2013**, *42*, 168–177. [CrossRef]
8. Fonseca, A.; Gorayeb, R.; Canavarro, M.C. Women's help-seeking behaviours for depressive symptoms during the perinatal period: Socio-demographic and clinical correlates and perceived barriers to seeking professional help. *Midwifery* **2015**, *31*, 1177–1185. [CrossRef]
9. Bina, R. Predictors of postpartum depression service use: A theory-informed, integrative systematic review. *Women Birth* **2019**, *33*, e24–e32. [CrossRef]
10. Maloni, J.A.; Przeworski, A.; Damato, E.G. Web recruitment and internet use and preferences reported by women with postpartum depression after pregnancy complications. *Arch. Psychiatr. Nurs.* **2013**, *27*, 90–95. [CrossRef]
11. Riper, H.; Andersson, G.; Christensen, H.; Cuijpers, P.; Lange, A.; Eysenbach, G. Theme issue on e-mental health: A growing field in internet research. *J. Med. Internet Res.* **2010**, *12*, e74. [CrossRef]
12. Lal, S.; Adair, C.E. E-mental health: A rapid review of the literature. *Psychiatr. Serv.* **2014**, *65*, 24–32. [CrossRef] [PubMed]
13. Fonseca, A.; Gorayeb, R.; Canavarro, M.C. Women's use of online resources and acceptance of e-mental health tools during the perinatal period. *Int. J. Med. Inform.* **2016**, *94*, 228–236. [CrossRef] [PubMed]
14. Jannati, N.; Mazhari, S.; Ahmadian, L.; Mirzaee, M. Effectiveness of an app-based cognitive behavioral therapy program for postpartum depression in primary care: A randomized controlled trial. *Int. J. Med. Inform.* **2020**, *141*, 104145. [CrossRef] [PubMed]
15. Lee, E.W.; Denison, F.C.; Hor, K.; Reynolds, R.M. Web-based interventions for prevention and treatment of perinatal mood disorders: A systematic review. *BMC Pregnancy Childbirth* **2016**, *16*, 38. [CrossRef] [PubMed]

16. Nair, U.; Armfield, N.R.; Chatfield, M.D.; Edirippulige, S. The effectiveness of telemedicine interventions to address maternal depression: A systematic review and meta-analysis. *J. Telemed. Telecare* **2018**, *24*, 639–650. [CrossRef] [PubMed]
17. Danaher, B.G.; Milgrom, J.; Seeley, J.R.; Stuart, S.; Schembri, C.; Tyler, M.S.; Ericksen, J.; Lester, W.; Gemmill, A.; Kosty, D.B.; et al. MomMoodBooster web-based intervention for postpartum depression: Feasibility trial results. *J. Med. Internet Res.* **2013**, *15*, 1–20. [CrossRef]
18. O'Mahen, H.A.; Woodford, J.; McGinley, J.; Warren, F.C.; Richards, D.A.; Lynch, T.R.; Taylor, R.S. Internet-based behavioral activation—Treatment for postnatal depression (Netmums): A randomized controlled trial. *J. Affect. Disord.* **2013**, *150*, 814–822. [CrossRef]
19. Sheeber, L.B.; Seeley, J.R.; Feil, E.G.; Davis, B.; Sorensen, E.; Kosty, D.B.; Lewinsohn, P.M. Development and pilot evaluation of an internet-facilitated cognitive-behavioral intervention for maternal depression. *J. Consult. Clin. Psychol.* **2012**, *80*, 739–749. [CrossRef]
20. Andersson, G.; Titov, N. Advantages and limitations of Internet-based interventions for common mental disorders. *World Psychiatry* **2014**, *13*, 4–11. [CrossRef]
21. Schuster, R.; Pokorny, R.; Berger, T.; Topooco, N.; Laireiter, A.R. The advantages and disadvantages of online and blended therapy: Survey study amongst licensed psychotherapists in Austria. *J. Med. Internet Res.* **2018**, *20*, e11007. [CrossRef] [PubMed]
22. Van der Vaart, R.; Witting, M.; Riper, H.; Kooistra, L.; Bohlmeijer, E.T.; van Gemert-Pijnen, L.J. Blending online therapy into regular face-to-face therapy for depression: Content, ratio and preconditions according to patients and therapists using a delphi study. *BMC Psychiatry* **2014**, *14*, 355. [CrossRef] [PubMed]
23. Wentzel, J.; van der Vaart, R.; Bohlmeijer, E.T.; van Gemert-Pijnen, J.E. Mixing online and face-to-face therapy: How to benefit from blended care in mental health care. *JMIR Ment. Health* **2016**, *3*, 1–9. [CrossRef] [PubMed]
24. Erbe, D.; Eichert, H.C.; Riper, H.; Ebert, D.D. Blending face-to-face and internet-based interventions for the treatment of mental disorders in adults: Systematic review. *J. Med. Internet Res.* **2017**, *19*, 1–22. [CrossRef]
25. Mol, M.; van Genugten, C.; Dozeman, E.; van Schaik, D.J.; Draisma, S.; Riper, H.; Smit, J.H. Why uptake of blended internet-based interventions for depression is challenging: A qualitative study on therapists' perspectives. *J. Clin. Med.* **2020**, *9*, 91. [CrossRef]
26. Titzler, I.; Saruhanjan, K.; Berking, M.; Riper, H.; Ebert, D.D. Barriers and facilitators for the implementation of blended psychotherapy for depression: A qualitative pilot study of therapists' perspective. *Internet Interv.* **2018**, *12*, 150–164. [CrossRef]
27. Kooistra, L.C.; Ruwaard, J.; Wiersma, J.E.; van Oppen, P.; van der Vaart, R.; van Gemert-Pijnen, J.E.; Riper, H. Development and initial evaluation of blended cognitive behavioural treatment for major depression in routine specialized mental health care. *Internet Interv.* **2016**, *4*, 61–71. [CrossRef]
28. Høifødt, R.S.; Lillevoll, K.R.; Griffiths, K.M.; Wilsgaard, T.; Eisemann, M.; Kolstrup, N. The clinical effectiveness of web-based cognitive behavioral therapy with face-to-face therapist support for depressed primary care patients: Randomized controlled trial. *J. Med. Internet Res.* **2013**, *15*, e153. [CrossRef]
29. Kooistra, L.C.; Wiersma, J.E.; Ruwaard, J.; Neijenhuijs, K.; Lokkerbol, J.; van Oppen, P.; Smit, F.; Riper, H. Cost and effectiveness of blended versus standard cognitive behavioral therapy for outpatients with depression in routine specialized mental health care: Pilot randomized controlled trial. *J. Med. Internet Res.* **2019**, *21*, e14261. [CrossRef]
30. Fonseca, A.; Monteiro, F.; Alves, S.; Gorayeb, R.; Canavarro, M.C. Be a mom, a web-based intervention to prevent postpartum depression: The enhancement of self-regulatory skills and its association with postpartum depressive symptoms. *Front. Psychol.* **2019**, *10*, 265. [CrossRef]
31. Fonseca, A.; Pereira, M.; Araújo-Pedrosa, A.; Gorayeb, R.; Ramos, M.M.; Canavarro, M.C. Be a mom: Formative evaluation of a web-based psychological intervention to prevent postpartum depression. *Cogn. Behav. Pract.* **2018**, *25*, 473–495. [CrossRef]
32. Fourianalistyawati, E.; Uswatunnisa, A.; Chairunnisa, A. The role of mindfulness and self compassion toward depression among pregnant women. *Int. J. Public Health Sci.* **2018**, *7*, 162–167. [CrossRef]
33. Stotts, A.L.; Villarreal, Y.R.; Klawans, M.R.; Suchting, R.; Dindo, L.; Dempsey, A.; Spellman, M.; Green, C.; Northrup, T.F. Psychological flexibility and depression in new mothers of medically vulnerable infants: A mediational analysis. *Matern. Child Health J.* **2019**, *23*, 821–829. [CrossRef] [PubMed]

34. World Medical Association. Declaration of Helsinki—Ethical Principles for Medical Research Involving Human Subjects. Available online: https://www.wma.net/policies-post/wma-declaration-of-helsinki-ethical-principles-for-medical-research-involving-human-subjects/ (accessed on 7 September 2020).
35. American Psychological Association. *Publication Manual of the American Psychological Association*; American Psychological Association: Washington, DC, USA, 2020.
36. Wenzel, A.; Kleiman, K. *Cognitive Behavioral Therapy for Perinatal Distress*; Routledge: New York, NY, USA, 2014.
37. Pugh, N.E.; Hadjistavropoulos, H.D.; Dirkse, D. A randomised controlled trial of therapist-assisted, internet-delivered cognitive behavior therapy for women with maternal depression. *PLoS ONE* **2016**, *11*, e0149186. [CrossRef]
38. Beck, J.S. *Cognitive Therapy: Basics & Beyond*; Guilford Press: New York, NY, USA, 1995.
39. Shiffman, S. *Ecological Momentary Assessment*; Oxford Handbooks Online: Oxford, UK, 2014.
40. Areias, M.E.G.; Kumar, R.; Barros, H.; Figueiredo, E. Comparative incidence of depression in women and men, during pregnancy and after childbirth: Validation of the Edinburgh postnatal depression scale in Portuguese mothers. *Br. J. Psychiatry* **1996**, *169*, 30–35. [CrossRef]
41. Pais-Ribeiro, J.; Silva, I.; Ferreira, T.; Martins, A.; Meneses, R.; Baltar, M. Validation study of a Portuguese version of the hospital anxiety and depression scale. *Psychol. Health Med.* **2007**, *12*, 225–237. [CrossRef]
42. Laranjeira, C.A. Translation and adaptation of the fatigue severity scale for use in Portugal. *Appl. Nurs. Res.* **2012**, *25*, 212–217. [CrossRef]
43. Ferreira, P.L.; Ferreira, L.N.; Pereira, L.N. Contribution for the validation of the Portuguese version of EQ-5D. *Acta Med. Port.* **2013**, *26*, 664–675.
44. Rodrigues, D.; Lopes, D. The investment model scale (IMS): Further studies on construct validation and development of a shorter version (IMS-S). *J. Gen. Psychol.* **2013**, *140*, 16–28. [CrossRef]
45. Barnes, C.R.; Adamson-Macedo, E.N. Perceived maternal parenting self-efficacy (PMP S-E) tool: Development and validation with mothers of hospitalized preterm neonates. *J. Adv. Nurs.* **2007**, *60*, 550–560. [CrossRef]
46. Nazaré, B.; Fonseca, A.; Canavarro, M.C. Avaliação da ligação parental ao bebé após o nascimento: Análise fatorial confirmatória da versão portuguesa do postpartum bonding questionnaire (PBQ). *Laboratório Psicol.* **2012**, *10*, 47–61.
47. Moreira, H.; Gouveia, M.J.; Canavarro, M.C. A bifactor analysis of the difficulties in emotion regulation scale-short form (DERS-SF) in a sample of adolescents and adults. *Curr. Psychol.* **2020**, 1–26. [CrossRef]
48. Castilho, P.; Pinto-Gouveia, J.; Duarte, J. Evaluating the multifactor structure of the long and short versions of the self-compassion scale in a clinical sample. *J. Clin. Psychol.* **2015**, *71*, 856–870. [CrossRef] [PubMed]
49. Pinto-Gouveia, J.; Gregório, S.; Dinis, A.; Xavier, A. Experiential avoidance in clinical and non-clinical samples: AAQ-II Portuguese version. *Int. J. Psychol. Psychol. Ther.* **2012**, *12*, 139–156.
50. Soares, L.; Lemos, M.S. *Escala de Motivação para a Terapia (Versão Portuguesa)*; Faculdade de Psicologia e de Ciências da Educação da Universidade do Porto: Porto, Portugal, 2003; documento não publicado.
51. Ramos, M.A.T. Análise das Características Psicométricas da Versão Portuguesa do Working Alliance Inventory—Short Revised. Master's Thesis, Universidade do Minho, Guimarães, Portugal, 2008.
52. Bouwmans, C.; De Jong, K.; Timman, R.; Zijlstra-Vlasveld, M.; Van der Feltz-Cornelis, C.; Tan, S.S.; Hakkaart-van Roijen, L. Feasibility, reliability and validity of a questionnaire on healthcare consumption and productivity loss in patients with a psychiatric disorder (TiC-P). *BMC Health Serv. Res.* **2013**, *13*, 217. [CrossRef]
53. Eysenbach, G.; CONSORT EHEALTH-Group. CONSORT-EHEALTH: Improving and standarding evaluation reports of web-based and mobile health interventions. *J. Med. Internet Res.* **2011**, *13*, e126. [CrossRef]
54. Schuster, R.; Schreyer, M.L.; Kaiser, T.; Berger, T.; Klein, J.P.; Moritz, S.; Laireiter, A.; Trutschnig, W. Effects of intense assessment on statistical power in randomized controlled trials: Simulation study on depression. *Internet Interv.* **2020**, *20*, 100313. [CrossRef]
55. Demirci, J.R.; Bogen, D.L. Feasibility and acceptability of a mobile app in an ecological momentary assessment of early breastfeeding. *Matern. Child Nutr.* **2017**, *13*, e12342. [CrossRef]
56. Wenze, S.J.; Miller, I.W. Use of ecological momentary assessment in mood disorders research. *Clin. Psychol. Rev.* **2010**, *30*, 794–804. [CrossRef]

57. SPMS. *Ehealth em Portugal: Visão 2020*; SPMS: Lisboa, Portugal, 2015.
58. European Commission. eHealth Action Plan 2012–2020—Innovative Healthcare for the 21st Century, Communication from the Commission to the European Parliament, the Council, the European Economic and Social Committee and the Committee of the Regions. Available online: http://ec.europa.eu/health/ehealth/docs/com_2012_736_en.pdf (accessed on 7 September 2020).

Publisher's Note: MDPI stays neutral with regard to jurisdictional claims in published maps and institutional affiliations.

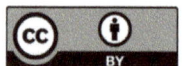

© 2020 by the authors. Licensee MDPI, Basel, Switzerland. This article is an open access article distributed under the terms and conditions of the Creative Commons Attribution (CC BY) license (http://creativecommons.org/licenses/by/4.0/).

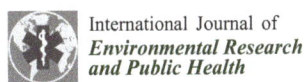

Article

Feasibility and Clinical Usefulness of the Unified Protocol in Online Group Format for Bariatric Surgery Candidates: Study Protocol for a Multiple Baseline Experimental Design

Alba Quilez-Orden [1,2], Vanesa Ferreres-Galán [3] and Jorge Osma [1,2,*]

1. Department of Psychology and Sociology, University of Zaragoza, 44003 Teruel, Spain; aquilez@iisaragon.es
2. Health Research Institute of Aragón, 50009 Zaragoza, Spain
3. Mental Health Unit of the Regional Hospital of Vinaròs, 12500 Castellón, Spain; ferreres_van@gva.es
* Correspondence: osma@unizar.es; Tel.: +34-97-864-5390

Received: 25 June 2020; Accepted: 20 August 2020; Published: 25 August 2020

Abstract: Obesity is currently becoming a serious global public health problem due to its high prevalence and continuous increase. This condition is associated with different physical and mental health problems. The presence of emotional disorders (anxiety, depression and related disorders) among candidates for bariatric surgery is very high and predicts worse physical and psychological results. The present study aims to explore the feasibility and clinical usefulness of the Unified Protocol, a transdiagnostic emotion regulation-based intervention, delivered in an online group format to patients with emotional disorder diagnosis or symptoms, who are waiting for bariatric surgery. We will conduct a pilot study with a repeated single-case experimental design (multiple baseline design) in a public mental health service. The sample will consist of 60 participants, who will be randomized to three baseline conditions: 8, 12 or 15 evaluation days before the intervention. Diagnostic criteria, symptomatology and body mass index are the primary outcome measures, and we will include affectivity, personality, quality of life, body image, eating behavior and surgical complications like secondary measures. An analysis of treatment satisfaction will be also performed. Assessment points will include pre-treatment, baseline, treatment, post-treatment, and follow-ups every three months until two years after post-treatment. The results obtained in this study may have important clinical, social and economic implications for public mental health.

Keywords: emotional disorders; transdiagnostic; online group format; unified protocol; bariatric surgery; obesity

1. Introduction

Obesity is a chronic disease characterised by an increase in body fatness, which is usually estimated by body mass index (BMI) calculated as measured body weight (kg) divided by measured height squared (m^2) [1]. Obesity is currently becoming a serious global public health problem due to its high prevalence and increase in recent years [2]. In Spain alone, 25% of the population is obese or overweight, and the expectations are alarming. It is expected that in 2030, up to 80% of Spanish men and 55% of women will be obese or overweight, exceeding 27.2 million of people [3].

The causes of obesity are complex and multifactorial [1], and this condition is associated with different health problems, such as myocardial infarction, hypertension, stroke, dyslipidemia, diabetes mellitus, or obstructive sleep apnea [4–6]. All these alterations affect the quality of life and can disturb important areas of functioning (e.g., physical function, vitality, social functioning and emotional role) [7,8]. In addition to all of these complications, people with obesity experience significant psychological difficulties [7]. Due to all of these health implications, obesity represents a challenge to the countries' economies [9]. As of 2016 in Spain, the obesity cost meant almost two billion euros of extra expenses for the National Health System [3].

For all these reasons (high prevalence and associated costs), many efforts have been made to find treatments for obesity and weight loss, which include lifestyle interventions, pharmacological interventions, surgical interventions, and endoscopic bariatric procedures [7]. Bariatric surgery (BS) is the most commonly performed procedure worldwide [10] and the most effective intervention for individuals with severe obesity (BMI greater than 40 kg/m^2) [11], and includes a group of surgical procedures performed to facilitate weight loss, such as open or laparoscopic roux-en-Y gastric bypass, sleeve gastrectomy, and adjustable gastric banding. The most obvious and studied benefits of BS refer to physical issues, specifically weight loss and improvement of obesity-related physical comorbidities; however, between 10% and 25% of patients who undergo BS show suboptimal weight loss, and it is estimated that they regain approximately 10% of their weight during the first decade after the intervention [12]. Regarding the psychological benefits of BS, limited and inconclusive results have been found [13]. Some systematic reviews have reported improvements after BS, especially in depressive symptoms, but also limited only to the first months after the intervention, and they tend to reappear after the first two years [10].

Some studies have questioned whether previous psychopathology history could influence the results obtained by BS [2]. This topic is especially relevant because the percentage of psychopathology among people waiting for BS (between 20.9% and 55.5%) [12] is much higher than in the general population (between 12.53% and 13.87%) [14]. Specifically, the group of emotional disorders (ED), which includes anxiety and mood disorders, eating disorders, and related disorders ([15]; Supplementary Materials), are the most prevalent disorders among BS candidates: eating disorders (50%), mood disorders (31.5%), anxiety disorders (24%), and substance use related disorders (10%) [12]. It has been concluded that the presence of EDs among candidates for BS predicts worse results in the long term [11], furthermore, a meta-analysis states that the prevalence of suicide mortality is up to 1.8%, and the prevalence of suicide is up to 0.3% after bariatric surgery [16].

As we can observe, psychological evaluation and intervention play a fundamental role in the multidisciplinary work performed with these patients before and after BS although, until now, it has not received much attention [12]. Improvements in eating psychopathology (e.g., binge eating, emotional eating, body image dissatisfaction) have been reported from psychological interventions using psychoeducation, goal setting, self-monitoring, normalized eating, stimulus control, cognitive restructuring, and relapse prevention [11]. Cognitive–behavioral therapy (CBT) is the one that accumulates the most evidence of the improvement of eating behaviors (e.g., binge eating and emotional eating) and psychological functioning (e.g., quality of life, depression, and anxiety symptoms) [11]. Despite the good outcomes achieved, these CBT interventions have been developed to treat specific disorders (e.g., eating disorders or anxiety disorders), and this fact raises some limitations. First, clinicians' great effort to specialize in a range of different interventions; second, the increased costs for health systems and clinicians in training, and as a consequence, the difficulties in dissemination and implementation of the CBT interventions [17]. Furthermore, if we consider that the most prevalent disorders among patients with obesity are EDs [12], there are additional limitations to specific CBT interventions. This is because in the case of these disorders, comorbidity is very high, and subclinical symptoms or unspecified disorders usually arise [18]. These comorbid conditions make it even more difficult to choose the best specific CBT treatment in each case [19].

To address all the limitations of the specific CBT treatments previously discussed, in recent years, different CBT interventions from a transdiagnostic approach have been developed and tested. In this sense, the Unified Protocol for the transdiagnostic treatment of EDs (UP) is a CBT emotion-based intervention designed to treat the etiological and maintenance mechanisms shared by all EDs [20]. This intervention focuses on a wide range of emotional psychopathology, considering comorbid disorders and subclinical or unspecified symptoms, reducing treatment times and costs, and improving response to treatment [17].

The UP is made up of eight treatment modules, five of which are considered core modules because they are focused on training different specific emotion-regulation skills [21]. Despite that the UP is a protocolized intervention, it is also flexible and versatile, allowing clinicians to use some of the modules or to change modules' order to personalize the UP to their patients [22]. Its main objective is to enhance emotion-regulation strategies to all people presenting emotional dysregulation problems [15]. To date, the UP has shown a significant improvement in pre-treatment symptoms and has obtained effect sizes that are at least comparable to existing specific CBT interventions, in on-site and online formats [23]. Beyond the mood or anxiety disorders per se, the UP has been applied to different health problems, such as cancer [24], HIV [25], or irritable bowel syndrome [26]. Despite the positive data on the effectiveness of the UP for the treatment of EDs in different health conditions, we have found no studies about its clinical utility to improve anxiety and depressive symptoms or EDs in patients with obesity who are waiting for BS.

As mentioned, the UP can be applied in various formats, such as onsite or online (both individual and group). Regarding online interventions in mental health (e-Health), there is an important amount of evidence over the last 15 years informing that online treatments are effective to treat a wide range of mental health disorders and that they can be as effective as onsite treatments [27]. We also know that online interventions do not negatively affect the therapeutic relationship [28] and that the users generally show high levels of acceptance and satisfaction with this delivery format [29]. The use of Information and Communication Technologies (ICTs) reduces the burden on health professionals and users, facilitating data collection and accessibility to Treatment [30]. In fact, different studies have shown the need to develop technology-based interventions to increase accessibility to treatment for BS candidates because their obesity condition significantly affects their mobility, and that makes it difficult for them to attend weekly sessions on-site [31]. Another practical benefit of delivering online psychological interventions is related to the current situation caused by the Covid-19 pandemic because the online format (e.g., emails, videoconference, etc.) will allow phycologists to continue their interventions and/or the follow-up assessments in case of new mobility restrictions [32]. Finally, the online group format can offer additional advantages to the online format itself, as it facilitates social support among the participants in the therapy and also allows them to share experiences and learn from each other [33].

Therefore, the general objective of this study is to analyze the feasibility and clinical usefulness of the UP, applied in an online group format, in a mental health setting of the National Health System to candidates for BS who have at least one diagnosis of ED or emotional symptoms.

The specific objectives pursued are: to evaluate adherence to treatment and clinical improvement in the primary and secondary measures after applying the UP and to study its long term clinical usefulness until two years after the intervention. Thus, the main hypotheses proposed for this study are: (1) statistically significant differences (reliable change index; RCI) will be obtained between the scores obtained at the pre-treatment, baseline, and post-treatment on the primary and secondary measures; (2) the improvements obtained after the application of the UP will be maintained in the long term (follow-ups of up to two years); (3) participants in the pilot study will report high adherence rates and high satisfaction scores regarding the treatment delivery format and its components.

2. Materials and Methods

This is a pilot study using a repeated single-case experimental design (multiple baseline design) to explore the feasibility and clinical usefulness of a transdiagnostic emotion-based online group intervention (UP) for BS candidates with EDs or subclinical anxious or depressive symptoms attended to in a public mental health service. We have chosen this design for three reasons: (1) the unit of intervention and unit of data analysis is an individual case, specifically a cluster of participants; (2) the case provides its own control for comparison purposes because a number of variables are measured before the intervention and compared with measures during and after the intervention and (3) the variable is repeatedly measured within and across different conditions or levels of the independent variable. Furthermore, and because our main objective is to answer the question "Is the Unified Protocol able to improve the emotional state of people waiting for BS?", we chose a multiple baseline design to improve experimental control throughout replication, introducing the independent variable at different points in time. The fundamental idea of choosing this type of design is that each of the participants can be their own control group [34].

The multiple baseline design involves the application of the treatment variable in a staggered way over time, through different observational units. This design is suitable for health services research interventions that are focused on changing patient behavior. This methodology facilitates a systematic comparison of pre-intervention and post-intervention measures [35], and conducting a preliminary assessment of a novel intervention [36]. Like randomized controlled trials (RCTs), the multiple baseline design can demonstrate that a significant change in behaviour has occurred and that is result of the intervention. One of the main limitations is that each participant must show changes only when the intervention is applied, and this issue, at a practical level is complicated, can make it difficult for the researcher to draw clear conclusions about the impact of the intervention. In order to reduce this limitation and improve the internal validity, researchers start treatment at different times across settings, behaviors, or people [37]. The multiple baseline design has advantages over the RCTs because this design requires fewer population groups and communities and they may act as their own controls [35]. In this sense, researchers often use this design with several people at once addressing the issue of external validity [37].

In the present investigation, all consecutive patients who are selected to undergo BS and who present anxiety or depressive symptoms or at least one diagnosis of ED, will be asked to participate. Once inclusion criteria are met (see "Inclusion and exclusion criteria" section), each patient will be randomly assigned to one of the multiple baseline conditions: 8, 12, or 15 evaluation days before the intervention. These multiple baseline conditions have been chosen following the current guides for single-case designs [34,38].

A random assignment will be carried out to reduce the threat of selection, and the fact of choosing three conditions is one of the established standards for this type of designs in order to reduce the threat of ambiguous temporal precedence and maturation [38]. Furthermore, the fact that all three conditions involve evaluation periods of 8, 12 and 15 days is due to the established standard of having a minimum of five data points in each phase to reduce the threat of attrition [38]. By choosing at least eight, we make sure to meet it even considering the probability that participants will forget to fill out the assessment one day. Actually, the reason for choosing those days is the temporal stability of the variables that we measured through the study.

In addition, the intervention will begin in a staggered manner with individual sessions (to reduce the threat of the history) and to reduce the threat of testing, a pre-treatment assessment will be performed prior to starting the baseline, to consider that the assessment process itself can have therapeutic effects on participants [38].

The study includes five assessment moments (pre-treatment, baseline, treatment, post-treatment, and follow-up, one every three months until two years after treatment completion). The flow chart of the study design is shown in Figure 1.

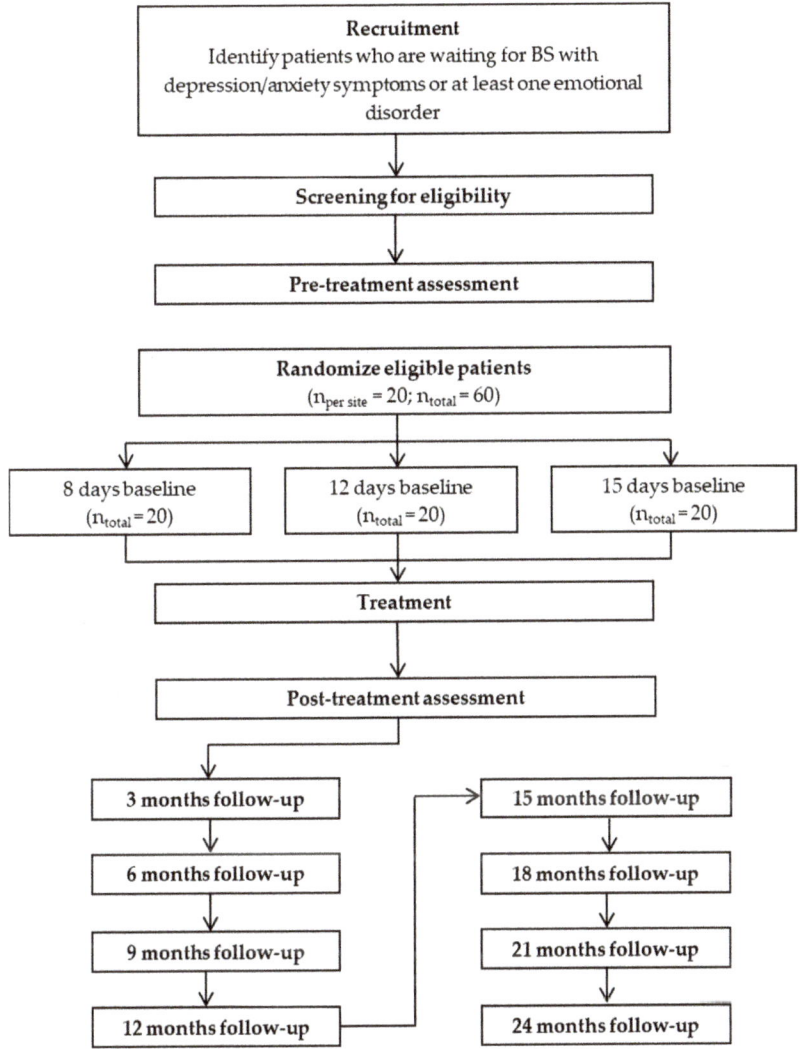

Figure 1. Study flow chart. BS: Bariatric surgery.

2.1. Sample and Recruitment

The study recruitment will start in September 2020 until December 2024. The study will be conducted in a public mental health center in Spain (Mental Health Unit of the Regional Hospital of Vinaròs, Castellón). Participants will be people over 18 years of age who have anxious or depressive symptoms, or at least one diagnosis of EDs according to Diagnostic and Statistical Manual of Mental Disorders five edition criteria [39] and who have been selected for a subsequent BS.

To calculate the sample size, we drew on a study that proposed stepwise rules of thumb for pilot studies based on the target effect size and the size of the future trial [40]. Previous works that study the efficacy of CBT procedures either in person or online have shown large variations in effect sizes, obtaining mainly medium to large effect sizes [41,42]. Taking these data into account, and expecting a 90% powered main trial and assuming a sample loss of 35% [43] we established a sample size of 20 participants per experimental condition for the present study, that is, a total sample of 60 participants.

2.2. Procedure

The participants who are referred to the mental health unit for having fulfilled the requirements to be candidates for BS, will be evaluated to see if they meet the rest of the inclusion criteria for this study. In Table 1, it can be seen the selection criteria used to choose the appropriate candidates to receive the BS. These criteria are based on the European Guidelines for Obesity Management in Adults, which indicates that a comprehensive obesity management can only be accomplished by a multidisciplinary obesity management team [44].

Table 1. Inclusion criteria and main contraindications for BS.

Inclusion Criteria
- BMI >40 or 35 with associated major comorbidities
- Age between 18 and 65 years
- Long-standing obesity (3–5 years)
- Failure in dietary attempts and treatments under control
- Absence of anesthetic contraindication and acceptable surgical risk
- Not having endocrine causes of obesity
- Understanding of the weight loss process, associated problems and the stated objective
- Commitment to adhere to the monitoring standards
Contraindications
Relative
- Clearly unfavorable family environment
- Personality disorder
- Psychogenic vomiting
- Hyperphagia in other psychological disorders or other eating disorders
- Mild intellectual disability
- Psychotic disorders without positive symptoms
- Any psychiatric illness that significantly hinders the good follow-up and completion of the guidelines and medical indications for this process and may worsen the patient's state of health
Absolute
- Drug dependency
- Moderate or severe intellectual disability
- Psychotic disorder with positive symptoms
- Bulimia nervosa

Participants' evaluation and selection will be carried out by the clinical psychologists and psychiatrists of the mental health unit of the Regional Hospital of Vinaròs (Castellón). The clinical psychologists who will participate in this trial will be in charge of collecting all the information from the participants (alphanumeric codes assigned to the participants will be entered to safeguard their anonymity). The coded information will be given to the author J.O. to introduce it in the database and then, returned to the center.

Participants who have received the approval for BS by the multidisciplinary health team and also have met the inclusion criteria by the clinician (see "Eligibility criteria" section), will be invited to participate in the study through an informative document. They will also be provided with confidentiality and informed consent documents. After accepting to participate, an email will be sent to participants with a link through which they will be able to complete the pre-treatment evaluation on the Qualtrics survey platform [45]. Then, they will be informed by phone of the experimental condition to which they will have been randomly assigned, which may be 8, 12, or 15 days baseline assessment, and they will then complete online the baseline assessment protocol on the same platform [45]. Randomization to the different baselines will be done with randomizer software (www.randomizer.org). Randomization will be performed by a researcher unrelated to the study using the computer-generated sequence mentioned. In the program, the researcher will generate one set of 60 numbers, which will have a one to three range. Participants will be randomly assigned to the 8, 12 or 15 baseline days.

The baseline and psychological intervention will be conducted between the period of acceptance for BS and the BS implementation, that last approximately one year in public health settings. The intervention will be carried out in an online group format through the Cisco Webex platform. The UP will be applied in twelve weekly 2-h online group sessions. To comply with the experimental design of the multiple baseline, when each participant completes the baseline evaluation, they will receive the first online session in individual format (to receive the first session in stages), then they will continue with the second session and the rest of the treatment in group format. The content of each session is shown in Table 2. Participants will receive the therapy support manual [11]. The online group will consist of five to eight participants, one therapist (V.F.-G.), and one co-therapist (A.Q.-O.). For ethical reasons, if any of the patients feel uncomfortable during the study with the online group format, they may leave the group and receive individual onsite attention (treatment as usual). In this case, the content and estimated number of sessions will be the same, although the frequency will be stipulated by the mental health unit depending on its possibilities.

Table 2. Treatment content split by session.

Session Number	Content
Session 1	Setting Goals and Maintaining Motivation
Session 2	Understanding your Emotions: What is an Emotion?
Session 3	Understanding your Emotions: Following the ARC (Antecedent, Response, Consequence)
Session 4	Mindful Emotion Awareness—I
Session 5	Mindful Emotion Awareness—II
Session 6	Cognitive Flexibility—I
Session 7	Cognitive Flexibility—II
Session 8	Countering Emotional Behaviors
Session 9	Understanding and Confronting Physical Sensations
Session 10	Putting it into Practice: Emotion Exposures—I
Session 11	Putting it into Practice: Emotion Exposures—II
Session 12	Recognizing Accomplishments and Looking to the Future

The study plans to conduct a follow-up assessment every three months until two years after treatment completion. All follow-ups will be conducted online. Considering the time interval of the baseline, the psychological intervention and the BS procedure, the two first follow-ups (three and six months after intervention) will be conducted before BS, and the rest will be conducted after BS. In addition, at the baseline and during treatment, the participants must fill out an online survey made up of 14 questions that will ask about the intensity of the emotions of happiness, sadness, anxiety, other emotions, difficulties in emotion regulation, body image, and emotional eating. Through this weekly evaluation, we expect to observe how the participants evolve in the different variables throughout the different treatment modules.

2.3. Eligibility Criteria

The inclusion criteria for participation in the project will be: (1) being over 18 years of age; (2) being a BS candidate; (3) presenting anxious or depressive symptomatology (moderate scores on the Beck Depression Inventory-II [46,47] and/or Beck Anxiety Inventory [48,49]) or meeting the criteria for at least one ED (anxiety, mood, and related disorders) on the International Neuropsychiatric Interview (MINI; [50]); (4) speaking Spanish or Catalan fluently; (5) committing to attend the sessions; (6) understanding and accepting the contents of the informed consent, expressed by signing it; (7) having Internet to fulfill the protocol assessments and to participate in the online intervention and (8) agreeing to maintain the prescribed medication (including dosage) if any, during the evaluation period and treatment. If medication stability is not possible, the participant's data will be treated separately in the analyses.

The protocol also includes one exclusion criteria that may interfere: (1) having a severe condition that would require being prioritized for treatment, so that an interaction between the two interventions cannot be ruled out. These include a severe mental disorder (bipolar disorder, personality disorder, schizophrenia, or an organic mental disorder), suicide risk at the time of assessment, or substance use in the last three months (excluding cannabis, coffee, and/or nicotine).

2.4. Ethics

All participants who meet the inclusion criteria will sign the personal data protection document before randomization so that they have a notion of whom and for what purpose this study's results will be used. Participants will be also informed of what the treatment consists of before starting it, as well as the duration and phases of the study (informed consent). Direct participation in the study will be voluntary. Participants will not obtain any financial or material compensation, and their participation will not imply any risk for them. The UP has already demonstrated its efficacy in previous experimental and quasi-experimental studies with different health problems (see "Introduction" section).

Data management will be carried out following the Spanish Royal Decree 1720/2008, of 19 January, which approves the Regulations for the development of the Organic Law 15/1999, of 13 December, on the protection of personal data [51]. The treatment, communication, and transfer of personal data will follow the provisions of the Declaration of Helsinki [52] in Law 14/2007 on biomedical research. As of 25 May 2018, the new legislation on personal data in the EU is fully applicable, specifically Regulation (EU) 2016/679 of the European Parliament and of the Council of 27 April 2016, on Data Protection (GDRP; General Data Protection Regulation). Under the aforementioned legislation, participants can exercise their rights of access, modification, opposition, and cancellation of data, for which they must contact their health professional of reference.

The data collected for the study will be identified by an alphanumeric code, and only the health professionals collaborating in the study will be able to relate these data to the participants and their corresponding medical records. Therefore, the identity of the participants in the study will not be revealed to any person, with exceptions in case of a medical emergency or legal requirement.

The study already has the approval by the Ethical Research Committee of the General University Hospital of Castellón (CEIm; CI/HIP version 1.0 de 20/07/2019). In addition, the protocol study has been registered at https://clinicaltrials.gov/ (6 March 2020; NCT04421443).

2.5. Measures

The evaluation protocol will be administered online by Qualtrics survey [45] at five different moments: pre-treatment, baseline, treatment, post-treatment, and follow-ups every three months until two years after the intervention. Assessment instruments will include demographic characteristics (age, sex, education, marital status, and employment status), a diagnostic interview, and well-established questionnaires for both primary and secondary outcomes. Next, the primary and secondary outcomes that will be evaluated at the pre, post-treatment, and follow-up periods will be described, and later the specific measures that will be used for the baseline evaluation and during the treatment will be specified. Table 3 shows the distribution of the measures that will be administered during the study.

Table 3. Distribution of the variables administered throughout the intervention.

Measures	Pre-Treatment	Baseline	Treatment	Post-Treatment	Follow-Ups [1]
Demographic characteristics	X				
MINI	X			X	X
BDI-II	X			X	X
BAI	X			X	X
BMI	X	X	X	X	X
PANAS	X			X	X
NEO-FFI	X			X	X
QLI	X			X	X
EuroQol	X			X	X
MI	X			X	X
DERS	X			X	X
BEAQ	X			X	X
PHLMS	X			X	X
ERQ	X			X	X
Surgical Complications	X				
BITE	X			X	X
BSQ	X			X	X
EES	X			X	X
OASIS			X		
ODSIS			X		
OESIS			X		
PESIS			X		
STQ				X	X
Baseline assessment battery [2]		X			
Assessment battery during treatment [3]			X		

Note: MINI: International Neuropsychiatric Interview; BDI-II: Beck Depression Inventory-II; BAI: Beck Anxiety Inventory; BMI: Body Mass Index; PANAS: Positive and Negative Affect Scale; NEO-FFI: NEO Five-Factor Inventory; QLI: Quality of Life Index; MI: Maladjustment Inventory; DERS: Difficulties in Emotion Regulation Scale; BEAQ: Brief Experiential Avoidance Questionnaire; PHLMS: Philadelphia Mindfulness Scale; ERQ: Emotion Regulation Questionnaire; BITE: Bulimic Investigatory Test; BSQ: Body Satisfaction Questionnaire; EES: Emotional Eating Scale; OASIS: Overall Anxiety Severity and Impairment Scales; ODSIS: Overall Depression Severity and Impairment Scales; OESIS: Other Emotions Severity and Impairment Scale; PESIS: Positive Emotion Severity and Impairment Scale; STQ: Satisfaction with Treatment Questionnaire. [1] Quarterly follow-ups up to two years after treatment; [2] For more information about the specific items that make up the baseline assessment battery see section "Baseline assessment"; [3] For more information about the specific items that make up the assessment during treatment battery see section "Assessment during treatment".

2.5.1. Primary Outcomes

Primary and secondary diagnosis according to the DSM-5 criteria will be evaluated with the International Neuropsychiatric Interview (MINI [50]). Subclinical symptoms of anxiety and depression will be evaluated through the Beck Depression Inventory-II (BDI-II [46,47]) and the Beck Anxiety Inventory (BAI [48,49]). The weight gain or loss of the participants will be evaluated through the Body Mass Index (BMI).

2.5.2. Secondary Outcomes

Secondary outcomes can be grouped around: affectivity, personality traits, quality of life and interference, emotion regulation, aspects related to surgical complications, eating behaviors and body image, and satisfaction with and evaluation of the treatment received.

To assess affectivity, the Positive and Negative Affect Scale (PANAS [53,54]) will be administered to evaluate positive and negative affect. Personality will be measured with the NEO Five-Factor Inventory (NEO-FFI [55]), which offers a rapid and general measure of the Big Five personality traits of which we will only assess Neuroticism and Extraversion. The Quality of Life Index (QLI [56]) will be used to evaluate several aspects related to quality of life (i.e., physical disability, emotional well-being, self-care and independent functioning, occupational functioning, interpersonal functioning, social–emotional support, community and services support, personal fulfillment, spiritual fulfillment, and overall quality of life). EuroQol [57,58] is a generic instrument that will be used to measure health-related quality of life. It has five dimensions (mobility, personal care, daily activities, pain, and anxiety/depression), and a general state of health perceived through a visual analog scale. Similarly, the Maladjustment Inventory (MI [59]) will be used to evaluate the extent to which the subject's current problems impact negatively on different areas of daily life, namely, work, social life, leisure time, relationship with the partner, family life, and overall adjustment in daily activities.

Regarding emotion regulation, it will be assessed using the Difficulties in Emotion Regulation Scale (DERS [60,61]), which presents five dysregulation dimensions: emotional lack of control, emotional rejection, life interference, lack of emotional attention, and emotional confusion. In addition, to assess the different emotion regulation skills that will be trained through the UP, we will use the Brief Experiential Avoidance Questionnaire (BEAQ [62,63]), which is a self-report questionnaire with 15 items that measure experiential avoidance; the Philadelphia Mindfulness Scale (PHLMS [64,65]), which is a 20-item questionnaire that assesses two mindfulness constructs: awareness and acceptance and the Emotion Regulation Questionnaire (ERQ [66,67]), which is a self-report questionnaire commonly used to assess two emotion-regulation strategies: cognitive reappraisal (six items) and expressive suppression (four items).

To assess surgical complications, the professional will be asked to refer the participant to the mental health unit a report describing the course of the operation and the recovery from it. Specific measures related to eating disorders will also be used, such as the Bulimic Investigatory Test (BITE [68,69]), which is a self-report questionnaire used to evaluate the presence and severity of bulimic symptomatology, and cognitive and emotional signs and symptoms associated with binge eating; the Body Satisfaction Questionnaire (BSQ [70,71]), which is a self-applied scale used to evaluate the fear of gaining weight, feelings of low self-esteem because of one's appearance, the desire to lose weight, and body dissatisfaction, and Emotional Eating Scale (EES [72]), which is a 25-item self-report assessing a person's tendency to cope with negative affect through eating. Participants' weight will be checked monthly to calculate their body mass index (BMI).

Additionally, we created an ad hoc questionnaire to evaluate the participants' evaluation of and satisfaction with the treatment received, the Satisfaction with Treatment Questionnaire (STQ). The Evaluation of the UP Components section consists of nine items that evaluate the extent to which the participants consider that the UP in general, and each of its components in particular, were useful to help them to regulate their emotions adaptively; the Satisfaction with Treatment section presents seven items that evaluate participants' overall satisfaction with the treatment received. In both sections, higher scores show higher levels of positive evaluation and satisfaction. A total of 12 items will also be added to assess the participants' opinion of the online evaluation through Qualtrics and of the Cisco Webex platform used to carry out the online evaluation. At the end of the questionnaire, six open-ended questions appear in which the participants can qualitatively express their opinion of different aspects of the treatment received and the delivery format.

All measures used in the study have been standardized in Spanish. Administration time is between 30 and 40 min for the MINI and approximately 90 min for the primary and secondary outcomes conjointly.

2.5.3. Baseline Assessment

To facilitate the daily baseline assessment, we have summarized in one item the variable we want to evaluate, for example, the emotion regulation strategies. For this purpose, we have chosen the item with the greatest factor load for each variable [73]. Specifically, participants will answer a battery of 19 questions: six questions about the presence and intensity of specific emotions (e.g., happiness, sadness, anxiety); five questions to assess the five subscales of the Difficulties in Emotion Regulation Scale (DERS [60,61]), which are emotional lack of control, emotional rejection, life interference, lack of emotional attention, and emotional confusion (e.g., "During this day, to what extent have you paid attention to your feelings?"); two questions that refer to the two subscales of the Emotion Regulation Questionnaire (ERQ [66,67]), which are reappraisal and suppression (e.g.," During this day, to what extent have you been able to control your emotions by changing the way you think about the situation you were in?"); two questions that refer to the two subscales of the Philadelphia Mindfulness Scale (PHLMS [64,65]), which are acceptance and awareness (e.g., "During this day, when your emotions have changed, to what extent have you been aware of it immediately?"); one question to assess experiential avoidance based on the Brief Experiential Avoidance Questionnaire (BEAQ [62,63]) ("During this day, would you say that one of your biggest goals has been to be free of any painful emotion?"); one question from the Emotional Eating Scale (EES [72]) regarding the impulse to eat as a consequence of having experienced an intense emotion ("During this day, to what extent have you felt the urge to eat as a result of experiencing intense emotions?") and one last question from the Body Satisfaction Questionnaire (BSQ [70,71]), which asks about the extent to which the participant has been satisfied with their body image ("During this day, how satisfied have you been with your body image?").

2.5.4. Assessment during Treatment

The assessment during treatment battery involves continuing to fill in the same baseline questions once a week. In addition, before starting each online session, participants will be asked to fill in an emotional scale to assess its presence, intensity, and interference during the last week. Participants can choose the emotion or emotions that should be assessed. The UP offers four different emotional rating scales: The Overall Anxiety and Depression Severity and Impairment Scales (OASIS; ODSIS [74–76]), Other Emotions Severity and Impairment Scale (e.g., guilt, shame, or anger) (OESIS [77]), and a Positive Emotion Severity and Impairment Scale (e.g., happiness) (PESIS [77]; Supplementary Materials). All of them are used in the UP to help patients to continuously monitor the scores throughout the sessions and their progress over the treatment.

2.6. Data Analysis

The analyses will be carried out with the statistical package IBM SPSS Statistics version 22.0 for Windows [78]. First, the sociodemographic characteristics of the sample will be analyzed with descriptive statistics, calculating the mean and standard deviation of the scores in the different questionnaires administered. Next, a missing-value analysis and the Little Missing Completely At Random (MCAR) test will be performed to determine whether or not the distribution of missing values is random, and therefore whether the last observation made (LOCF) can be used. Internal consistency will be explored using Cronbach's alpha.

As the sample size is expected to be less than 50, the normal distribution of the variables will be verified with the Shapiro–Wilk normality test. Depending on the result of this test, parametric or non-parametric repeated measures analysis will be carried out to verify whether or not the differences in the scores of the variables measured at different times are statistically significant. In case the variables follow a normal distribution, parametric repeated measures analysis will be carried out, specifically the Multivariate Analysis of Variance (ANOVA), and in case the variables do not follow a normal distribution, non-parametric repeated measures analysis will be carried out, specifically the Friedman test. If the repeated measures analysis show statistically significant differences between the evaluation time points, post-hoc comparisons will be carried out to correct the level of significance to avoid increasing the type I error. Thus, regarding adjustment for multiple comparisons, the Bonferroni correction will be carried out in case of having performed parametric analysis, and the Wilcoxon signed rank test in case of having performed non-parametric analysis in the comparison of means. More detailed information on this has been added in the data analysis section, explaining step by step which statistical analyzes will be carried out.

Finally, the Reliable Change Index (RCI), which assesses the clinically significant change obtained to determine in which variables the scores have approached those of the normative sample, will be calculated. A clinically significant change will be considered if the RCI score obtained is equal to or greater than 1.96 [79].

Another aspect that we consider important to analyze is how the participants change their scores in each of the variables evaluated based on the content addressed each module. For this purpose, a visual analysis of the changes in the scores will be carried out, to see how the slopes change in the different phases of the study (evaluation and treatment), and in the different modules within the treatment. This visual analysis has been used in previous studies [21]. To carry out this visual analysis, the data from 19 questions that the participants will fill in weekly will be used.

Attendance at sessions will also be recorded to calculate the attendance rate, which will be used as an indicator of viability and acceptance of treatment by users. For the same purpose, quantitative and qualitative analyses will be carried out. At the quantitative level, the participants' evaluation of and satisfaction with the treatment received will be evaluated using an ad hoc designed questionnaire (see "Measures" section). Qualitatively, participants will be asked to answer six main questions about treatment, and their answers will be analyzed by selecting and classifying the information through a segmentation process, identifying key themes and categories of analysis [80].

3. Expected Results

Based on the reviewed bibliography, the type of design of the present study, the proposed objectives and the characteristics of the intervention that will be carried out, we hope that the results will reveal the feasibility and clinical usefulness of the UP applied in an online group format, in a mental health setting of the national health system for candidates of BS who have at least one diagnosis of ED or emotional symptoms. The concrete results that are expected to reach this conclusion are shown in more detail in Table 4.

Table 4. Main expected outcomes. UP: Unified Protocol for the transdiagnostic Treatment of Eds.

Clinical Usefulness of the UP for Bariatric Surgery Candidates
Group Results: - Depending on the characteristics of the sample obtained (we will check if the parametric assumptions are met), the results of the parametric/non-parametric tests that allow comparing the group scores between the different time points are expected to show statistically significant differences in the desired direction.
Individual Results: - To obtains statistically significant differences (Reliable Change Index; RCI) between the scores obtained at the pre-treatment, baseline, and post-treatment on the primary and secondary measures. - A maintaining of improvements obtained after the application of the UP in the long term (follow-ups of up to two years), with statistically significant differences (Reliable Change Index; RCI) between the scores obtained at the pre-treatment/post-treatment and follow-ups on the primary and secondary measures.
In both cases, the expected directions for the different variables are: - An increase for the variables positive affect, extraversion, quality of life and health-related quality of life. - A decrease for the variables negative affect, neuroticism, interference of symptoms, emotional dysregulation, bulimic symptomatology, dissatisfaction with body image and emotional eating. Feasibility of the UP for Bariatric Surgery Candidates - High session attendance rates. - High scores on the STQ both in the questions that refer to the treatment itself and its different modules, and in the questions that refer to the group and online format.

Reporting of results will follow the Consolidated Standards of Reporting Trials (CONSORT) recommendations, specifically its extension for designs N-of-one Trials [81].

4. Discussion

Obesity and being overweight have become a serious public health problem due to their high prevalence and associated costs [2,9]. EDs are highly present in people with obesity [7], and this can interfere with a commitment to voluntary weight loss [82] and it is also associated with worse post-intervention outcomes [11]. An intervention based on emotion-regulation training could help those patients to achieve both aims, to lose weight before the BS to prevent surgery problems and the emergence of emotional symptoms after the BS, maintaining their emotional and physical achievements over time. In addition to the clinical implications, the results derived from this study may also have an important economic impact. Thus, health policies and the managing of this health condition in public health settings could be also influenced.

To prove this, longitudinal studies are needed and some limitations regarding the interventions (specific CBT versus transdiagnostic intervention) and the delivery formats (onsite versus online) must be considered. The use of the UP in an online group intervention format in a public mental health setting with people waiting for BS has the following benefits:

1. It can allow clinicians to use a single treatment for those candidates who present different EDs, with comorbidity, and also with subclinical symptoms or unspecified disorders [15].
2. In other public health systems similar to the Spanish one, where onsite specific CBT is the most common delivery format, and therapy sessions occur at long intervals (e.g., more than a month) due to waiting lists, a UP online group intervention can help to increase the frequency of sessions and reduce costs because there are more patients treated simultaneously (five to eight patients in the same group), which can facilitate better patient care.
3. Thanks to the online format, this intervention will facilitate access to psychological interventions in those candidates who face mobility challenges due to their obesity condition [31]. This innovative approach would be in line with the goals of the World Health Organization proposed in the mental health action plan to use electronic technologies to expand the delivery of mental health care [83].
4. The fact of receiving quarterly follow-ups up to two years after treatment allows guaranteeing the prevention of relapses and maintaining the results, especially beyond the year and a half or two years, which is the moment in which the literature recognizes that pre-BS problems tend to reappear [42].
5. Furthermore, this advantage offered by long term relapse prevention follow-ups leads to a condition of reduced healthcare costs that are associated with the care of comorbid health problems in this type of patients [3].
6. And finally, it is known that group therapy provides benefits to the patient that are not obtained with individual treatment, such as reducing isolation, facilitating social support, and learning from the experiences of others [33], which could improve its efficiency.

Our study also has some limitations. First, some people who are going to undergo BS will prefer individual treatment, which could be a barrier to enroll those participants in our study (e.g., abandonment or decrease in UP satisfaction and effectiveness). In this case, it could be explained to the patient that group treatment resulted in greater weight losses than individual treatment, even for those clients with a preference for individual therapy and that matching clients with their preferences for individual or group therapy did not enhance treatment outcome either in terms of weight loss or improvements in psychological functioning [84]. Furthermore, a study in a sample of people with EDs diagnosis attended to in public mental health settings in Spain found that the majority of participants preferred receiving psychological treatment in an individual format, followed by group format, and, rarely, in an online format, so it will be necessary to explain to patients the advantages and disadvantages of receiving psychotherapy through individual, group, or online format to help them to decide whether or not to participate in this study [85]. In this sense, the arguments that must be strengthened to justify a group application, in addition to those mentioned previously, are the possibility of sharing experiences, the opportunity to learn from others and receive comments and support and for the online format, convenience [85]. The second main limitation, is that, due to this being a pilot study, the results must be interpreted with caution, as further RCT studies with greater rigor will be required. In this sense, it should be noted that this kind of study is an advisable cost-effective method to preliminarily examine the efficacy, feasibility and/or implementation of recent intervention programs or applications with different samples [86].

Despite the aforementioned limitations, the present study may have different implications. At the research level, it will be the first pilot study aimed at evaluating the feasibility and clinical utility of an online group format of a transdiagnostic intervention for the treatment of ED in public settings in Spain with people waiting for BS, allowing us to increase the evidence on UP's effectiveness, flexibility, and versatility. At a clinical level, the results of the study will reveal whether UP can improve emotional symptoms in candidates and, therefore, improve the effects of BS in the long term. This would have important implications for patients, as it could achieve much more notable improvements after the intervention, and would serve to prevent relapses that generally appear in the long term around two years after BS.

5. Conclusions

In sum, the present study supports the idea of the need to test new forms of psychological interventions with patients waiting for BS [12]. This would allow us to improve the previous psychopathology, and, therefore, to potentiate the effects of BS in the short and long term [2].

The UP may be a good treatment option, considering that it is directed at EDs (which are the most prevalent in people with obesity problems) [12], and that it allows addressing comorbidity, subclinical symptoms, and unspecified disorders [15].

In addition, its application through an online group format can provide extra advantages, as it allows access to treatment for people with mobility problems, something very common among candidates for BS [31], and also fosters social support among the members of the group [33].

Based on all this, the results of the development of this study may have important implications for the National Health System, which will be able to meet the psychological needs of patients with obesity problems, improving their quality of life before the intervention, and enhancing its results in the long term, which will mean a reduction in costs to the system and more specialized and multidisciplinary care for patients who are in this situation.

Supplementary Materials: Unified Protocol for Transdiagnostic Treatment of Emotional Disorders (therapist guide and workbook) are available at https://www.oxfordclinicalpsych.com/view/10.1093/med-psych/9780190685973.001.0001/med-9780190685973; https://www.oxfordclinicalpsych.com/view/10.1093/med-psych/9780190686017.001.0001/med-9780190686017. Both Spanish versions are available at https://www.alianzaeditorial.es/libro/manuales/protocolo-unificado-para-el-tratamiento-transdiagnostico-de-los-trastornos-emocionales-manual-del-terapeuta-david-h-barlow-9788491814795/; https://www.alianzaeditorial.es/libro/manuales/protocolo-unificado-para-el-tratamiento-transdiagnostico-de-los-trastornos-emocionales-manual-del-paciente-david-h-barlow-9788491814818/.

Author Contributions: Conceptualization, J.O.; methodology, J.O. and A.Q.-O.; description of the analysis, A.Q.-O.; resources, J.O. and V.F.-G.; writing—original draft preparation, A.Q.-O.; writing—review and editing, J.O., A.Q.-O. and V.F.-G.; supervision, J.O.; funding acquisition, J.O. All authors have read and agreed to the published version of the manuscript.

Funding: Funding for the study was provided by the Aragon Government (Department of Innovation, Research and University), and the European Regional Development Fund (ERDF) "Building Europe from Aragon" (research team S31_20D).

Acknowledgments: We would like to thank all mental health professionals working at the General University Hospital of Vinaròs in Castellón (Spain) for its commitment to ongoing scientific research in clinical and health psychology.

Conflicts of Interest: The authors declare no conflict of interest.

References

1. Yumuk, V.; Tsigos, C.; Fried, M.; Schindler, K.; Busetto, L.; Micic, D.; Toplak, H. European Guidelines for Obesity Management in Adults. *Obes. Facts* **2015**, *8*, 402–424. [CrossRef] [PubMed]
2. Oltmanns, J.R.; Rivera, J.; Cole, J.; Merchant, A.; Steiner, J.P. Personality psychopathology: Longitudinal prediction of change in body mass index and weight post-bariatric surgery. *Health Psychol.* **2020**, *39*, 245–254. [CrossRef] [PubMed]

3. Hernáez, A.; Zomeño, M.D.; Dégano, I.R.; Pérez-Fernández, S.; Goday, A.; Vila, J.; Civeira, F.; Moure, R.; Marrugat, J. Exceso de peso en España: Situacioón actual, proyecciones para 2030 y sobrecoste directo estimado para el Sistema Nacional de Salud [Excess Weight in Spain: Current Situation, Projections for 2030, and Estimated Direct Extra Cost for the Spanish Health Sy. *Span. J. Cardiol.* **2019**, *72*, 916–924. [CrossRef]
4. Castaneda, D.; Popov, V.B.; Wander, P.; Thompson, C.C. Risk of Suicide and Self-harm Is Increased After Bariatric Surgery—A Systematic Review and Meta-analysis. *Obes. Surg.* **2019**, *29*, 322–333. [CrossRef]
5. De Luca, M.; Angrisani, L.; Himpens, J.; Busetto, L.; Scopinaro, N.; Weiner, R.; Sartori, A.; Stier, C.; Lakdawala, M.; Bhasker, A.G.; et al. Indications for Surgery for Obesity and Weight-Related Diseases: Position Statements from the International Federation for the Surgery of Obesity and Metabolic Disorders (IFSO). *Obes. Surg.* **2016**, *26*, 1659–1696. [CrossRef]
6. OECD/European Union. *Health at a Glance: Europe 2018: State of Health in the EU Cycle*; OECD Publishing, Paris/European Union: Brussels, Belgium, 2018. [CrossRef]
7. Spirou, D.; Raman, J.; Smith, E. Psychological outcomes following surgical and endoscopic bariatric procedures: A systematic review. *Obes. Rev.* **2020**, e12998. [CrossRef]
8. Dixon, J.B.; Dixon, M.E.; O'Brien, P.E. Depression in Association With Severe Obesity. *Arch. Intern. Med.* **2003**, *163*, 2058. [CrossRef]
9. OECD. *The Heavy Burden of Obesity: The Economics of Prevention, OECD Health Policy Studies 2019*; OECD: Paris, France, 2019. [CrossRef]
10. Jumbe, S.; Hamlet, C.; Meyrick, J. Psychological Aspects of Bariatric Surgery as a Treatment for Obesity. *Curr. Obes. Rep.* **2017**, *6*, 71–78. [CrossRef]
11. Lauren, A.D.; Sijercic, I.; Cassin, S.E. Preoperative and post-operative psychosocial interventions for bariatric surgery patients: A systematic review. *Obes. Rev.* **2020**, e12926. [CrossRef]
12. Sarwer, D.B.; Heinberg, L.J. A Review of the Psychosocial Aspects of Clinically Severe Obesity and Bariatric Surgery. *Am. Psychol. Assoc.* **2020**, *75*, 252–264. [CrossRef]
13. Geller, S.; Dahan, S.; Levy, S.; Goldzweig, G.; Hamdan, S.; Abu-Abeid, S. Body Image and Emotional Eating as Predictors of Psychological Distress Following Bariatric Surgery. *Obes. Surg.* **2019**. [CrossRef] [PubMed]
14. Institute for Health Metrics and Evaluation. Global Health Data Exchange. Available online: http://ghdx.healthdata.org/gbd-results-tool (accessed on 5 May 2020).
15. Barlow, D.H.; Farchione, T.J.; Sauer-Zavala, S.; Murray-Latin, H.; Ellard, K.K.; Bullis, J.R.; Bentley, K.H.; Boettcher, H.T.; Cassiello-Robbins, C. *Unified Protocol for Transdiagnostic Treatment of Emotional Disorders: Therapist Guide*, 2nd ed.; Oxford University Press: New York, NY, USA, 2018.
16. Lim, R.B.C.; Zhang, M.W.B.; Ho, R.C.M. Prevalence of all-cause mortality and suicide among bariatric surgery cohorts: A meta-analysis. *Int. J. Environ. Res. Public Health* **2018**, *15*, 1519. [CrossRef] [PubMed]
17. Barlow, D.H.; Farchione, T.J.; Bullis, J.R.; Gallagher, M.W.; Murray-Latin, H.; Sauer-Zavala, S.; Bentley, K.H.; Thompson-Hollands, J.; Conklin, L.R.; Boswell, J.F.; et al. The unified protocol for transdiagnostic treatment of Emotional Disorders compared with diagnosis-specific protocols for anxiety disorders: A randomized clinical trial. *JAMA Psychiatry* **2017**, *74*, 875–884. [CrossRef] [PubMed]
18. Brown, T.; Campbell, L.; Lehman, C.; Grisham, J.; Mancill, R. Current and Lifetime Comorbidity of the DSM-IV Anxiety and Mood Disorders in a Large Clinical Sample. *J. Abnorm. Psychol.* **2001**, *110*, 585–599. [CrossRef] [PubMed]
19. McManus, F.; Shafran, R.; Cooper, Z. What does a 'transdiagnostic approach have to offer the treatment of anxiety disorders? *Br. J. Clin. Psychol.* **2010**, *49*, 491–505. [CrossRef] [PubMed]
20. Brown, T.A.; Barlow, D.H. A proposal for a dimensional classification system based on the shared features of the DSM-IV Anxiety and Mood Disorders: Implications for Assessment and Treatment. *Psychol. Assess.* **2009**, *21*, 256–271. [CrossRef]
21. Sauer-Zavala, S.; Cassiello-Robbins, C.; Conklin, L.R.; Bullis, J.R.; Thompson-Hollands, J.; Kennedy, K.A. Isolating the Unique Effects of the Unified Protocol Treatment Modules Using Single Case Experimental Design. *Behav. Modif.* **2017**, *41*, 286–307. [CrossRef]
22. Sauer-Zavala, S.; Cassiello-Robbins, C.; Ametaj, A.A.; Wilner, J.G.; Pagan, D. Transdiagnostic Treatment Personalization: The Feasibility of Ordering Unified Protocol Modules According to Patient Strengths and Weaknesses. *Behav. Modif.* **2019**, *43*, 518–543. [CrossRef]
23. Sakiris, N.; Berle, D. A systematic review and meta-analysis of the Unified Protocol as a transdiagnostic emotion regulation based intervention. *Clin. Psychol. Rev.* **2019**, *72*, 1017–1051. [CrossRef]

24. Weihs, K.L.; McConnell, M.H.; Wiley, J.F.; Crespi, C.M.; Sauer-Zavala, S.; Stanton, A.L. A Preventive Intervention to Modify Depression Risk Targets after Breast Cancer Diagnosis: Design and Single-Arm Pilot Study. *Psychooncology* **2019**, *28*, 880–887. [CrossRef]
25. Parsons, J.T.; Rendina, H.J.; Moody, R.L.; Gurung, S.; Starks, T.J.; Pachankis, J.E. Feasibility of an Emotion Regulation Intervention to Improve Mental Health and Reduce HIV Transmission Risk Behaviors for HIV-Positive Gay and Bisexual Men with Sexual Compulsivity. *Aids Behav.* **2017**, *21*, 1540–1549. [CrossRef] [PubMed]
26. Johari-Fard, R.; Ghafourpour, R. The effectiveness of Unified Treatment approach on quality of life and symptoms of patients with irritable bowel syndrome referred to gastrointestinal clinics. *Int. J. BodyMind Cult.* **2015**, *2*, 85–94.
27. Andersson, G. Internet-Delivered Psychological Treatments. *Annu. Rev. Clin. Psychol.* **2016**, *12*, 157–179. [CrossRef] [PubMed]
28. Andersson, G. Using the Internet to provide cognitive behaviour therapy. *Behav. Res. Ther.* **2009**, *47*, 175–180. [CrossRef]
29. Andrews, G.; Cuijpers, P.; Craske, M.G.; McEvoy, P.; Titov, N. Computer therapy for the anxiety and depressive disorders is effective, acceptable and practical health care: A meta-analysis. *PLoS ONE* **2010**, *5*. [CrossRef]
30. Andreu-pejó, L.; Martínez-borba, V.; Suso-ribera, C.; Osma, J. Can we predict the evolution of depressive symptoms, adjustment, and perceived social support of pregnant women from their personality characteristics? A technology-supported longitudinal study. *Int. J. Environ. Res. Public Health* **2020**, *17*, 3439. [CrossRef]
31. King, W.C.; Engel, S.G.; Elder, K.A.; Chapman, W.H.; Eid, G.M.; Wolfe, B.M.; Belle, S.H. Walking capacity of bariatric surgery candidates. *Surg. Obes. Relat. Dis.* **2012**, *8*, 48–59. [CrossRef]
32. Wind, T.R.; Rijkeboer, M.; Andersson, G.; Riper, H. The COVID-19 pandemic: The 'black swan' for mental health care and a turning point for e-health. *Internet Interv.* **2020**, *20*, 100317. [CrossRef]
33. Yalom, I.D.; Leszcz, M. *The Theory and Practice of Group Therapy*, 5th ed.; IUP: New York, NY, USA, 2005.
34. Kratochwill, T.R.; Hitchcock, J.H.; Horner, R.H.; Levin, J.R.; Odom, S.L.; Rindskopf, D.M.; Shadish, W.R. Single-Case Intervention Research Design Standards. *Remed. Spec. Educ.* **2012**, *34*, 26–38. [CrossRef]
35. Hawkins, N.G.; Sanson-Fisher, R.W.; Shakeshaft, A.; D'Este, C.; Green, L.W. The multiple baseline design for evaluating population-based research. *Am. J. Prev. Med.* **2007**, *33*, 162–168. [CrossRef]
36. Barlow, D.H.; Nock, M.K.; Hersen, M. *Single Case Experimental Designs: Strategies for Studying Behavior Change*, 3rd ed.; Allyn & Bacon: Boston, MA, USA, 2009.
37. Barlow, H.D.; Durand, V.M.; Hofmann, S.G. *Abnormal Psychology: An Integrative Approach*, 8th ed.; Cengage Learning: Boston, MA, USA, 2018.
38. Kratochwill, T.R.; Hitchcock, J.; Horner, R.H.; Levin, J.R.; Odom, S.L.; Rindskopf, D.M.; Shadish, W.R. Single-Case Design Technical Documentation. *What Work. Clear. House* **2010**. [CrossRef]
39. American Psychiatric Association. *Diagnostic and Statistical Manual of Mental Disorders*, 5th ed.; American Psychiatric Association: Arlington, VA, USA, 2013.
40. Bell, M.L.; Whitehead, A.L.; Julious, S.A. Guidance for using pilot studies to inform the design of intervention trials with continuous outcomes. *Clin. Epidemiol.* **2018**, *10*, 153–157. [CrossRef] [PubMed]
41. Cassin, S.; Sockalingam, S.; Du, C.; Wnuk, S.; Hawa, R.; Parikh, S.V. A pilot randomized controlled trial of telephone-based cognitive behavioural therapy for preoperative bariatric surgery patients. *Behav. Res. Ther.* **2016**, *80*, 17–22. [CrossRef] [PubMed]
42. Sockalingam, S.; Leung, S.E.; Hawa, R.; Wnuk, S.; Parikh, S.V.; Jackson, T.; Cassin, S.E. Telephone-based cognitive behavioural therapy for female patients 1-year post-bariatric surgery: A pilot study. *Obes. Res. Clin. Pract.* **2019**, *13*, 499–504. [CrossRef]
43. Andersson, G.; Cuijpers, P. Internet-based and other computerized psychological treatments for adult depression: A meta-analysis. *Cogn. Behav. Ther.* **2009**, *38*, 196–205. [CrossRef]
44. Martín, E.; Ruiz-Tovar, J.; Sánchez, R. *Vía Clínica de Cirugía Bariátrica 2017*; Im3mediA comunicación: Albacete, Spain, 2017.
45. *Qualtrics (Version 2.16)*; Qualtrics software: Provo, UT, USA, 2017.
46. Beck, A.T.; Steer, R.A.; Brown, G.K. *Manual for the Beck Depression Inventory-II*; Psychological Corporation: San Antonio, TX, USA, 1996.

47. Sanz, J.; Perdigón, A.L.; Vázquez, C. The Spanish adaptation of the Beck's Depression Inventory-II (BDI-II): Psychometric properties in the general population. *Clin. Salud* **2003**, *14*, 249–280.
48. Beck, A.T.; Steer, R. *Beck Anxiety Inventory Manual*; Psychological Corporation: San Antonio, TX, USA, 1993.
49. Magán, I.; Sanz, J.; García-Vera, M.P. Psychometric properties of a Spanish version of the Beck Anxiety Inventory (BAI) in general population. *Span. J. Psychol.* **2008**, *11*, 626–640. [CrossRef]
50. Sheehan, D.V. *Mini International Neuropsychiatric Interview 7.0. (MINI 7.0)*; Medical Outcomes Systems: Jacksonville, FL, USA, 2015.
51. Ministerio de Justicia. Real Decreto 1720/2008, de 19 de Enero, Para la Aprobación de la Ley Orgánica 15/1999 de Protección de Datos de Carácter Personal. *Boletín Oficial del Estado*, 19 January 2008; pp. 4103–4136.
52. Asociación Medica Mundial Declaración de Helsinki. Principios éticos Para las Investigaciones Con Seres Humanos. In Proceedings of the 59th Asamblea General, Seúl, Korea, 18 October 2008.
53. Watson, D.; Clark, L.A.; Tellegen, A. Development and validation of brief measures of positive and negative affect: The PANAS scales. *J. Personal. Soc. Psychol.* **1988**, *54*, 1063–1070. [CrossRef]
54. Sandín, B.; Chorot, P.; Lostao, L.; Joiner, T.E.; Santed, M.A.; Valiente, R.M. Escalas PANAS de Afecto Positivo y Negativo: Validación factorial y convergencia transcultural. *Psicothema* **1999**, *11*, 37–51.
55. Costa, P.T.; McCrae, R.R. *Revised NEO Personality Inventory (NEO-PI-R) and NEO Five-Factor Inventory (NEO-FFI)*; TEA Ediciones: Madrid, Spain, 1999.
56. Mezzich, J.E.; Ruipérez, M.A.; Pérez, C.; Yoon, G.; Liu, J.; Mahmud, S. The Spanish Version of the Quiality of Life Index. *J. Nerv. Ment. Dis.* **2000**, *188*, 301–305. [CrossRef]
57. Brooks, R. EuroQol: The current state of play. *Health Policy* **1996**, *37*, 53–72. [CrossRef]
58. Badia, X.; Roset, M.; Montserrat, S.; Herdman, M.; Segura, A. La versión española del EuroQol: Descripción y aplicaciones EuroQol Spanish Version: Description and Aplications. *Clin. Med.* **1999**, *112*, 79–86.
59. Echeburúa, E.; Corral, P.; Fernández-Montalvo, J. Maladjustment Inventory (MI): Psychometric properties in clinical contexts. *Análisis Modif. Conducta* **2000**, *26*, 325–340.
60. Gratz, K.L.; Roemer, L. Multidimensional assessment of emotion regulation and dysregulation: Development, factor structure, and initial validation of the difficulties in emotion regulation scale. *J. Psychopathol. Behav. Assess.* **2004**, *26*, 41–54. [CrossRef]
61. Hervás, G.; Jódar, R. The Spanish version of the Difficulties in Emotion Regulation Scale. *Clin. Salud* **2008**, *19*, 139–156.
62. Gámez, W.; Chmielewski, M.; Kotov, R.; Ruggero, C.; Suzuki, N.; Watson, D. The Brief Experiential Avoidance Questionnaire: Development and initial validation. *Psychol. Assess.* **2014**, *26*, 35–45. [CrossRef]
63. Vázquez-Morejón, R.; León, J.M.; Martín, A.; Vazquez, A.J. Validation of a spanish version of the brief experiential avoidance questionnaire (BEAQ) in clinical population. *Psicothema* **2019**, *31*, 335–340. [CrossRef]
64. Cardaciotto, L.; Herbert, J.D.; Forman, E.M.; Moitra, E.; Farrow, V. The assessment of present-moment awareness and acceptance: The Philadelphia Mindfulness Scale. *Assessment* **2008**, *15*, 204–223. [CrossRef]
65. Tejedor, R.; Feliu-Soler, A.; Pascual, J.C.; Cebolla, A.; Portella, M.J.; Trujols, J.; Soriano, J.; Pérez, V.; Soler, J. Psychometric properties of the Spanish version of the Philadelphia Mindfulness Scale. *Rev. Psiquiatr. Salud Ment.* **2014**, *7*, 157–165. [CrossRef]
66. Gross, J.J.; John, O.P. Individual differences in two emo- tion regulation processes: Implications for affect, relationships, and well-being. *J. Personal. Soc. Psychol.* **2003**, *85*, 348–362. [CrossRef]
67. Cabello, R.; Salguero, J.M.; Fernández-Berrocal, P.; Gross, J.J. A Spanish adaptation of the Emotion Regulation Questionnaire. *Eur. J. Psychol. Assess.* **2013**, *29*, 234–240. [CrossRef]
68. Henderson, M.; Freeman, C.P.L. A self-rating scale for bulimia the 'bite'. *Br. J. Psychiatry* **1987**, *150*, 18–24. [CrossRef] [PubMed]
69. Moya, T.R.; Bersabé, R.; Jiménez, M. Fiabilidad y validez del test de investigación bulímica de Edimburgo (BITE) en una muestra de adolescentes españoles; Reliability and validity of the Bulimic Investigatory Test Edinburgh (BITE) in a sample of Spanish adolescents. *Psicol. Conduct.* **2004**, *12*, 447–461.
70. Cooper, P.J.; Taylor, M.J.; Cooper, Z.; Fairburn, C.G. The development and validation of the Body Shape Questionnaire. *Int. J. Eat. Disord.* **1987**, *6*, 485–494. [CrossRef]
71. Raich, R.M.; Mora, M.; Soler, A.; Avila, C.; Clos, I.; Zapater, L. Adaptación de un instrumento de evaluación de la insatisfacción corporal; Adaptation of a body dissatisfaction assessment instrument. *Clin. Health* **1996**, *7*, 51–66.

72. Arnow, B.; Kenardy, J.; Agras, W. The Emotional Eating Scale: The development of a measure to assess coping with negative affect by eating. *Int. J. Eat. Disord.* **1995**, *18*, 79–90. [CrossRef]
73. Suso-Ribera, C.; Castilla, D.; Zaragozá, I.; Ribera-Canudas, M.V.; Botella, C.; García-Palacios, A. Validity, Reliability, Feasibility, and Usefulness of Pain Monitor, a Multidimensional Smartphone App for Daily Monitoring of Adults with Heterogeneous Chronic Pain. *Clin. J. Pain* **2018**, *34*, 900–908. [CrossRef]
74. Norman, S.B.; Cissel, S.H.; Means-Christensen, A.J.; Stein, M.B. Development and validation of an Overall Anxiety Severity and Impairment Scale. *Depress. Anxiety* **2006**, *23*, 245–249. [CrossRef]
75. Bentley, K.H.; Gallagher, M.W.; Carl, J.R.; Barlow, D.H. Development and validation of the Overall Depression Severity and Impairment Scale. *Psychol. Assess.* **2014**, *26*, 815–830. [CrossRef]
76. Osma, J.; Quilez-Orden, A.; Suso-Ribera, C.; Peris-Baquero, O.; Norman, S.B.; Bentley, K.H.; Sauer-Zavala, S. Psychometric properties and validation of the Spanish versions of the overall anxiety and depression severity and impairment scales. *J. Affect. Disord.* **2019**, *252*, 9–18. [CrossRef]
77. Barlow, D.; Sauer-Zavala, S.; Farchione, T.; Murray, H.; Ellard, K.; Bullis, J.; Castellano-Robbins, C. *The Unified Protocol for Transdiagnostic Treatment of Emotional Disorders: Client Workbook*, 2nd ed.; Oxford University Press: New York, NY, USA, 2018.
78. IBM Corp. *IBM SPSS Statistics for Windows*; Version 22.0 2013; IBM: Armonk, NY, USA, 2013.
79. Jacobson, N.S.; Truax, P. Clinical significance: A statistical approach to defining meaningful change in psychotherapy research. *J. Consult. Clin. Psychol.* **1991**, *59*, 12–19. [CrossRef]
80. De Andrés Pizarro, J. El análisis de estudios cualitativo. *Aten. Primaria* **2000**, *25*, 42–46. [CrossRef]
81. Shamseer, L.; Sampson, M.; Bukutu, C.; Schmid, C.H.; Nikles, J.; Tate, R.; Johnston, B.C.; Zucker, D.; Shadish, W.R.; Kravitz, R.; et al. Consort extension for reporting N-of-1 trials (CENT) 2015: Explanation and elaboration. *J. Clin. Epidemiol.* **2016**, *76*, 18–46. [CrossRef]
82. Welbourn, R.; Dixon, J.; Barth, J.H.; Finer, N.; Hughes, C.A.; le Roux, C.W.; Wass, J. NICE-Accredited Commissioning Guidance for Weight Assessment and Management Clinics: A Model for a Specialist Multidisciplinary Team Approach for People with Severe Obesity. *Obes. Surg.* **2016**, *26*, 649–659. [CrossRef] [PubMed]
83. World Health Organization. *Mental Health Action Plan 2013–2020*; World Health Organization: Geneva, Switzerland, 2013.
84. Renjilian, D.A.; Perri, M.G.; Nezu, A.M.; McKelvey, W.F.; Shermer, R.L.; Anton, S.D. Individual versus group therapy for obesity: Effects of matching participants to their treatment preferences. *J. Consult. Clin. Psychol.* **2001**, *69*, 717–721. [CrossRef] [PubMed]
85. Osma, J.; Suso-Ribera, C.; Peris-Baquero, O.; Gil-Lacruz, M.; Pérez-Ayerra, L.; Ferreres-Galan, V.; Torres-Alfosea, M.A.; López-Escriche, M.; Domínguez, O. What format of treatment do patients with emotional disorders prefer and why? Implications for public mental health settings and policies. *PLoS ONE* **2019**, *14*, e0218117. [CrossRef] [PubMed]
86. Osma, J.; Sánchez-Gómez, A.; Peris-Baquero, O. Applying the unified protocol to a single case of major depression with schizoid and depressive personality traits. *Psicothema* **2018**, *30*, 364–369. [CrossRef]

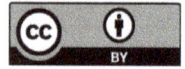

© 2020 by the authors. Licensee MDPI, Basel, Switzerland. This article is an open access article distributed under the terms and conditions of the Creative Commons Attribution (CC BY) license (http://creativecommons.org/licenses/by/4.0/).

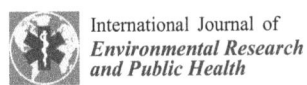

Article

Telemonitoring in Chronic Pain Management Using Smartphone Apps: A Randomized Controlled Trial Comparing Usual Assessment Against App-Based Monitoring with and without Clinical Alarms

Carlos Suso-Ribera [1,*], Diana Castilla [2,3], Irene Zaragozá [3], Ángela Mesas [4], Anna Server [4], Javier Medel [4] and Azucena García-Palacios [1,3]

1. Department of Basic and Clinical Psychology and Psychobiology, Universitat Jaume I, 12071 Castellón, Spain; azucena@uji.es
2. Department of Personality, Assessment, and Psychological Treatments, Universidad de Valencia, 46010 Valencia, Spain; diana.castilla@uv.es
3. Ciber Fisiopatologia Obesidad y Nutricion (CB06/03 Instituto Salud Carlos III) (Ciber Physiopathology Obesity and Nutrition, CB06/03 Instituto Salud Carlos III Health Institute), 28029 Madrid, Spain; irenezaragoza@gmail.com
4. Pain Clinic, Vall d'Hebron Hospital, 08035 Barcelona, Spain; amesas@vhebron.net (Á.M.); aserver@vhebron.net (A.S.); fjmedel@vhebron.net (J.M.)
* Correspondence: susor@uji.es; Tel.: +34-964-387-643

Received: 18 June 2020; Accepted: 7 September 2020; Published: 9 September 2020

Abstract: Background. The usefulness of mHealth in helping to target face-to-face interventions for chronic pain more effectively remains unclear. In the present study, we aim to test whether the Pain Monitor mobile phone application (app) is well accepted by clinicians, and can help improve existent medical treatments for patients with chronic musculoskeletal pain. Regarding this last goal, we compared three treatment conditions, namely usual treatment, usual treatment with an app without alarms and usual treatment with an app with alarms. All treatments lasted one month. The three treatments were compared for all outcomes, i.e., pain severity and interference, fatigue, depressed mood, anxiety and anger. Methods. In this randomized controlled trial, the usual monitoring method (i.e., onsite; $n = 44$) was compared with daily ecological momentary assessment using the Pain Monitor app—both with ($n = 43$) and without alarms ($n = 45$). Alarms were sent to the clinicians in the presence of pre-established undesired clinical events and could be used to make treatment adjustments throughout the one-month study. Results. With the exception of anger, clinically significant changes (CSC; 30% improvement) were greater in the app + alarm condition across outcomes (e.g., 43.6% of patients experienced a CSC in depressed mood in the app + alarm condition, which occurred in less than 29% of patients in the other groups). The clinicians were willing to use the app, especially the version with alarms. Conclusions. The use of apps may have some benefits in individual health care, especially when using alarms to tailor treatments.

Keywords: chronic pain; smartphone app; telemonitoring; ecological momentary assessment; randomized controlled trial

1. Introduction

Chronic Pain: A Major Public Health Challenge

Chronic pain is a multidimensional, distressing experience that can occur with or without tissue damage and persists over extended periods of time (at least three months) [1]. This disease is a public health problem worldwide [2]. Specifically, it is currently estimated that chronic pain affects between 20% and 30% of the adult population worldwide [3–8] and up to 70% of adults older than 65 years [9]. As a consequence, chronic pain has become the most expensive disease in the world [10] and accounts for up to 2% of the annual European gross domestic product [11]. Additionally, with the age distribution shifting towards the elderly [12], the economic burden of this disease is likely to increase in the coming years.

In this scenario, various efforts have been made to improve chronic pain treatments in recent decades. However, existing reviews only provide modest support for the most popular chronic pain treatments, including medical interventions, physical therapy, psychological treatment—or a combination of these [13–15]. Several factors, such as patient characteristics, unexplored genetic or biomechanical mechanism factors or the experience of therapists, could help explain the modest effectiveness of existing treatments for chronic pain. However, some authors have suggested that inadequate monitoring of patient progress and response to treatment is likely to be, at least in part, responsible for the limited impact of current therapies for chronic pain [16,17].

Due to its chronic nature, management of chronic pain often requires prolonged and regular contact with the health care system [18]. In this sense, it is important to note that a move towards self-management will be needed, rather than relying on the care of health professionals [19]. However, in doing so, monitoring could still remain a challenge because limited resources and existing waiting lists in public health settings limit the quality of patient monitoring in chronic pain settings [20,21]. For example, pain treatment follow-up is still predominantly discrete during on-site appointments. This is problematic because pain-related variables, such as pain intensity, mood, and fatigue can vary across and within days [22,23], even in patients with chronic pain such as osteoarthritis [24], rheumatic diseases [25], multiple sclerosis [23] and fibromyalgia [26].

The aforementioned variability of symptoms in patients with chronic pain means that a single measure may not be representative of the entire experience. Furthermore, retrospective pain assessment leads to recall bias and reduces accuracy [27]. This could be minimized with paper diaries. However, research has shown that the use of paper diaries is problematic due to participant noncompliance (missing data and back-filling) and errors associated with manual data entry [28,29]. Additionally, neither episodic on-site assessment nor paper diaries permit timely communication and response to undesired events experienced by the patient during the course of treatment [20].

Another problem related to the current model of care in chronic pain refers to decision-making in the face of unwanted events. Specifically, the current approach to care requires patients to judge when an undesired event is problematic and what is the preferred action to take in the face of that event [30–32]. This approach is problematic, as some patients may tolerate serious or even urgent problems (e.g., tachycardia, severe drowsiness, or persistent vomiting, diarrhea or urine retention) for too long, while others may seek care for symptoms that are less urgent or not problematic (e.g., very mild or short-term). For patients with chronic pain, an added problem is that patients combine appointments with their general practitioner, emergency services and specialized pain clinics for the treatment of their pain and related symptoms [33]. This practice is likely to be problematic, as the alternation of different specialized and nonspecialized services could lead to unpredictable treatment plans in response to unwanted events.

Telemonitoring with episodic phone calls, which is becoming an increasingly common practice, also only partially solves the aforementioned problems. First, because undesired events (e.g., side medication effects or decreased treatment effectiveness) can occur at different treatment stages [34], which means that control calls will often occur before or long after unwanted events occur. Additionally, because such phone calls require the active participation of a healthcare professional, which makes this procedure resource-consuming and ineffective [18].

Taking all the previous into account, it has been argued that our societies will not be able to sustain the current model of care for this condition [20,21,35,36], especially due to the aging of the population and the dramatic increase in the prevalence of this disease in the elderly [9]. Indeed, this appears to be true now more than ever as a result of the COVID-19 crisis, imposed restrictions on circulation and saturation of health systems [37]. Our team has already achieved some important goals in the design, development and implementation of a new tool, namely a smartphone app called Pain Monitor, which facilitates regular assessment of patient outcomes using mobile technology and minimal healthcare professional involvement in assessment. The app, which has been developed by a multidisciplinary team including physicians, nurses, psychologists and engineers following guidelines on pain research and eHealth [38–41], was found to have valid content (i.e., comparable to well-established paper-and-pencil measures) and high patient acceptability (i.e., response rates greater than 70% for daily responses over a period of one month) [42]. While important milestones have been achieved, the utility of the app in terms of increased treatment effectiveness (e.g., further reduction in pain severity and associated symptoms) remains unclear.

In fact, although it has been argued that mobile technology (mHealth)—especially the use of smartphone apps—facilitates this paradigm shift towards telemonitoring in chronic pain care, reviews on this topic have evidenced that randomized controlled trials (RCT) evaluating the usefulness of these tools are lacking in the chronic pain literature [39,41,43–45]. Therefore, the current investigation constitutes an important step forward into the literature on this important public health condition. In particular, the goal of the present study is to test whether incorporating the Pain Monitor app into routine medical treatment results in better pain-related outcomes in patients with chronic musculoskeletal pain. As a secondary objective, we want to investigate the opinion of healthcare professionals on the app (the patients' opinion was already evaluated in the validation study [42]), which is key for future implementation [46].

This RCT had three conditions, i.e., usual treatment (TAU) with the usual assessment method (episodic, combined on-site and by phone call), TAU with app-based assessment without clinical alarms and TAU with app-based assessment with clinical alarms. Eligible patients were adults with chronic musculoskeletal pain, the most common chronic pain condition, which included pain in the bones, muscles, nerves, ligaments or tendons [47]. As recommended in the guidelines, we focus not only on the effectiveness of mHealth in pain severity levels [38]. In particular, outcomes also include interference of pain on functioning, fatigue and mood (depression, anxiety and anger).

The study goal is to compare the response to one month of usual pain treatment for patients in the three monitoring conditions, namely usual episodic monitoring, monitoring with an app without clinical alarms and monitoring with an app with clinical alarms. All patients received the usual treatment for their pain, so differences in outcomes (pain severity and interference, fatigue and mood) across outcomes were expected to occur as a consequence of the assigned monitoring condition. Another goal was to investigate the opinions about the app of health professionals involved in the study (e.g., in charge of disseminating the study, helping download the app and proposing the treatment).

We expected that the use of the app with alarms that were sent to the healthcare professional in the presence of unwanted clinical events would allow a quick detection of patient suffering (see the alarms in Appendix A), including severe pain levels, side medication effects, high interference of pain on functioning and psychological distress, as well as a quick reaction to these events. As a consequence of the above, we anticipated that patients in the app + alarm condition (telemonitoring) would report a greater reduction in pain severity, pain interference, fatigue, depressed mood, anxiety and anger. Additionally, we expected that patients in this condition would also experience unwanted clinical events (e.g., poor treatment response or undesired clinical events associated with treatment onset) for a shorter time compared to treatment as usual or treatment as usual with the app, but without alarms. In relation to the professionals' opinion on the app, we expected that the professionals would experience some burden as they help patients to download the app and respond to alarms. However, we also anticipated that they would perceive the app to be useful and would be willing to use it in the future, preferably the version with alarms.

2. Materials and Methods

The study protocol—including a description of the planned procedures and analyses—was published before starting the recruitment [18]. However, we summarize the main study characteristics, as well as any deviations from the original plan, in the next lines.

The study started in late 2017 and ended in late 2018. All procedures were approved by the ethical review board of the Vall d'Hebron Hospital in Barcelona on 25th, June 2017 and registered on clinicaltrials.gov on 25th, July 2017 (NCT03247725).

2.1. Design

This is a superiority RCT with three conditions: (1) treatment as usual (TAU); (2) TAU + daily assessment using the Pain Monitor app (TAU + app); or (3) TAU + daily assessment using the Pain Monitor app with alarms (TAU + app + alarm). Because we want to ensure that telemonitoring and not the daily response to pain-related items in the app is responsible for patient benefits, we allocated patients using the app into two conditions: telemonitoring (i.e., use of the app with alarms to the physician in the presence of unwanted events detected by the app) and daily app use without alarms. Patients were randomly assigned to the study condition before agreeing to participate. Randomization was performed by an independent researcher with an online randomization tool. There was no allocation ratio. The patients' treating physicians performed the enrollment and assignment to previously randomized conditions. Patients were assigned to conditions based on a random allocation sequence. If they refused to participate because of the assigned condition, the TAU was offered, but they were excluded from the study.

Patients and treating physicians were not blinded to allocation. In the case of patients, this was done for ethical and safety reasons, especially for those using the app without alarms, as they needed to know that the app would not report any adverse event to the physicians. Regarding the medical staff, blinding was not possible because the clinicians had to know that they would receive alarms from a subset of patients, and they had to check their electronic clinical records to decide whether a change in the treatment was required after receiving an alarm. Most assessments were completed by patients, who, as noted earlier, were not blind to their assigned condition for ethical and safety reasons. The only evaluation that was conducted by health professionals, i.e., the follow-up assessment in the TAU group, was as well not blinded. There are several reasons to explain why assessment was not blinded in this case either. For example, calling the patient required accessing to patient personal data, which is restricted to health professionals. Additionally, the TAU condition aimed at recreating the usual practice at the pain clinic, which implies that a health professional is in charge of patient episodic monitoring between appointments. All the physicians at the pain clinic participated in the study, so calls could not be performed by a clinical external to the study and blinded to the patients' condition.

2.2. Participants

The study was advertised by physicians at the pain unit of the Vall d'Hebron Hospital, a tertiary care hospital in Barcelona. The study was presented to all consecutive patients with chronic pain that met the inclusion criteria. Eligibility included being over 18 years of age, not presenting any psychological disorders or problems with language that would make participation difficult, having a mobile phone with Android operating system, accepting the assigned condition and signing the informed consent form. There were no exclusion criterion in terms of previous or existing treatment for pain at study onset or treatment changes during the study, so that the study was as naturalistic as possible, and the sample representative of patients treated at the clinic. In relation to the limitation to Android operating systems, note that by the time the study was conducted the app was only available for Android for economic reasons, as this is the operating system used by more than 90% of phones in Spain [48].

Sample size was calculated a priori with the statistical software G*Power [49] considering previous studies on complications of pain treatments [30,50]. We expected that the rapid detection of such problems using alarms would result in moderate between-group differences in primary outcomes (see below). Taking 80% power, an alpha level of 0.05 and an expected Cohen's d of 0.5, we calculated that 50 participants would be needed in each condition.

2.3. Interventions

All patients received the same intervention (TAU). This consisted of the usual medical treatment for their pain at the pain unit according to the usual practice at the pain clinic and pain guidelines [51,52]. The treatment could include medication (e.g., opioids, antidepressants or anticonvulsants), more invasive techniques (e.g., infiltration) or a combination of both. This treatment was proposed during the first appointment at the clinic (day of baseline assessment). However, if only an infiltration was proposed, because this could only be scheduled one or two weeks later, baseline assessment was postponed until the infiltration was performed. This was done to ensure that baseline assessment occurred on the day of initiation of treatment, regardless of the prescribed treatment.

The prescribed treatment (TAU) remained unchanged during the whole study duration (one month), except when an alarm was received by the clinicians (TAU + app + alarm condition only). Only in this scenario, phone calls were made by the physicians to explore whether a treatment change was required. Alarms were notified to the clinicians on the following working day after their occurrence. These were expected to be responded to on the same day or the next two days, depending on the severity of the alarm.

The duration of the study was set to one month since treatment onset because the clinicians considered that this is a critical period in which most problems with the treatment occur (e.g., poor effect on outcomes or side effects).

2.4. Pain Monitor App

Pain Monitor is a mobile phone app developed for Android, in which patients are asked to respond twice daily during 30 days (morning and evening, at flexible times from 10 am to 12 am and from 7 pm to 9 pm). A reminder is sent to the participant at 10 am and 7 pm and again 90 min later if a response had not been provided. The app incorporates different algorithms which allow sending clinical alarms to professionals (consult Appendix A to see a summary of the parameters that these algorithms follow). The alarms included in this study were established by the medical staff in a joined decision based in clinical experience and research data. The assessment protocol used in the app was validated in a previous study which allowed a reduction of items which can be more effectively used in ecological momentary assessments [42].

In accordance with recommendations from RCT guidelines in pain settings [38], outcomes included pain severity and side effects of the medication (primary outcomes), as well as fatigue, pain interference and mood states, namely depression, anxiety and anger (secondary outcomes). All these items used a 11-point numerical rating scale where 0 indicated the less severe symptomatology (e.g., no pain or sadness) and 10 reflected the most severe levels of symptoms (e.g., most intense pain or sadness). Pain interference on functioning was composed of 4 items, namely interference of pain on sleep, work/housework, leisure and social interactions. Similar to the brief pain inventory [53], an overall interference score was computed as a mean of these items to obtain a measure of overall interference of pain on functioning. For all items, with the exception of pain interference, patients were asked to report on their current status (i.e., current pain severity, fatigue and mood). For interference of pain on functioning, patients were asked to report the experienced interference during the night (interference of pain on sleep) or during the day (interference on work/housework, leisure and social interactions).

In past research, single items for each of these constructs were validated to be used in the Pain Monitor app [42]. To do so, a single item for each construct was correlated with well-established measures of pain severity, pain interference, fatigue and mood. Specifically, pain severity and interference items were validated against the brief pain inventory [53], while fatigue and mood items were validated against the Profile of Mood States [54], the hospital anxiety and depression scale for depression and anxiety [55] and the Beck depression inventory-II for depression [56]. The correlations were found to be significant and moderate in strength. The validated app items can be found in the current study protocol, which can be accessed for free [18]. For the present study purposes, only a subset of the full protocol was used. See items used in the RCT in Appendix B.

The list of adverse symptoms included the most frequent side effects of treatments for pain [52,57,58]. Note that the item that evaluated these physical symptoms did not explicitly refer to side medication effects. This was done to avoid inducing the idea that, if experienced, symptoms were due to the proposed treatment. Thus, the item stated "Please, indicate which of the following symptoms you experienced today (select only those that you do not normally experience)." Note that, even if patients experienced unusual symptoms after treatment onset, these cannot be only attributed to pain treatment, as they could be a consequence of many other factors (e.g., an infection, stress, hormonal changes, etc.).

Daily symptoms were only tracked in the TAU + app and TAU + app + alarm conditions, because these were assessed with the app. Tacking daily symptoms in the TAU group would have required daily calls, which was not feasible and would largely imply a deviation from usual practice at the clinic.

All conditions (TAU, TAU + app and the TAU + app + alarm) completed the aforementioned measures (i.e., single items on pain severity, side effects of the medication, fatigue, pain interference and mood) at baseline (the same day treatment was proposed) and the end of the study (30 days after). However, patients in the TAU + app and the TAU + app + alarm conditions also responded to the protocol twice daily. This was done to control for the effect of daily measuring (TAU + app) and to generate the alarms (TAU + app + alarm). The protocol was automatically prompted in the morning and in the evening to reduce the reliance on the patient's memory.

Patients in the TAU condition completed the protocol as usual, i.e., with paper and pencil at baseline and by phone at the end of study (30 days later). This second measurement was not done face-to-face because patients are usually scheduled no earlier than 4–5 months after the previous appointment. In the TAU follow-up assessment, one of the pain clinic physicians, AM, made the phone calls to the participants. If patients were unavailable, they were called daily for up to three consecutive days. If no response was obtained, this was considered a missing value. The other two groups (TAU + app and TAU + app + alarms) were assessed with the Pain Monitor app at all times. The comparability of the paper-and-pencil and app assessments was not conducted here because the validity of the current assessment protocol across measurement modalities was already performed in past research [42].

The participating clinicians helped patients download the app during the initial appointment and provided support during this first use (completion of baseline evaluation). Patients also received the contact information from the lead researcher, CSR, in case technical problems occurred with the app.

In addition to patient measurement, we explored the professionals' experience with the app. Consistent with the technology acceptance model [59], we evaluated perceived utility ("To what extent do you believe the app is useful for pain management?"), acceptability ("To what extent did you experience burden due to the alarms generated by the app?") and intention to use ("To what extent would you like to use the app with alarms in the future?"). All physicians participating in the study and working at the pain clinic ($n = 6$) were invited to participate in this survey at the end of the study. All questionnaires were anonymized.

2.5. Data Analysis

First, a descriptive analysis of the sample (i.e., age, sex, marital status, job status, educational level, pain localization and pain duration), including the study flow chart, was conducted. This included an analysis of means and standard deviations for age and percentages for the remaining variables.

Next, we investigated whether randomization resulted in comparable groups in terms of study outcomes (multivariate analysis of variance, MANOVA).

Originally, we planned to explore between and within changes in all study outcomes using a repeated measures MANOVA. However, during the review process it was noted that nonparametric statistics should be used due to the ordinal nature of the measures used (11-point numerical rating scales) [60]. Therefore, we calculated a Kruskal–Wallis H test to compare the change in outcomes under three conditions, as a well as a Friedman test to investigate baseline-to-follow-up changes for each condition. Both analyses were complementary, since the Kruskal–Wallis test provides evidence on between-group differences and the Friedman test reports on within-group evolution. In the Kruskal–Wallis test, the dependent variables were change scores (e.g., end of study pain severity—baseline pain severity) because the test cannot be computed with repeated measures. In Friedman's test, analyses were computed separately for each condition because between-group changes cannot be investigated. Due to multiple comparisons, a more restrictive alpha level of 0.01 was set for the analyses.

Again different from that which was planned, we added an analysis of clinically meaningful improvements at the individual level due to insufficient power and loss in sample size (see the results section). This analysis is recommended in guidelines for pain trials and a reduction in 30% of severity of symptoms is argued to be a useful benchmark, representing at least moderate clinically significant changes (CSC) for the individuals [61,62]. Therefore, a CSC in an outcome for a given individual occurred if follow-up scores (e.g., one month after treatment, i.e., end of study) improved when compared to baseline scores by at least 30% of baseline score. For example, a baseline pain level of 5 and a follow-up pain level of 3 would represent a positive CSC reduction (the follow-up pain level is smaller than $5 - 5 \times 0.3 = 3.5$). Note that this 30% benchmark is only a recommended value based on past research with different outcomes and response scales, including 11-point numeric rating scales as the ones used in the present study [62]. However, change scores have ranged from 30% to 60% across investigations depending on the outcomes and the measures used [61], so the generalizability of our findings should be taken with caution.

As a final step, an analysis of variance (ANOVA) was computed to compare the number of side effects experienced by patients in the app + alarm and patients in the app without alarm conditions. This was followed by an analysis of frequencies of the types of alarms received and the clinicians' opinion about the app. As planned, interim analyses were not conducted because no harm was expected from adding the app to TAU [18].

2.6. Trial Registration and Ethics

Trial registration code in ClinicalTrials.gov is NCT03247725. The ethics committee of the Vall d'Hebron Hospital approved the present study and its procedures (code PR(ATR)381/2015).

3. Results

The study flowchart is shown in Figure 1. The initial recruitment plan included 150 chronic pain patients (at least 50 were needed per condition). Because we anticipated some attrition due to the longitudinal nature of the study and the occurrence of technological problems, we recruited 165 patients which were randomly assigned to conditions prior to recruitment. This resulted in 56 patients in the TAU condition, 56 in the TAU + app condition and 53 in the TAU + app + alarms condition. Finally, data were obtained from 44 patients in the TAU condition, 45 patients in the TAU + app condition and 43 patients in the TAU + app + alarm condition, which corresponds to 78.6%, 80.4% and 81.1% of the initial sample, respectively. In the TAU condition, attrition was mainly due to the fact that patients failed to respond to follow-up assessment phone calls (for each patient, up to six phone calls were made over three consecutive days to obtain the follow-up assessment). In the two app conditions, attrition was mainly a result of problems with the phone (e.g., lack of memory or buying a new smartphone during the study due to a failure or malfunction of the old one).

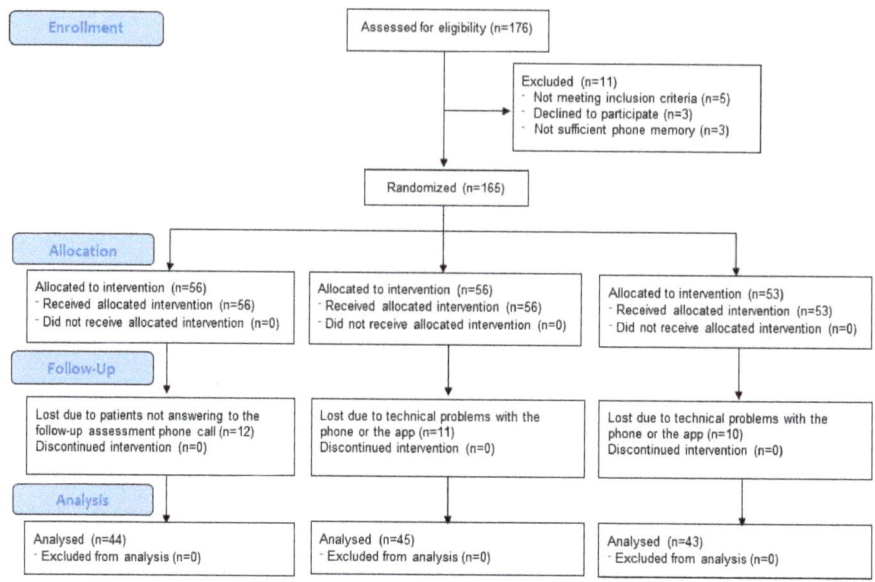

Figure 1. Study flowchart.

Overall, the response to the prompted daily questions in app was good (on average, patients responded to 77.0% of daily evaluations) and comparable to past research [42]. Note that an alarm was set to indicate when a patient was not responding to the app items (e.g., over two consecutive missing days), so that the principal investigator, CSR, could call patients and explore reasons for missing data (e.g., technical problems or lack of time or motivation).

3.1. Sample Characteristics

Patients had a mean age of 52.1 years (range = 23–82, SD = 11.2) and the majority were women (73.8%). Most of the participants were married or in a relationship (73.2%). One third of the patients were working at the time of assessment (34.4%). The rest of the participants were on temporary sick leave (20.6%), had compensation for permanent disability (19.1%) or were retired (11.5%), unemployed (7.6%) or homemakers (6.9%). Regarding educational level, 33.1% had only completed primary education, 32.3% had completed secondary studies, and 34.6% had completed tertiary education (technical or university studies).

Patients had musculoskeletal pain, most frequently pain in the low back or in the neck. Patients had been experiencing pain for between 6 months and 1 year (9.9%), 1–5 years (37.2%), 5–10 years (24.0%) or over 10 years (28.9%).

3.2. Baseline Differences in Study Variables

A MANOVA was conducted to investigate whether the randomization had effectively resulted in comparable patient profiles at baseline. The results supported the success of randomization. Specifically, baseline pain severity ($F = 1.65$, $p = 0.196$), pain interference ($F = 1.58$, $p = 0.211$), fatigue ($F = 0.42$, $p = 0.656$), sadness ($F = 0.22$, $p = 0.806$), anxiety ($F = 1.01$, $p = 0.368$) and anger ($F = 0.42$, $p = 0.656$) were comparable across conditions. The same occurred with sociodemographic characteristics, namely age ($F = 2.33$, $p = 0.101$), gender ($\chi^2 = 1.86$, $p = 0.395$), marital status ($\chi^2 = 7.9$, $p = 0.660$), educational level ($\chi^2 = 4.72$, $p = 0.318$), job status ($\chi^2 = 7.59$, $p = 0.669$) and pain duration ($\chi^2 = 3.16$, $p = 0.789$).

3.3. Changes in Pain Severity, Pain Interference, Fatigue and Mood across Treatment Conditions

As explained in the data analysis section and the beginning of the results section, two analytical approaches were followed due to sample size and reduced power. The first was the planned analysis of differences at the group level (Kruskal–Wallis and Friedman test). As indicated in Table 1, the Friedman test indicated that a treatment main effect was not observed for any outcome in the TAU and the TAU + app conditions. Only in the TAU + app + alarm condition a change (e.g., reduction) in pain interference was revealed ($Z = -3.32$, $p < 0.001$). The Kruskal–Wallis test revealed that none of the change scores differed across conditions (all $p > 0.01$).

In addition to changes at the group level, we also investigated changes at the individual level by means of an analysis of CSC (i.e., improvement of 30% or more with respect to baseline scores). The results are reported on Table 2. Again, the statistical analyses did not indicate significant differences in the proportion of clinically improved patients across conditions. However, this may again be due to insufficient sample size. Note, however, that the proportion of patients showing a CSC in outcomes was consistently higher in the TAU + app + alarm condition, with the only exception of anger, where the numbers were similar in the previous and the TAU condition. For example, 33.3% of patients in the TAU + app + alarm condition experienced a CSC reduction in pain severity after one month of treatment, while only half of this proportion improved in the other two conditions (15.4 in TAU and 16.7 in TAU + app). Similarly, a CSC in sadness was obtained by 43.6% of patients in the TAU + app + alarm condition and less than 30% of patients in the other two groups. Comparable results were revealed for pain interference, fatigue and anxiety, always in favor of the TAU + app + alarm condition.

Table 1. Group-level changes in study outcomes across conditions.

Outcomes	TAU			TAU + App			TAU + App + Alarm			Kruskal-Wallis Test
	Baseline Mean (SD)	Follow-Up Mean (SD)	Friedman Z	Baseline Mean (SD)	Follow-Up Mean (SD)	Friedman Z	Baseline Mean (SD)	Follow-Up Mean (SD)	Friedman Z	Chi-Squared
Pain severity	6.28 (0.34)	5.90 (0.37)	−1.25	5.56 (0.33)	5.50 (0.36)	−0.22	5.58 (0.34)	5.14 (0.37)	−1.22	1.60
Pain interference	5.81 (0.37)	5.42 (0.38)	−0.83	4.94 (0.37)	4.75 (0.38)	−0.30	5.13 (0.37)	4.28 (0.38)	−3.32 **	4.61
Fatigue	6.41 (0.37)	5.85 (0.39)	−1.94	4.94 (0.36)	4.65 (0.37)	−1.07	5.44 (0.37)	5.14 (0.39)	−2.05	1.19
Sadness	4.26 (0.43)	4.13 (0.42)	−0.25	3.94 (0.41)	3.69 (0.40)	−0.78	4.11 (0.43)	3.47 (0.42)	−1.76	1.79
Anxiety	3.89 (0.48)	5.03 (0.45)	−2.07	3.20 (0.45)	3.50 (0.42)	−0.63	3.70 (0.47)	3.35 (0.44)	−0.75	6.55
Anger	2.73 (0.43)	3.60 (0.46)	−1.29	2.57 (0.42)	3.29 (0.45)	−1.65	2.51 (0.43)	2.60 (0.46)	−0.19	0.55

TAU—treatment as usual. ** $p < 0.001$.

Table 2. Percentage of participants showing a clinically significant improvement in study outcomes across conditions.

Outcomes	TAU	TAU + App	TAU + App + Alarm	χ^2	p
Pain severity	15.4	16.7	33.3	4.65	0.098
Pain interference	17.5	20.0	38.5	5.27	0.072
Fatigue	17.9	14.3	25.6	1.74	0.419
Sadness	26.3	28.6	43.6	3.13	0.209
Anxiety	16.2	21.4	30.8	2.36	0.308
Anger	25.0	14.3	23.7	1.70	0.427

TAU—treatment as usual.

3.4. Differences in Frequency of Experienced Physical Symptoms

As noted earlier, the daily frequency of undesired and unusual physical symptoms was evaluated with the app only, so these were not assessed in the TAU condition for reasons of feasibility and fidelity to usual practice. The ANOVA results indicated that the average daily number of unwanted symptoms was slightly, but not significantly higher (F = 1.49, p = 0.226) in the group without alarms (mean = 1.47, SD = 0.64) compared to the group with alarms (mean = 1.33, 0.38).

In total, 51 alarms were received in the TAU + app + alarm condition. The most frequent were related to recurrent headache (n = 11), gait instability (n = 10), interference of pain on sleep (n = 5), urine retention (n = 4), very severe pain levels that do not improve with treatment (n = 3) and sleepiness (n = 3). These data were collected by the app daily based on patient self-reports. In total, 93% of alarms were considered sufficiently relevant to call the patient and further investigate whether an action (e.g., a change in the medication) was required.

3.5. Professionals' Experience with the App

As indicated in Table 3, the pain clinic physicians (n = 6) generally perceived that the app was useful for pain management (e.g., increased treatment safety and effectiveness) and for their own comfort as health care providers. Importantly, they were keener on using the app version with alarms than the version without alarms.

Table 3. Physician opinions about the mHealth solution.

To What Extent the App …	Completely Disagree	Slightly Disagree	Neither Agree Nor Disagree	Slightly Agree	Completely Agree
Was useful for pain management	0	0	0	3	3
Increases treatment safety	0	0	0	4	2
Increases treatment effectiveness	0	0	1	5	0
Gives me comfort	0	1	1	3	1
Is useful for me as a professional	0	0	0	4	2
Can be useful for patients	0	0	0	2	4
With alarms is something I want To use in the future	0	0	0	4	2
Without alarms is something I want to use in the future	0	2	1	2	1
Alarms impact daily job burden	0	4	1	0	1
Has an impact on burden (help patient downloading the app)	2	2	1	1	0

We also investigated burden. On average, the physicians perceived that helping the patient download the app and guiding them during the first use required 13 min (7–20 min range, median = 15 min) and responding to all daily alarms (e.g., looking at the patient's medical record and calling them) required 28 min in total (10–45-min range; median = 27.5 min). As reported in Table 3, the burden was generally perceived as low or average.

4. Discussion

The present study aimed to compare the effectiveness of three monitoring approaches in patients with chronic pain, namely usual episodic monitoring, monitoring with an app without clinical alarms and monitoring with an app with clinical alarms. For one month, all patients received the usual treatment for their pain, but different effects on outcomes (pain severity and interference, fatigue, depression, anxiety and anger) were expected to emerge across monitoring conditions. Another goal was to investigate the opinion of health professionals about the app.

In relation to the first goal and contrary to our expectations, monitoring with the app and alarms did not have a significantly greater impact on outcomes compared to the usual monitoring method or the app without alarms condition, both at the group and individual level. However, consistent with our hypotheses there was only a reduction in pain interference in the group of patients using the app with clinical alarms for telemonitoring. In addition, the analyses at the individual level showed that the proportion of patients reporting a clinically meaningful reduction (i.e., over 30%) in almost all outcomes, namely pain severity, pain interference, fatigue, depression and anxiety, was higher in patients who were monitored using the app with alarms. Regarding the second objective, the healthcare professionals involved generally perceived that the app was useful for pain management in the sense that it improved treatment safety and effectiveness. They also believed that it increased their sense of comfort as healthcare providers. Importantly, they were more satisfied with the version of the app that included alarms. Regarding the burden of using the app, they reported that helping patients download the app and respond to alarms required some extra time, but they found this burden to be low or moderate.

For several years, it has been argued that eHealth and particularly mHealth will inevitably change our health systems in general [63] and pain management in particular [45]. To date, the focus of existing eHealth and mHealth solutions in pain settings has been mostly placed on self-administered treatments, mostly of psychological or alternatively of physical therapy nature [64–66]. While developing alternatives to face-to-face multidimensional treatments for chronic pain is indeed important, most patients still advocate individual, face-to-face treatments [67] and the first-line intervention for patients with chronic pain, namely medical treatment, will probably continue to require some patient-professional face-to-face interaction. Thus, the development of tools that improve face-to-face interventions and allow for a rapid adaptation of treatments as a function of patient evolution during treatment, as in measurement-based care [68], should be a major focus of research in chronic pain settings. This study may provide some novel insights about the potential utility, as well as the implementation challenges of this new approach to monitoring. In fact, to the best of our knowledge, this is the first randomized controlled trial that explored the utility of telemonitoring adults with chronic pain between onsite appointments using a smartphone app.

One of the findings regarding the implementation of mHealth in chronic pain management was that this system was well accepted by the pain physicians involved, which is critical for implementation purposes [69]. Importantly, they preferred the app version that included alarms, even when these generated some burden. While these results are encouraging, a lesson learned based on this perceived burden is that, if mHealth telemonitoring is to be implemented in the future, it may be advisable to allocate some time for clinicians to assist patients with the first app use, as well as to check daily alarms and call patients to make treatment adjustments. This will be especially relevant if a similar technology is to be implemented in routine care for all patients (note that, on average, it took around 30 min for each alarm, considering the time to check the electronic medical record, call the patient and make adjustments to the treatment if necessary). This time, however, clinicians found it beneficial—as indicated by reports showing overall low burden and high perceived usefulness of alarms. Additionally, these costs in terms of time spent dealing with alarms must be weighed against the potential costs of not receiving such alarms (e.g., patients attending the emergency services or taking ineffective medications). While acknowledging the previous positive findings in terms of clinician's acceptability and the potential benefits of using alarms, it is important to note that conclusions about the actual sustainability and cost-effectiveness of this new approach to monitoring at a large scale should be taken with caution.

In relation to the utility of this new approach to monitoring, one of the main study goals was to explore whether the inclusion of telemonitoring (app with alarms) would lead to improved outcomes thanks to a rapid detection of poor treatment response, chronic low mood or high interference of pain on functioning. One problem was sample loss. Thus, even though a visual inspection of mean-level differences across conditions suggested somewhat larger improvements in the app + alarm condition in pain interference, sadness and anxiety, these results should not be overemphasized. Even the fact that pain interference only significantly improved in the app + alarm condition should be interpreted with caution due to sample size loss during the study. An interesting and more promising finding, however, was the fact that the percentage of patients reporting a clinically meaningful improvement in almost all outcomes, i.e., pain severity, pain interference, fatigue, sadness and anxiety was always higher in the app + alarm condition. This is important because, different from the analysis of changes at the group mean level, CSC is explored at the individual level. As noted in past research, while "managers and trialists may be happy for treatments to work on average, patients expect their doctors to do better than that" [70]. At the individual level, our results support the idea that the use of the app with alarms may indeed result in more patients benefiting from medical treatment. For example, while 15.4% and 16.7% of patients in the TAU and TAU + app conditions showed a clinically significant reduction in pain severity, twice the number of patients in the TAU + app + alarm condition (33.3%) showed such reductions.

An important finding in the present study was that the use of the app with alarms as adjunct to medical treatments for pain may as well provide some benefits on the functioning and mental well-being of individuals, again when explored at the individual level. Chronic pain is a very disabling and mentally distressing experience. Not surprisingly, musculoskeletal diseases, which were the type of conditions included in the present study, have become the leading cause of sick leave in Europe and account for approximately half of work-related illnesses [12] and the prevalence of anxiety and mood disorders in patients with chronic pain is two-to-three times higher than in the general population [71]. While the impact of pain on the physical functioning status and mental well-being of individuals is patent, the first-line treatments for the disease, namely medical interventions, have shown to exert a modest effect on daily functioning and, especially, on the mental health status of individuals, even when pain is effectively reduced [72–74]. Therefore, the finding that the use of the app with alarms resulted in a larger number of patients reporting improved pain interference with functioning, fatigue and mental well-being, is encouraging. Note for example, that depression and anxiety levels were meaningfully reduced in 43.6% and 30.8% of patients in the app + alarm condition, while reductions in depression and anxiety in the other two conditions occurred in less than 29% and 22% of patients, respectively. Again, note that these results refer to the percentage of patients with clinically significant improvements. By contrast, the analyses at the group level indicated that the effect of the condition was insufficient to reveal group differences with the recruited sample, even when pain interference only significantly improved in the app + alarm condition.

In addition to exploring the effectiveness of usual medical treatment in several conditions, this study aimed to investigate whether physical symptoms rarely experienced by the patient before treatment onset were minimized in the app + alarm condition compared to the group using the app without alarms. Of course, one thing to keep in mind is that there is no guarantee that these physical symptoms are actually due to the recently proposed pain treatment. By mentioning that patients should only report symptoms that they do not usually experience, we expected to reduce possible misinterpretation of symptoms. However, it is also possible for patients to experience unusual symptoms for reasons other than the onset of a new pain treatment (e.g., an infection, hormonal changes or a stressful daily event, to name some examples). This limitation is difficult to address, so the results regarding the number of daily symptoms should be taken with caution. While acknowledging the previous, an important finding was that algorithms can be effectively created so that the determination of when an event becomes alarming (e.g., experiencing nausea or dizziness for a given number of days) no longer depends solely on the interpretation of the patient. Of course, reporting of symptoms rather than signs requires patient self-report. However, the contribution of the present study is that an algorithm can be used to effectively send an alarm to professionals, so that action can be taken. Note that these alarms could be generated because of the ecological momentary assessment with the app, which current and past research has revealed to be feasible in terms of patient response rates [42].

As a final remark, which may be important for implementation purposes, the study revealed that patient follow-up using phone calls was difficult and technical and phone-related problems are likely to occur when implementing mHealth. In relation the former, calling patients in the TAU condition for follow-up assessment was very time consuming and largely ineffective. Specifically, if often took several calls to get in contact with the participants and these were not always available to complete the survey at the time of the call. This occurred despite the fact that patients were informed that a follow-up call would be made one month after the baseline assessment. This supports the need for more flexible and patient-dependent assessment tools, such as smartphone apps. In this sense, patient daily self-monitoring eliminated the need for physician active monitoring, so only when the app algorithm detected an undesired event, this was notified to the physician and only then a phone call was made. In relation to technical problems, such as app malfunctioning or problems with the patients' phone, such as crashing or low battery or memory, these did occur in the study and resulted in almost 20% of loss in sample size. Recent research into telemonitoring in chronic pain states that these technical problems are something we will probably have to accept [37]. One lesson we learned, however, is that the inclusion of an alarm that sends a notification when patient responses are missing for a number of days (e.g., two in the present study) may be a good strategy to minimize technical problems. This strategy was implemented in the present investigation and it helped us identify some technical problems (e.g., patients that changed their phone or patients that were not receiving the push notifications). These problems would have probably remained undetected otherwise. Similar to past research [75], a technical team will probably be needed to address such technical problems if technological solutions are to be implemented in routine care. In addition to using alarms, another option to minimize missing data are to create a plan to maintain the app after the initial development is completed, which may help reduce technical problems associated with operating system updates [76].

To the best of our knowledge, this is the first study to use an alarm-based telemonitoring system in a randomized controlled trial in chronic pain settings. Some study limitations, including loss of sample due to technical or phone-related problems or the reduced power in the analyses have been already discussed. However, in relation to sample size it is important to mention that the anticipation of a 10% drop-out was clearly insufficient. At least 25% should have been expected based on our results. We expect that this will help researchers when calculating the required sample size for similar future studies. It is also important to acknowledge additional shortcomings, such as the reliance on subjective outcomes only (e.g., the inclusion of wearable devices could have provided more objective data on physical functioning) and the focus on musculoskeletal pain only, which prevents us from generalizing the findings to specific populations or to all chronic pain populations. In relation to wearable devices, however, it is important to note that their inclusion in routine practice may be less ecological than the use of smartphones since the latter are much more frequently utilized by the population. Another shortcoming that should be acknowledged is that the required sample size was obtained based on an uncorrected alpha level of 0.05. Corrections such as Bonferroni–Holm [77] should be considered in future similar investigations conducting multiple comparisons as this may significantly impact on sample size requirements. For instance, by correcting the alpha level to 0.01 due to multiple comparisons in the present study, the sample size needed would have increased from 150 to 222. Furthermore, in relation to sample size, it is important to note that the patient's ability to use the technology was not evaluated in the present investigation because excellent usability findings had already been reported in the original validation study [42]. Therefore, it is difficult to know to what extent technical ability impacted on study completion and, ultimately, on the final sample size. Additionally, as mentioned earlier during the text, the selection of a 30% cutoff to determine the benchmark for a clinically significant change may also have influenced the results. It is possible that more restrictive benchmarks would have resulted in different percentages of change across conditions and, therefore, to different conclusions. The inclusion of a midpoint response, as in the "Neither agree nor disagree" option in the healthcare professionals' questionnaire, may have also been problematic. In this sense, even though the use of a midpoint response may be useful when participants are ambivalent or neutral, they may also be used when participants have no opinion or when they want to provide a response that is socially desirable [78]. In addition, the use of midpoint responses negatively impacts score reliability [79]. In the present study, the prevalence of midpoint responses was 8.3%, which appears to be an acceptable level of uncertainty according to past research [80]. However, future research should consider whether the inclusion of such midpoint response options is crucial for the study's needs and should preferably include a very clear midpoint response or a response scale without midpoints [78]. Finally, because no analysis of costs was made, it is difficult to know to what extent the implementation of mHealth was cost-effective. This should be addressed in future hybrid designs.

5. Conclusions

The present study may contribute to the field of mHealth in chronic pain in a number of ways. First, the study showed that mobile apps can be effectively implemented for patient monitoring. In this sense, the Pain Monitor app allowed us to collect a large number of data associated with pain and treatment in an automated way. This information has never before been collected with this level accuracy (i.e., daily assessment as opposed to the traditional retrospective assessment). This is important given the heterogeneity both in the etiology and the treatment of chronic pain, as ecological momentary assessment could help us obtain a more accurate picture of treatment response which may help guide interventions in a more effective manner [42]. Second, this RCT may serve guide future research in a more effective matter as it provided data on the impact that telemonitoring is likely to have on physical and mental health outcomes in patients with musculoskeletal chronic pain. Third, it showed that, if effective, telemonitoring is more likely to have an impact on outcomes if an alarm system that allows for a rapid response to unwanted events occurs, which suggests that daily assessment only is not likely to be sufficient to have an impact on outcomes. Finally, the lessons learned in terms of physicians' burden and technology problems and solutions may help researchers, clinicians and policy makers interested in the field of mHealth.

Author Contributions: Conceptualization, C.S.-R., D.C., I.Z., Á.M., A.S., J.M. and A.G.-P.; methodology, C.S.-R., D.C., I.Z., Á.M., A.S., J.M. and A.G.-P.; software, A.G.-P., C.S.-R., I.Z. and D.C.; validation, C.S.-R., Á.M., A.S. and J.M.; formal analysis, C.S.-R.; investigation, C.S.-R., Á.M., A.S. and J.M.; resources, C.S.-R., D.C., I.Z., Á.M., A.S., J.M. and A.G.-P.; data curation, I.Z., D.C. and C.S.-R.; writing—original draft preparation, C.S.-R.; writing—review and editing, C.S.-R., D.C., I.Z., Á.M., A.S., J.M. and A.G.-P.; visualization, C.S.-R.; supervision, A.G.-P., C.S.-R. and Á.M.; project administration, A.G.-P., C.S.-R. and Á.M.; funding acquisition, A.G.-P., D.C., I.Z. and C.S.-R. All authors have read and agreed to the published version of the manuscript.

Funding: This research was funded by Jaume I University, Grant Number POSDOC/2016/15 and The Valencian Community Government, Grant Number GV_2019_095. The APC was funded by The Valencian Community Government, Grant Number GV_2019_095.

Conflicts of Interest: The authors declare no conflict of interest.

Appendix A

Alarms Generated by the Pain Monitor App

- Morning pain > 7 during 5 consecutive days
- Evening pain > 7 during 5 consecutive days
- Morning sadness >7 during 5 consecutive days
- Evening sadness >7 during 5 consecutive days
- Morning anxiety >7 during 5 consecutive days
- Evening anxiety >7 during 5 consecutive days
- Vomiting during 2 consecutive days
- Tachycardia during 2 consecutive days
- Blurred vision during 2 consecutive days
- Headache during 2 consecutive days
- Dry mouth during 2 consecutive days
- Constipation during 5 consecutive days
- Drowsiness during 5 consecutive days

- Nausea during 3 consecutive days
- Itching during 3 consecutive days
- Diarrhea during 2 consecutive days
- Fever during 2 consecutive days
- Facial redness during 2 consecutive days
- Urine retention during 2 consecutive days
- Unsteady walking during 3 consecutive days
- Excessive sweating during 7 consecutive days
- Dizziness during 3 consecutive days
- Do not take the medication and there is no intention to take it
- Number of rescue medication > 3
- Sleep interference > 7
- Missing data = 2 consecutive days

Appendix B

Items in the Pain Monitor App Used in the Randomized Controlled Trial

Appendix B.1

Sociodemographic Items (Assessed Once, the First Day of App Use):

1. Please indicate your date of birth (DD/MM/YYYY)
2. What type of user are you?
    a. I am a person with chronic pain
    b. I do not have chronic pain, but I want to see the app
3. Please indicate your gender:
    a. Male
    b. Female
4. Please indicate your type of pain. You may select more than one option:
    a. Fibromyalgia
    b. Low back pain
    c. Cervical pain
    d. Rheumatoid arthritis
    e. Osteoarthritis; Headache
    f. Neuropathic pain
    g. Cancer pain
    h. None of the above.
5. If you selected "None of the above" please indicate your type of pain. Otherwise, leave this question blank. Press OK to continue.
6. Please indicate the location where your pain is more intense:
    a. Head
    b. Shoulder
    c. Neck
    d. High back
    e. Lower back

- f. Arm
- g. Elbow
- h. Wrist
- i. Hand
- j. Abdomen
- k. Chest
- l. Buttock
- m. Hip
- n. Leg
- o. Knee
- p. Foot
- q. Whole body
- r. Somewhere not listed

7. Who is currently treating your pain? You may select more than one option:

    - a. General practitioner
    - b. Rheumatologist
    - c. Orthopedic specialist
    - d. Rehabilitation physician
    - e. Psychiatrist
    - f. Pain Unit
    - g. Neurosurgeon
    - h. Neurologist
    - i. Oncologist
    - j. Another professional.

8. When did your current pain start?

    - a. Less than one year ago
    - b. Between 1 and 5 years ago
    - c. Between 5 and 10 years ago
    - d. More than 10 years ago

9. What is your current treatment for pain? You may select more than one option:

    - a. Physiotherapy
    - b. Pharmacotherapy
    - c. Infiltrations
    - d. Psychological treatment
    - e. Natural / alternative treatments
    - f. My pain is not being treated

10. Did you start a new treatment for pain in the last month?

    - a. Yes
    - b. No

11. Please select the treatment/s you started in the last month. You may select more than one option:

    - a. Physiotherapy
    - b. Pharmacotherapy
    - c. Infiltrations

d. Psychological treatment
e. Natural / alternative treatments
f. I have not started a new treatment

12. What is your marital status?

    a. Single
    b. Married
    c. In a relationship
    d. Divorced
    e. Separated
    f. Widowed

13. What is your job status?

    a. Active worker
    b. Sick leave
    c. Permanent disability
    d. Unemployed
    e. Homemaker
    f. Retired
    g. Student

14. What is the highest level of education you have completed?

    a. No studies
    b. Less than high school
    c. High school graduate
    d. Technical training
    e. University degree

15. Do you currently have a diagnosis of depression by a physician or a psychologist?

    a. Yes
    b. No

16. Do you currently have a diagnosis of anxiety by a physician or a psychologist?

    a. Yes
    b. No

Appendix B.2

Outcomes (Assessed Twice per Day)

1. Please indicate the intensity of your CURRENT PAIN: 0 No pain ———10 Extreme pain
2. Please indicate the intensity of your CURRENT FATIGUE: 0 No fatigue ———10 Extreme fatigue
3. Please indicate the intensity of your CURRENT SADNESS: 0 No sadness ——— 10 Extremely sad
4. Please indicate the intensity of your CURRENT ANXIETY: 0 No anxiety ——— 10 Extremely anxious
5. Please indicate the intensity of your CURRENT ANGER: 0 No anger ——— 10 Extremely angry

Appendix B.3

Items Used for Generating Alarms Only (Assessed Once Daily, in the Evening Except for Pain Interference on Sleep Which Was Evaluated in the Morning Assessment)

1. Did your PAIN interfere with the quality of your SLEEP LAST NIGHT? 0 No interference —— 10 Maximum interference
2. Did your PAIN interfere with your SOCIAL INTERACTIONS TODAY? 0 No interference —— 10 Maximum interference
3. Did your PAIN interfere with the quality of your LEISURE ACTIVITIES TODAY? 0 No interference —— 10 Maximum interference
4. Did your PAIN interfere with your USUAL WORK or HOUSEWORK TODAY? 0 No interference —— 10 Maximum interference
5. Did you experience any of these symptoms TODAY? You may select more than one option. Only select symptoms that were not present before pain treatment onset:

    a. Nausea
    b. Vomiting
    c. Tachycardia
    d. Constipation
    e. Drowsiness / sedation
    f. Blurred vision
    g. Dry mouth
    h. Headache
    i. None of the above

6. Did you experience any of these symptoms TODAY? You may select more than one option. Only select symptoms that were not present before pain treatment onset:

    a. Dizziness
    b. Itching
    c. Diarrhea
    d. Gait instability
    e. Excessive sweating
    f. Fever
    g. Urine retention
    h. Facial redness
    i. A different symptom
    j. None of the above

7. Did you take your prescribed medication TODAY?

    a. Yes
    b. No, but I will do it later
    c. No and I do not plan to take it
    d. I have not been prescribed a pain medication

8. How many times did you take a rescue medication TODAY?

    a. 0
    b. 1
    c. 2
    d. 3
    e. 4
    f. 5
    g. 6

h. 7
i. 8
j. 9
k. 10
l. More than 10

References

1. de C. Williams, A.C.; Craig, K.D. Updating the definition of pain. *Pain* **2016**, *157*, 2420–2423. [CrossRef] [PubMed]
2. Bevan, S.; Quadrello, T.; Mcgee, R.; Mahdon, M.; Vavrovsky, A.; Barham, L. *Fit for Work Pain-European Report*; The Work Fundation: London, UK, 2009.
3. Breivik, H.; Collett, B.; Ventafridda, V.; Cohen, R.; Gallacher, D. Survey of chronic pain in Europe: Prevalence, impact on daily life, and treatment. *Eur. J. Pain* **2006**, *10*, 287–333. [CrossRef] [PubMed]
4. Johannes, C.B.; Le, T.K.; Zhou, X.; Johnston, J.A.; Dworkin, R.H. The prevalence of chronic pain in United States adults: Results of an Internet-based survey. *J. Pain* **2010**, *11*, 1230–1239. [CrossRef] [PubMed]
5. Wong, W.S.; Fielding, R. Prevalence and characteristics of chronic pain in the general population of Hong Kong. *J. Pain* **2011**, *12*, 236–245. [CrossRef] [PubMed]
6. Fayaz, A.; Croft, P.; Langford, R.M.; Donaldson, L.J.; Jones, G.T. Prevalence of chronic pain in the UK: A systematic review and meta-analysis of population studies. *BMJ Open* **2016**, *6*, e010364. [CrossRef] [PubMed]
7. Azevedo, L.F.; Costa-Pereira, A.; Mendonça, L.; Dias, C.C.; Castro-Lopes, J.M. Epidemiology of chronic pain: A population-based nationwide study on its prevalence, characteristics and associated disability in Portugal. *J. Pain* **2012**, *13*, 773–783. [CrossRef] [PubMed]
8. Reid, K.J.; Harker, J.; Bala, M.M.; Truyers, C.; Kellen, E.; Bekkering, G.E.; Kleijnen, J. Epidemiology of chronic non-cancer pain in Europe: Narrative review of prevalence, pain treatments and pain impact. *Curr. Med. Res. Opin.* **2011**, *27*, 449–462. [CrossRef] [PubMed]
9. Miró, J.; Paredes, S.; Rull, M.; Queral, R.; Miralles, R.; Nieto, R.; Huguet, A.; Baos, J. Pain in older adults: A prevalence study in the Mediterranean region of Catalonia. *Eur. J. Pain* **2007**, *11*, 83–92. [CrossRef] [PubMed]
10. Gaskin, D.J.; Richard, P. The economic costs of pain in the United States. *J. Pain* **2012**, *13*, 715–724. [CrossRef]
11. Bevan, S. Economic impact of musculoskeletal disorders (MSDs) on work in Europe. *Best Pract. Res. Clin. Rheumatol.* **2015**, *29*, 356–373. [CrossRef]
12. Bevan, S.; Quadrello, T.; Mcgee, R.; Mahdon, M.; Vavrovsky, A.; Barham, L. Fit for Work? Musculoskeletal Disorders in the European Workforce. Available online: http://www.bollettinoadapt.it/old/files/document/3704FOUNDATION_19_10.pdf (accessed on 15 February 2018).
13. Geneen, L.J.; Moore, R.A.; Clarke, C.; Martin, D.; Colvin, L.A.; Smith, B.H. Physical activity and exercise for chronic pain in adults: An overview of Cochrane Reviews. *Cochrane Database Syst. Rev.* **2017**, *1*, CD011279. [CrossRef] [PubMed]
14. Gatchel, R.; McGeary, D.; McGeary, C.; Lippe, B. Interdisciplinary chronic pain management: Past, present, and future. *Am. Psychol.* **2014**, *69*, 119–130. [CrossRef] [PubMed]
15. Hughes, L.S.; Clark, J.; Colclough, J.A.; Dale, E.; McMillan, D. Acceptance and commitment therapy (ACT) for chronic pain: A systematic review and meta-analyses. *Clin. J. Pain* **2017**, *33*, 552–568. [CrossRef] [PubMed]
16. Salaffi, F.; Sarzi-Puttini, P.; Atzeni, F. How to measure chronic pain: New concepts. *Best Pract. Res. Clin. Rheumatol.* **2015**, *29*, 164–186. [CrossRef] [PubMed]
17. Dansie, E.J.; Turk, D.C. Assessment of patients with chronic pain. *Br. J. Anaesth.* **2013**, *111*, 19–25. [CrossRef] [PubMed]
18. Suso-Ribera, C.; Mesas, Á.; Medel, J.; Server, A.; Márquez, E.; Castilla, D.; Zaragozá, I.; García-Palacios, A. Improving pain treatment with a smartphone app: Study protocol for a randomized controlled trial. *Trials* **2018**, *19*, 145. [CrossRef]
19. Mann, E.G.; LeFort, S.; VanDenKerkhof, E.G. Self-management interventions for chronic pain. *Pain Manag.* **2013**, *3*, 211–222. [CrossRef]

20. OECD; EU. *Health at a Glance: Europe 2016—State of Health in the EU Cycle*; OECD Publishing: Paris, France, 2016; ISBN 9789264265585.
21. Busse, R.; Blümel, M.; Scheller-Kreinsen, D.; Zentner, A. *Tackling Chronic Disease in Europe: Strategies, Interventions and Challenges*; WHO: Copenhagen, Denmark, 2010; Volume 20.
22. Kikuchi, H.; Yoshiuchi, K.; Miyasaka, N.; Ohashi, K.; Yamamoto, Y.; Kumano, H.; Kuboki, T.; Akabayashi, A. Reliability of recalled self-report on headache intensity: Investigation using ecological momentary assessment technique. *Cephalalgia* **2006**, *26*, 1335–1343. [CrossRef]
23. Kratz, A.L.; Murphy, S.L.; Braley, T.J. Ecological Momentary Assessment of Pain, Fatigue, Depressive, and Cognitive Symptoms Reveals Significant Daily Variability in Multiple Sclerosis. *Arch. Phys. Med. Rehabil.* **2017**, *98*, 2142–2150. [CrossRef]
24. Allen, K.D.; Coffman, C.J.; Golightly, Y.M.; Stechuchak, K.M.; Keefe, F.J. Daily pain variations among patients with hand, hip, and knee osteoarthritis. *Osteoarthr. Cartil.* **2009**, *17*, 1275–1282. [CrossRef]
25. Schneider, S.; Junghaenel, D.U.; Keefe, F.J.; Schwartz, J.E.; Stone, A.A.; Broderick, J.E. Individual differences in the day-to-day variability of pain, fatigue, and well-being in patients with rheumatic disease: Associations with psychological variables. *Pain* **2012**, *153*, 813–822. [CrossRef] [PubMed]
26. Bartley, E.J.; Robinson, M.E.; Staud, R. Pain and fatigue variability patterns distinguish subgroups of Fibromyalgia patients. *J. Pain* **2018**, *19*, 372–381. [CrossRef] [PubMed]
27. García-Palacios, A.; Herrero, R.; Belmonte, M.A.; Castilla, D.; Guixeres, J.; Molinari, G.; Banos, R.M.; Baños, R.M.; Botella, C.; Garcia-Palacios, A.; et al. Ecological momentary assessment for chronic pain in fibromyalgia using a smartphone: A randomized crossover study. *Eur. J. Pain* **2014**, *18*, 862–872. [CrossRef]
28. Kirchner, T.R.; Shiffman, S. Ecological Momentary Assessment. In *Wiley-Blackwell Handb. Addict. Psychopharmacology*; MacKillop, J., de Wit, H., Eds.; John Wiley & Sons: Hoboken, NJ, USA, 2013; pp. 541–565. [CrossRef]
29. Smyth, J.M.; Stone, A.A. Ecological momentary assessment research in behavioral medicine. *J. Happiness Stud.* **2003**, *4*, 35–52. [CrossRef]
30. Deyo, R.A.; Mirza, S.K.; Turner, J.A.; Martin, B.I. Overtreating chronic back pain: Time to back off? *J. Am. Board Fam. Med.* **2009**, *22*, 62–68. [CrossRef]
31. Dargan, P.J.; Simm, R.; Murray, C. New approaches towards chronic pain: Patient experiences of a solution-focused pain management programme. *Br. J. Pain* **2014**, *8*, 34–42. [CrossRef] [PubMed]
32. Fashler, S.R.; Cooper, L.K.; Oosenbrug, E.D.; Burns, L.C.; Razavi, S.; Goldberg, L.; Katz, J. Systematic review of multidisciplinary chronic pain treatment facilities. *Pain Res. Manag.* **2016**, *2016*, 5960987. [CrossRef]
33. Hong, J.; Reed, C.; Novick, D.; Happich, M. Costs associated with treatment of chronic low back pain: An analysis of the UK general practice research database. *Spine (Phila. Pa. 1976)* **2013**, *38*, 75–82. [CrossRef]
34. Breivik, H.; Borchgrevink, P.C.; Allen, S.M.; Rosseland, L.A.; Romundstad, L.; Breivik Hals, E.K.; Kvarstein, G.; Stubhaug, A. Assessment of pain. *Br. J. Anaesth.* **2008**, *101*, 17–24. [CrossRef]
35. World Health Organization. *Innovative Care for Chronic Conditions*; WHO: Geneva, Switzerland, 2002.
36. Christensen, H.; Hickie, I.B. Using e-health applications to deliver new mental health services. *Med. J. Aust.* **2010**, *192*, 53–56. [CrossRef]
37. Eccleston, C.; Blyth, F.M.; Dear, B.F.; Fisher, E.A.; Keefe, F.J.; Lynch, M.E.; Palermo, T.M.; Reid, M.C.; de C. Williams, A.C. Managing patients with chronic pain during the COVID-19 outbreak. *Pain* **2020**, *161*, 889–893. [CrossRef] [PubMed]
38. Dworkin, R.H.; Turk, D.C.; Farrar, J.T.; Haythornthwaite, J.A.; Jensen, M.P.; Katz, N.P.; Kerns, R.D.; Stucki, G.; Allen, R.R.; Bellamy, N.; et al. Core outcome measures for chronic pain clinical trials: IMMPACT recommendations. *Pain* **2005**, *113*, 9–19. [CrossRef] [PubMed]
39. Rosser, B.A.; Eccleston, C. Smartphone applications for pain management. *J. Telemed. Telecare* **2011**, *17*, 308–312. [CrossRef] [PubMed]
40. Kaiser, U.; Kopkow, C.; Deckert, S.; Neustadt, K.; Jacobi, L.; Cameron, P.; De Angelis, V.; Apfelbacher, C.; Arnold, B.; Birch, J.; et al. Developing a core outcome-domain set to assessing effectiveness of interdisciplinary multimodal pain therapy. *Pain* **2017**, *1*, 673–683. [CrossRef] [PubMed]
41. Portelli, P.; Eldred, C. A quality review of smartphone applications for the management of pain. *Br. J. Pain* **2016**, *10*, 135–140. [CrossRef]

42. Suso-Ribera, C.; Castilla, D.; Zaragozá, I.; Ribera-Canudas, M.V.; Botella, C.; García-Palacios, A. Validity, reliability, feasibility, and usefulness of Pain Monitor. A multidimensional smartphone app for daily monitoring of adults with heterogeneous chronic pain. *Clin. J. Pain* **2018**, *34*, 900–908. [CrossRef]
43. Alexander, J.; Joshi, G. Smartphone applications for chronic pain management: A critical appraisal. *J. Pain Res.* **2016**, *9*, 731–734. [CrossRef]
44. Wallace, L.S.; Dhingra, L.K. A systematic review of smartphone applications for chronic pain available for download in the United States. *J. Opioid Manag.* **2014**, *10*, 63–68. [CrossRef]
45. Sundararaman, L.V.; Edwards, R.R.; Ross, E.L.; Jamison, R.N. Integration of Mobile Health Technology in the Treatment of Chronic Pain. *Reg. Anesth. Pain Med.* **2017**, *42*, 488–498. [CrossRef]
46. Lemey, C.; Larsen, M.E.; Devylder, J.; Courtet, P.; Billot, R.; Lenca, P.; Walter, M.; Baca-García, E.; Berrouiguet, S. Clinicians' concerns about mobile ecological momentary assessment tools designed for emerging psychiatric problems: Prospective acceptability assessment of the memind app. *J. Med. Internet Res.* **2019**, *21*, e10111. [CrossRef]
47. Araya Quintanilla, F.; Cuyul Vásquez, I.A. Influence of psychosocial factors on the experience of musculoskeletal pain: A literature review. *Rev. Soc. Española Dolor* **2018**, *26*, 44–51. [CrossRef]
48. Ericsson Mobility Report. 2016. Available online: https://www.ericsson.com/en/mobility-report/reports (accessed on 8 September 2020).
49. Faul, F.; Erdfelder, E.; Lang, A.-G.; Buchner, A. G*Power 3: A flexible statistical power analysis program for the social, behavioral, and biomedical sciences. *Behav. Res. Methods* **2007**, *39*, 175–191. [CrossRef] [PubMed]
50. Furlan, A.D.; Sandoval, J.A.; Mailis-gagnon, A.; Tunks, E. Opioids for chronic noncancer pain: A meta-analysis of effectiveness and side effects. *Can. Med. Assoc. J.* **2006**, *174*, 1589–1594. [CrossRef] [PubMed]
51. Turk, D.C.; Wilson, H.D.; Cahana, A. Treatment of chronic non-cancer pain. *Lancet* **2011**, *377*, 2226–2235. [CrossRef]
52. Attal, N.; Cruccu, G.; Baron, R.; Haanpää, M.; Hansson, P.; Jensen, T.S.; Nurmikko, T. EFNS guidelines on the pharmacological treatment of neuropathic pain: 2010 revision. *Eur. J. Neurol.* **2010**, *17*, 1113-e88. [CrossRef]
53. Cleeland, C.S.; Ryan, K.M. Pain assessment: Global use of the brief pain inventory. *Ann. Acad. Med. Singapore* **1994**, *23*, 129–138. [PubMed]
54. McNair, D.; Lorr, M.; Droppleman, L. *Profile of Mood States*; Educational and Industrial Testing Service: San Diego, CA, USA, 1971.
55. Zigmond, A.S.; Snaith, R.P. The hospital anxiety and depression scale. *Acta Psychiatr. Scand.* **1983**, *67*, 361–370. [CrossRef]
56. Beck, A.; Ward, C.H.; Mendelson, M.; Mock, J.; Erbauch, J. An inventory for measuring depression. *Arch. Gen. Psychiatry* **1961**, *4*, 561. [CrossRef]
57. Trescot, A.; Glaser, S.E.; Hansen, H.; Benyamin, R.; Patel, S.; Manchikanti, L. Effectiveness of opioids in the treatment of chronic non-cancer pain. *Pain Physician* **2008**, *11*, 181–200.
58. Varrassi, G.; Müller-Schwefe, G.; Pergolizzi, J.; Orónska, A.; Morlion, B.; Mavrocordatos, P.; Margarit, C.; Mangas, C.; Jaksch, W.; Huygen, F.; et al. Pharmacological treatment of chronic pain—The need for CHANGE. *Curr. Med. Res. Opin.* **2010**, *26*, 1231–1245. [CrossRef]
59. Davis, F.D.; Bagozzi, R.P.; Warshaw, P.R. User Acceptance of computer technology: A comparison of two theoretical models. *Manag. Sci.* **1989**, *35*, 982–1003. [CrossRef]
60. Kersten, P.; White, P.J.; Tennant, A. Is the pain visual analogue scale linear and responsive to change? An exploration using rasch analysis. *PLoS ONE* **2014**, *9*, e99485. [CrossRef] [PubMed]
61. Scott, W.; Wideman, T.H.; Sullivan, M.J.L. Clinically meaningful scores on pain catastrophizing before and after multidisciplinary rehabilitation: A prospective study of individuals with subacute pain after whiplash injury. *Clin. J. Pain* **2014**, *30*, 183–190. [CrossRef] [PubMed]
62. Ostelo, R.W.J.G.; Deyo, R.A.; Stratford, P.; Waddell, G.; Croft, P.; Von Korff, M.; Bouter, L.M.; de Vet, H.C. Interpreting change scores for pain and functional status in low back pain. *Spine (Phila. Pa. 1976)*. **2008**, *33*, 90–94. [CrossRef]
63. Borrelli, B.; Ritterband, L.M. Special issue on ehealth and mhealth: Challenges and future directions for assessment, treatment, and dissemination. *Health Psychol.* **2015**, *34*, 1205–1208. [CrossRef]
64. Thurnheer, S.E.; Gravestock, I.; Pichierri, G.; Steurer, J.; Burgstaller, J.M. Benefits of mobile apps in pain management: Systematic review. *JMIR mHealth uHealth* **2018**, *6*, e11231. [CrossRef]

65. Martorella, G.; Boitor, M.; Berube, M.; Fredericks, S.; Le May, S.; Gélinas, C. Tailored web-based interventions for pain: Systematic review and meta-analysis. *J. Med. Internet Res.* **2017**, *19*, e385. [CrossRef]
66. Mehta, S.; Peynenburg, V.A.; Hadjistavropoulos, H.D. Internet-delivered cognitive behaviour therapy for chronic health conditions: A systematic review and meta-analysis. *J. Behav. Med.* **2019**, *42*, 169–187. [CrossRef]
67. Osma, J.; Suso-Ribera, C.; Martínez-Borba, V.; Barrera, A.Z. Content and format preferences of a depression prevention program: A study in perinatal women. *An. Psicol.* **2020**, *36*, 56–63. [CrossRef]
68. Gual-montolio, P.; Martínez-borba, V.; Bretón-lópez, J.M.; Osma, J. How Are Information and Communication Technologies Supporting Routine Outcome Monitoring and Measurement-Based Care in Psychotherapy? A Systematic Review. *Int. J. Environ. Res. Public Health* **2020**, *17*, 3170. [CrossRef]
69. Peters, D.H.; Tran, N.T.; Adam, T. Implementation research in health: A practical guide. Alliance for Health Policy and Systems Research, World Health Organization: Geneva, Switzerland, 2013; p. 69. ISBN 978-92-4-150621-2.
70. Evans, J.G. Evidence-based and evidence-biased medicine. *Age Ageing* **1995**, *24*, 461–463. [CrossRef] [PubMed]
71. Pereira, F.G.; França, M.H.; de Paiva, M.C.A.; Andrade, L.H.; Viana, M.C. Prevalence and clinical profile of chronic pain and its association with mental disorders. *Rev. Saude Publica* **2017**, *51*, 96. [CrossRef] [PubMed]
72. da C. Menezes Costa, L.; Mahera, C.G.; McAuleya, J.H.; Hancock, M.J.; Smeets, R.J.E.M. Self-efficacy is more important than fear of movement in mediating the relationship between pain and disability in chronic low back pain. *Eur. J. Pain* **2011**, *15*, 213–219. [CrossRef]
73. Sullivan, M.J.L.; Adams, H.; Horan, S.; Maher, D.; Boland, D.; Gross, R. The role of perceived injustice in the experience of chronic pain and disability: Scale development and validation. *J. Occup. Rehabil.* **2008**, *18*, 249–261. [CrossRef]
74. Suso-Ribera, C.; Jornet-Gibert, M.; Ribera-Canudas, M.V.; McCracken, L.M.; Maydeu-Olivares, A.; Gallardo-Pujol, D.; Maydeu-Olivares, A.; Gallardo-Pujol, D. A reduction in pain intensity is more strongly associated with improved physical functioning in frustration tolerant individuals. *J. Clin. Psychol. Med. Settings* **2016**, *23*, 192–206. [CrossRef]
75. Lubans, D.R.; Smith, J.J.; Skinner, G.; Morgan, P.J. Development and implementation of a smartphone application to promote physical activity and reduce screen-time in adolescent boys. *Front. Public Health* **2014**, *2*, 1–11. [CrossRef]
76. Price, M.; Yuen, E.K.; Goetter, E.M.; Herbert, J.D.; Forman, E.M.; Acierno, R.; Ruggiero, K.J. mHealth: A mechanism to deliver more accessible, more effective mental health care. *Clin. Psychol. Psychother.* **2014**, *21*, 427–436. [CrossRef]
77. Holm, S. A simple sequential rejective method procedure. *Scand. J. Stat.* **1979**, *6*, 65–70.
78. Nadler, J.T.; Weston, R.; Voyles, E.C. Stuck in the middle: The use and interpretation of mid-points in items on questionnaires. *J. Gen. Psychol.* **2015**, *142*, 71–89. [CrossRef]
79. Weems, G.H.; Onwuegbuzie, A.J. The impact of midpoint responses and reverse coding on survey data. *Meas. Eval. Couns. Dev.* **2001**, *34*, 166–176. [CrossRef]
80. Garland, R. The mid-point on a rating scale: Is it desirable. *Mark. Bull.* **1991**, *2*, 66–70.

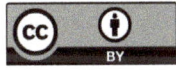

© 2020 by the authors. Licensee MDPI, Basel, Switzerland. This article is an open access article distributed under the terms and conditions of the Creative Commons Attribution (CC BY) license (http://creativecommons.org/licenses/by/4.0/).

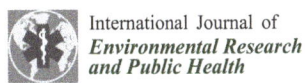

Article

Can We Predict the Evolution of Depressive Symptoms, Adjustment, and Perceived Social Support of Pregnant Women from Their Personality Characteristics? a Technology-Supported Longitudinal Study

Laura Andreu-Pejó [1,2], Verónica Martínez-Borba [1,2], Carlos Suso-Ribera [1] and Jorge Osma [2,3,*]

1. Nursing Department, Universitat Jaume I de Castelló, Castelló de la Plana, 12071 Valencia, Spain; pejo@uji.es (L.A.-P.); borba@uji.es (V.M.-B.); susor@uji.es (C.S.-R.)
2. Instituto de Investigación Sanitaria de Aragón, 50009 Zaragoza, Spain
3. Departmento de Psicología y Sociología, Universidad de Zaragoza, 44003 Teruel, Spain
* Correspondence: osma@unizar.es; Tel.: +34-97-8645-390 (ext. 861390)

Received: 24 April 2020; Accepted: 12 May 2020; Published: 14 May 2020

Abstract: *Background*: Research exploring the relationship between personality and important pregnancy outcomes (i.e., depressive symptoms, adjustment, and perceived social support) tends to be cross-sectional, arguably due to the difficulties of conducting longitudinal and mental health research in this population. The objective of this study is to use a web-based solution to longitudinally explore how personality traits are associated, not only with the co-occurrence of these outcomes but also with their evolution during pregnancy. Stability and change of these outcomes will also be investigated. *Methods*: The sample included 85 pregnant women attending several medical centers in Spain. The web-based assessment included sociodemographic and obstetric variables (ad hoc) and personality (at the second trimester only), and outcomes at both the second and the third trimester (i.e., depressive symptoms, adjustment, and perceived social support). *Results*: The results showed that adjustment worsened from the second to the third trimester of pregnancy. Neuroticism (N), low extraversion (E), and psychoticism (P) were cross-sectionally and longitudinally associated with outcomes. In addition, N and, to a lesser extent P, uniquely contributed to the evolution of these outcomes in the multivariate analyses, including autoregressions. *Conclusion*: Personality and especially N and P should be evaluated early during pregnancy mental health screening. The use of a web page appears to be a useful tool for that purpose. Technologies might also help disseminate mental health prevention programs for these women, which would be especially recommended for those with a personality profile characterized by high N and P and, to a lesser extent, low E.

Keywords: information and communication technologies; pregnancy; personality; depression; adjustment; social support

1. Introduction

Pregnancy is a period of great changes and demands for women and often challenges their ability to adapt to important physiological, social, and psychological changes and to continue to perform despite these difficulties [1]. Additionally, there is a large body of research suggesting that pregnant women may be particularly vulnerable to the detrimental effects of environmental stressors on their mental health [2], which altogether would explain the existence of high emotional distress and stress in this period of the woman's life [3]. For example, it is estimated that prenatal depression (PD) can affect up to 25%–38% of women worldwide [4]. In Spain, studies on the prevalence of

PD are scarce, although the available data indicates that at least 14.8% of women would experience moderate-to-severe symptoms of depression during pregnancy [5]. In addition, in Spain, the healthcare services provided to the perinatal women are mainly focused on the physical aspects related to pregnancy and postpartum, living aside the mental health aspects [6]. Thus, the study of mental well-being during the perinatal period and its predictors is relevant in this country if routine practices are to be changed. The clinical practice guidelines developed by the most prominent organizations in the field of perinatal mental health agree in emphasizing the importance of developing screening strategies that facilitate the detection of women who present risk factors for emotional problems throughout the perinatal period [7–10]. The risk factors for PD that are most frequently included in these clinical guidelines are current anxious and depressive symptoms, previous history of psychiatric problems, history of sexual abuse or child maltreatment, history of gender violence, adjustment problems with the partner, the experience of a traumatic birth, and the death of the baby during childbirth. In addition to these factors, there is evidence to suggest that certain normal personality traits, especially high neuroticism (N), high psychoticism (P), and low extraversion (E), are related to greater psychopathology in this population [11–13]. However, these guidelines do not yet support the need for the evaluation of these personality traits in pregnant women, which suggests that further research is needed in this field.

Regarding N, this is a personality trait characterized by the tendency to experience frequent and intense negative emotions in response to a stressful situation (e.g., pregnancy or childbirth). Furthermore, N is associated with a perception of ineffective coping. Thus, when N is high and persistent, processes such as worry, rumination, or emotional avoidance are likely to appear [14]. Interest in this personality trait, which is considered a widespread biological vulnerability factor for the etiology and maintenance of emotional disorders, including depression, has increased in recent years [15]. For example, Bunevicius et al. [16] found that high scores in N were, together with an unplanned and unwanted pregnancy, independent determinants of prenatal depressive disorders throughout pregnancy. In this same line, several authors have concluded that, of all personality dimensions, N could be considered the most important predictive risk factors for depression both in pregnancy and in the postpartum [13,17]. Additionally and linked with this tendency to experience negative emotions, N has been associated with low perceived social support [18] and poor adjustment to childbirth stressors [19].

Different to N, E refers to the tendency to experience positive emotions such as happiness, optimism, or enthusiasm and attitudes of security, activation, and interest for social interaction [20,21] and is associated with reduced vulnerability to affective disorders [22], increased social support [18], and successful adjustment to childbirth stressors [19]. In this sense, recent studies argue that low E, also known as introversion, would be a key personality trait associated with the onset of emotional disorders and poor adjustment during the perinatal period [23].

Finally, P is a personality trait that includes severe psychopathological conditions, such as deception or interpersonal alienation, to more frequent human expressions such as hostility, anger, and social isolation [24]. The literature exploring the role of P in pregnant women is scarce, but research so far supports the idea that high P poses a risk for perinatal women of PD [25]. The relationship between P and adjustment and social support during pregnancy remains unexplored. However, because P is inversely related to agreeableness [26], a key factor associated with perceived availability of social support [18] and effective coping use and adaptation during pregnancy [27], a negative impact of P on these outcomes would be expected.

To date, the relationship between personality and outcomes in perinatal research (i.e., depressive symptomatology and adaptation to the challenges associated with the perinatal period) has been predominantly explored using cross-sectional designs [13,16,17,25]. Consequently, little is actually known about the influence of normal personality traits (N, E, and P) in the evolution of depressive symptoms and adjustment of women during the perinatal period. Additionally, while it has been argued that poor social support, which is known to negatively impact mood and adjustment during the perinatal period [28,29], might be partly influenced by the personality profile of the mothers (i.e., high N, low E, and high P would arguably represent the high-risk profile) [13,17,20], this also remains unexplored during pregnancy. Note that social support and adjustment are key factors associated with well-being in the mother. Social support (i.e., perceived support from family, partners, and peers) is important both during pregnancy and at the postpartum, and low perceived support appears to add to the mental burden associated with the perinatal period (i.e., depression) [29]. Regarding maladjustment, this measure of poor emotional adaptation to the challenges that can occur during the perinatal period has been associated not only with suffering in the mother but also with internalizing problems in the baby [30]. In the light of the previous, the goal of the present investigation is to investigate whether the personality profile of prenatal women indeed predicts the evolution of depressive symptoms, adjustment to pregnancy, and social support perceived by these women using a longitudinal design.

As noted in the previous lines, there is an evident lack of longitudinal and prospective studies that try to clarify the role of personality traits and other psychosocial variables with respect to important perinatal outcomes, such as depressive symptoms and adjustment [31]. It is possible that this lack of longitudinal research is due to its high cost, especially in terms of time, because longitudinal research implies carrying out repeated evaluations during pregnancy. This might indeed problematic for public health systems since the time available for consultations is limited and estimated (i.e., 10–15 min per patient globally) [32]. Furthermore, reluctance to face-to-face psychological evaluations by women in the perinatal stage are frequent as a consequence of the stigma associated with mental illness [33].

The use of information and communication technologies (ICTs) might help overcome some of these limitations of traditional paper-and-pencil, face-to-face evaluations in the perinatal period. Briefly stated, repeated assessment using ICTs imposes less burden on healthcare professional and users, facilitates data collection since evaluations are carried out in the real context of women and traveling to the clinic for assessments is no longer needed, and minimizes stigmatization as they are perceived as being more anonymous and private [34]. Additionally, it is important to note that the use of ICTs in the general population has grown considerably in the past years. In 2008, 61% of homes in the European Union had access to the Internet. Now, in 2019, this has risen to 87% of homes [35]. Most importantly, in our field, 57% of pregnant women download health-related apps to seek information associated with pregnancy, which suggests that the use of ICTs in this field is growing significantly [36]. For this reason, the use of ICT in the field of mental health problems and maladjustment prevention [37], and specifically in the screening of depressive symptoms [38], is becoming increasingly popular and more feasible than ever. Particularly in Spain, where the public health system is very frequently used by the population, the implementation of such ICT solutions would be particularly useful to reduce the current burden associated with face-to-face assessments and interventions [36].

However, despite these promising benefits of ICT use in perinatal settings, most of the screening studies are cross-sectional and do not include the evaluation of risk factors for mental distress and poor adjustment to pregnancy [39]. From this need arises (Mamáfeliz (MMF; HappyMom)), a project that studies the risk factors for the development of perinatal emotional disorders longitudinally through the Internet (i.e., a web page). Thus, the main objective of this study is to explore how certain personality traits are associated, not only with the co-occurrence of depressive symptoms, maladjustment, and poor social support but also with their evolution during pregnancy. Importantly, a web application will be used for the longitudinal assessment of study variables. In addition to exploring the predictive role of personality on outcomes, we will also investigate the stability and change of depressive symptoms, adjustment, and social support during pregnancy. Stability and change will be investigated both at the order level (what is called "differential continuity") and at the group mean level (what is called "mean-level change"). We hypothesize scoring high in N and P will present a deterioration of depressive symptoms, adjustment, and perceived social support. By contrast, we anticipate that women scoring high in E will report an improvement in outcomes (i.e., reduction in depression and maladjustment and increase in social support). With respect to changes in outcomes, these will be investigated in an exploratory manner due to the limited literature in this regard.

2. Materials and Methods

2.1. Participants

The study sample consisted of 85 pregnant women who voluntarily agreed to participate in the project MMF and to be evaluated with a website throughout pregnancy. Women responded to two evaluations during pregnancy (completers), that is, between weeks 16–24 (Time 1) and weeks 30–36 of gestation (Time 2).

The mean age of the participants was 33.54 years (SD = 4.06; range 25–42). Of these, 94.1% were Spanish, 81.2% had a partner with whom they lived in the home, 94.1% had higher education, and 67.1% were working at the time of the first assessment. The sociodemographic characteristics of the participants are shown in Table 1.

Table 1. Sociodemographic characteristics of the sample (N = 85).

	Total
Nationality	
Spanish	94.1%
Latin American	2.4%
Western Europe	3.5%
Marital Status	
With a living partner	81.2%
Without a living partner	18.8%
Educational level	
≤12 years of education	5.9%
>12 years of education	94.1%
Employment situation	
Working	67.1%
Unemployment	20%
Sick leave	12.9%

2.2. Method

The study dissemination was made by the midwives of the collaborating centers. Study participation was offered to all pregnant women treated at the collaborating centers, which belong to the public or the private health network of MMF. The eligibility criteria were being a pregnant woman over 18 years of age, being fluent in Spanish, and having Internet access.

The collaborating healthcare personnel delivered the study information in writing along with a unique code for each participant to register into the program MMF. Thus, the entire study was conducted online. Once the participants accessed the application with their code, they had to read and accept the data protection and confidentiality documents and accept the informed consent form.

When the registration was completed, and the sociodemographic, obstetric, and medical data were filled, the evaluation of the main study variables began. Finally, the participants received a thank-you message, and they were informed that they would receive an email to complete the following evaluation in the following trimester.

The approval of the Ethics and Clinical Research Committees of all the collaborating centers was obtained.

2.3. Instruments

Sociodemographic, obstetric, and personality variables were assessed at Time 1 only (during the second trimester). Study outcomes (depressive symptoms, maladjustment, and social support) were evaluated longitudinally twice (during the second trimester and in the third trimester, to explore changes). Personality was only evaluated once to reduce the burden of assessment, because personality characteristics are relatively stable dispositions [40], and because the study focus was not on evaluating changes in personality but on predicting changes in outcomes based on baseline personality profiles.

Assessment of sociodemographic and obstetric variables (ad hoc items): Participants answered questions about their marital status, educational level, employment status, and economic level. They also responded to questions of an obstetric nature, such as the period of gestation, the history of abortion, pregnancy planning, and the level of pregnancy risk.

Revised Eysenck Personality Questionnaire (EPQ-RS) [41,42]: The EPQ-RS was administered to assess the three dimensions of normal personality from the Big Three's Eysenck model, namely neuroticism, extraversion, and psychoticism. This short version consists of 12 items per dimension in which every item evaluates a series of usual behaviors or ways of thinking or feeling. The questionnaire response format is "Yes" = 1 or "No" = 0, where higher scores represent a greater presence of the trait that it evaluates. Regarding their psychometric properties of the EPQ-RS, the three scales have an acceptable internal consistency in women, that is, a Cronbach's alpha of 0.82 for N, 0.79 for E, and 0.67 for P [42]. Similar results were found in our sample for N ($\alpha = 0.82$), E ($\alpha = 0.77$), and P ($\alpha = 0.60$).

Edinburgh Postnatal Depression Scale (EPDS) [43,44]: The EPDS consists of 10 items that evaluate the depressive symptoms experienced during the last seven days. Each item has four response options with a unique value that varies from 0 to 3. Items 1 and 2 are scored from 0 = "As much as always" to 3 = "Not at all", and items 3–10 are valued inversely, from 3 = "Yes, most of the time" to 0 = "No, never". The total score is obtained by summing the scores of all 10 items. Higher scores should be interpreted as indicating more severe depressive symptoms. The maximum total score is 30 points. The Spanish adaptation of the scale has obtained very good internal consistency estimates in pregnant women ($0.81 \leq \alpha \leq 0.85$, according to trimester during pregnancy) [43]. In our sample, good internal consistency was found both in the second ($\alpha = 0.86$) and the third ($\alpha = 0.85$) trimester of pregnancy.

Maladjustment Scale (MS) [45]. This scale consists of 5 items that evaluate to what extent the psychological distress experienced by the person affects different areas of daily life, that is work or studies, social activities, free time, family life, and relationship with their partner. In addition, the scale global item that refers to the overall degree of maladjustment. Each item is rated on a 6-point scale (0 = "None" to 5 = "Very Serious"). Higher scores represent higher maladjustment. Cronbach's alpha coefficient of the Spanish validation of the scale was 0.94 [45]. In our sample, good internal consistency was found both in the second ($\alpha = 0.85$) and the third ($\alpha = 0.82$) trimester of pregnancy.

Multidimensional scale of perceived social support (MSPSS) [46,47]. The MSPSS consists of 12 items evaluated on a 7-point Likert-type scale (1 = "Strongly disagree" to 7 = "Strongly agree"). The 12 items were designed to measure the perception of support in three areas: family (items 3, 4, 8, and 11), friends (items 6, 7, 9, and 12) and other significant persons (items 1, 2, 5, and 10). High scores indicate a greater perception of support received in each of the areas. In our study, we selected the family and friends scales to reduce the number of statistical analyses and to minimize the risk of multicollinearity problems. The use of the total score of the scale was discarded due to the interest in differentiating the support of the family from that of other agents, such as friends. The alpha coefficients of the family and friends scales were 0.89 and 0.92, respectively [47]. In our sample, good internal consistency was found both in the second ($\alpha = 0.94$) and the third ($\alpha = 0.94$) trimester in the family-scale. Similar results were found in the friends-scale both in the second ($\alpha = 0.97$) and the third ($\alpha = 0.95$) trimester.

2.4. Data Analysis

First, a descriptive analysis was made. Next, the change in the study variables was explored. Two different procedures were used to investigate the evolution of the study outcomes (i.e., depressive symptoms, adjustment, and social support) during pregnancy. On the one hand, the Student *t*-test for related samples was used to assess the change in mean scores (mean-level change). Additionally, Pearson's correlations were calculated to explore order changes between the two measurement times (differential continuity).

In order to explore the cross-sectional and prospective associations between baseline personality and outcomes, we first conducted a series of Pearson's correlations.

Finally, multivariate regression was carried out to explore to what extent the changes in study outcomes (i.e., depressive symptoms, adjustment, and perceived social support) at Time 2 (third trimester of pregnancy) were explained by personality factors, after controlling for important covariates (i.e., age the corresponding outcome at Time 1, that is during the second trimester of pregnancy). Age was included as a covariate because it has been related to psychosocial adjustment during the perinatal period in the literature [48]. A Holm–Bonferroni correction was used for all statistical analyses, which resulted in a *p*-value of 0.0125.

3. Results

3.1. Retention of the Participants Into the Online Assessment Program MMF

Regarding the participation of women in the online program MMF, 4500 women received codes to enroll in the program. Of these, 62.2% (n = 2797) effectively registered into the web, but only 5.9% (n = 266) participated at some point in the prenatal evaluation of the program. Finally, only 85 women completed both evaluations during the second and the third trimester during pregnancy. Figure 1 describes the flow diagram of study participation.

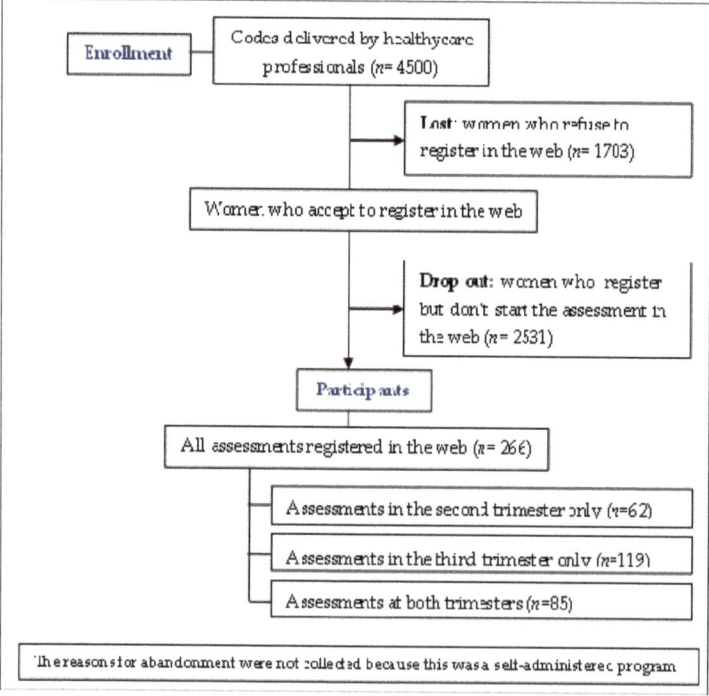

Figure 1. Flow chart of the participants in the study.

3.2. Descriptive Results of the Study Variables

Table 2 shows the means and standard deviations of the women's scores in the study variables, as well as a comparison with population normative scores. Overall, the women in our study showed a personality profile characterized by low N ($t = 7.17$, $p < 0.001$), average E ($t = 1.50$, $p = 0.135$), and low P ($t = 6.04$, $p < 0.001$). The levels of depressive symptoms during pregnancy in our sample were comparable to those of normative populations (all $p > 0.0125$). Perceived social support by family ($t = 3.59$, $p < 0.001$) and friends ($t = 4.55$, $p < 0.001$) was higher in our sample. Maladjustment scores could not be compared because normative scores do not exist for women.

Table 2. Descriptive statistics of study variables and comparison with normative scores.

Variables	N	Pregnant Women M (SD)	N	Reference Female Population M (SD)	t	p	d
Personality	85		583				
EPQ-RS (N)		3.8 (3.1)		6.6 (3.4)	7.169	<0.001	0.86
EPQ-RS (E)		8.7 (2.7)		8.2 (2.9)	1.498	0.135	0.18
EPQ-RS (P)		2.1 (1.8)		3.8 (2.5)	6.043	<0.001	0.78
Depressive symptoms	85		569				
EPDS (2nd T)		5.2 (4.6)		5.7 (3.9)	1.076	0.282	0.12
EPDS (3rd T)		4.7 (4.3)		5.7 (4.3)	1.999	0.046	0.23
Maladjustment	85						
MS		6.2 (5.3)		-	-	-	-
Social support	85		265				
MSPSS (Family)		6.5 (0.8)		6.0 (1.2)	3.592	<0.001	0.49
MSPSS (Friends)		6.3 (1.0)		5.6 (1.3)	4.549	<0.001	0.60

EPQ-RS = Eysenck Personality Questionnaire (N: neuroticism; E: extraversion; P: psychoticism); EPDS = Edinburgh Postnatal Depression Scale; T = trimester; MS = maladjustment scale; MSPSS = Multidimensional Scale of Perceived Social Support.

3.3. Evolution of Outcomes (Depressive Symptoms, Adjustment, and Perceived Social Support) During Pregnancy

Table 3 presents the means and standard deviations of study outcomes, as well as the analyses of change at the mean level and at the rank order level. Regarding mean values, only a significant increase in maladjustment was observed during pregnancy ($t = 4.83$, $p < 0.001$). Taking changes at the order level, the moderate-to-strong significant correlations should be interpreted as indicating some stability at the order level. Social support variables were the ones that remained more stable in terms of order (strong correlation).

Table 3. Evolution of study outcomes from the second (Time 1) to the third trimester (Time 2).

	Time 1		Time 2		t	95% CI	r
	M	SD	M	SD			
EPDS	5.2	4.6	4.7	4.3	−1.024	−1.42, 0.46	0.53 **
MS	6.2	5.3	8.9	5.4	4.832 **	1.59, 3.80	0.54 **
MSPSS (F)	6.5	0.8	6.4	1.0	−0.744	−0.15, 0.07	0.85 **
MSPSS (Fr)	6.3	1.0	6.1	1.0	−1.493	−0.29, 0.04	0.71 **

M = mean; SD = standard deviation; t = Student's t ; r = Pearson's correlation; EPDS = Edinburgh Postnatal Depression Scale; T = trimester; MS = maladjustment scale; MSPSS = Multidimensional Scale of Perceived Social Support; F = family; Fr = friends. * p (Holm Bonferroni sequential correction) < 0.0125; ** p < 0.001.

3.4. Bivariate Associations Between Personality Variables, Depressive Symptoms, Adjustment, and Perceived Social Support

Table 4 shows the bivariate associations between the main study variables. The results of the correlations between the variables evaluated at Time 1 (second trimester) showed that N was associated with greater depressive symptoms ($r = 0.61$, $p < 0.001$), greater maladjustment ($r = 0.29$, $p = 0.007$), and poorer perceived family ($r = -0.31$, $p = 0.004$) and friends support ($r = -0.34$, $p = 0.002$). Conversely, high levels in E were associated with a decreased depressive symptoms ($r = -0.43$, $p < 0.001$), reduced maladjustment ($r = -0.30$, $p = 0.006$), and increased perceived support by the family ($r = 0.34$, $p < 0.001$) and friends ($r = 0.34$, $p = 0.002$).

Table 4. Correlations between personality, age, and outcomes (i.e., depressive symptoms, adjustment, and social support).

	2	3	4	5	6	7	8	9	10	11	12
Second trimester											
1. Neuroticism	−0.36 **	0.19	−0.31 *	−0.34 *	0.61 **	0.29 *	0.10	−0.29 *	−0.48 **	0.54 **	0.46 **
2. Extraversion		−0.09	0.34 **	0.34 *	−0.43 **	−0.30 *	−0.12	0.28 *	0.38 **	−0.29 *	−0.36 **
3. Psychoticism			−0.34 *	−0.19	0.11	0.03	−0.09	−0.29 *	−0.34 *	0.33 *	0.08
4. Family support				0.65 **	−0.23	−0.20	−0.05	0.85 **	0.67 **	−0.33 *	−0.29 *
5. Friends support					−0.27	−0.18	0.04	0.60 **	0.71 **	−0.31 *	−0.16
6. Depression						0.67 **	0.13	−0.18	−0.28 *	0.53 **	0.48 **
7. Maladjustment							0.11	−0.13	−0.22	0.27	0.54 **
8. Age (third trimester)								−0.10	−0.04	0.18	0.15
9. Family support									0.71 **	−0.38 **	−0.27
10. Friends support										−0.47 **	−0.34 *
11. Depression											0.44 **
12. Maladjustment											

In bold, the intercorrelations between variables at the second trimester and their corresponding variable at the third trimester. * p (Holm Bonferroni sequential correction) < 0.0125; ** $p < 0.001$.

The cross-sectional associations between study variables evaluated in Time 2 (third trimester) showed family support ($r = -0.38$, $p < 0.001$) and friends support ($r = -0.47$, $p < 0.001$) were associated with decreased depressive symptoms. Support from friends ($r = -0.34$, $p = 0.001$) and depressive symptoms ($r = 0.44$, $p < 0.001$) were inversely associated with maladjustment.

Finally, the results of the longitudinal correlations showed that N at Time 1 was prospectively related to more severe depressive symptomatology ($r = 0.54$, $p < 0.001$), maladjustment ($r = 0.46$, $p < 0.001$), and poorer support from family ($r = -0.29$, $p = 0.008$) and friends ($r = -0.48$, $p < 0.001$) at Time 2. Similarly, P at Time 1 was related to greater depressive symptomatology ($r = 0.33$, p = 0.002) and less support from family members ($r = -0.29$, $p = 0.007$) and friends ($r = -0.34$, $p = 0.002$) at Time 2. Conversely, E at Time 1 was associated with less intense depressive symptoms ($r = -0.29$, $p = 0.008$) and maladjustment ($r = -0.36$, $p < 0.001$), as well as with increased support from the family ($r = 0.28$, $p = 0.010$) and friends ($r = 0.38$, $p < 0.001$) at Time 2.

Different to personality, age was not cross-sectionally or longitudinally related to outcomes (all $p > 0.050$).

3.5. Personality Factors as Predictors of Depressive Symptoms, Maladjustment, and Perceived Social Support Evolution During Pregnancy: Multivariate Analysis)

Table 5 presents the results of the multivariate regression analyzes. In order to decide whether potential covariates should be included in the regressions, we investigated the bivariate associations between economic level, abortion history, pregnancy risk, and history of childbirth. None of the correlations were significant and they were all very small in size (all $r < 0.20$, all $p > 0.05$), which might have been influenced by the low heterogeneity of responses (approximately 75% of women had moderately high economic levels, did not have previous abortions, and had very a low risk pregnancy and over 65% of them were primiparous). Thus, there was no evidence to support their inclusion in the multivariate regression and doing so would only increase the risk of multicollinearity.

Across personality variables, both N ($\beta = 0.40$, $t = 2.62$, $p < 0.001$, 95% CI = 0.10, 0.71) and P ($\beta = 0.58$, $t = 2.62$, $p < 0.001$, 95% IC = 0.10, 0.71) uniquely and significantly contributed to the prediction of depressive symptoms at a prospective level after controlling for the effect of baseline depressive symptoms. In relation to maladjustment, the only personality factor to prospectively and significantly contribute to this outcome above and beyond baseline maladjustment levels was N ($\beta = 0.50$, $t = 2.99$, $p < 0.0125$, 95% CI = 0.17, 0.84). Finally, and similar to depressive symptomatology, N ($\beta = -0.07$, $t = -2.65$, $p < 0.0125$, 95% CI = −0.12, −0.02) and P ($\beta = -0.10$, $t = -2.58$, $p < 0.0125$, 95% CI = −0.18, 0.02) were the personality dimensions to significantly and uniquely contribute to the prediction of perceived social support from friends at a prospective level and after controlling for baseline perceived friends support. Regarding perceived family support, the results did not indicate that personality variables contributed to the evolution of this outcome.

Table 5. Multivariate regression predicting study outcomes.

DV	Beta	t	95% CI	R^2 Change	F Change
Depression (T2)					
Block 1: depression (T1)	0.28	2.70 **	0.07, 0.50	0.279	32.15 **
Block 2: age (T1)	0.14	1.56	−0.04, 0.33	0.013	1.55
Block 3: personality (T1)				0.133	6.08 **
Neuroticism	0.40	2.62 **	0.10, 0.71		
Extraversion	−0.02	−0.16	−0.33, 0.28		
Psychoticism	0.58	2.84 **	0.17, 0.99		
Maladjustment (T2)					
Block 1: maladjustment (T1)	0.42	4.44 **	0.23, 0.60	0.291	34.09 **
Block 2: age (T1)	0.09	0.74	−0.15, 0.32	0.009	1.09
Block 3: personality (T1)				0.112	5.04 *
Neuroticism	0.50	2.99 *	0.17, 0.84		
Extraversion	−0.26	−1.35	−0.64, 0.12		
Psychoticism	0.03	0.12	−0.48, 0.55		
Family support (T2)					
Block 1: family support (T1)	0.95	12.48 **	0.80, 1.10	0.719	212.81 **
Block 2: age (T1)	−0.02	−1.03	−0.04, 0.01	0.004	1.08
Block 3: personality (T1)				0.001	0.06
Neuroticism	−0.06	−0.31	−0.05, 0.03		
Extraversion	−0.07	−0.31	−0.05, 0.04		
Psychoticism	−0.04	−0.12	−0.07, 0.06		
Social support friends (T2)					
Block 1: friends support (T1)	0.56	7.39 **	0.41, 0.71	0.506	84.95 **
Block 2 : age (T1)	−0.01	−0.68	−0.05, 0.02	0.005	0.82
Block 3: personality (T1)				0.100	6.73 **
Neuroticism	−0.07	−2.65 *	−0.12, −0.02		
Extraversion	0.03	1.15	−0.03, 0.09		
Psychoticism	−0.10	−2.58 *	−0.18, 0.02		

T1 = second trimester; T2 = third trimester. * p (Holm Bonferroni sequential correction) < 0.0125; ** p < 0.001.

4. Discussion

The present study aims at providing further evidence into the role of personality (N, E, and P) and important pregnancy outcomes, namely, depressive symptoms, adjustment to pregnancy challenges, and perceived social support. In order to achieve this goal and in order to address some limitations observed in the literature, this investigation included two major improvements compared to previous studies, namely, the implementation of a longitudinal design and the use of ICTs for assessment. Overall, the results indicated an important contribution of N and, to a lesser extent, P on the evolution of study outcomes, but failed to reveal a significant prospective association between E and outcomes when controlling for the remaining personality factors and baseline outcome scores. Additionally, while the inclusion of ICTs for technology made the longitudinal evaluation more feasible for healthcare professionals, response rates by participants were very poor, which will be discussed in more detail in the following lines.

Indeed, one of the strengths of the present study was the longitudinal investigation of the evolution of important perinatal outcomes. In this sense, the results showed that significant mean-level changes only occurred in maladjustment, so that women reported a poorer adaptation when comparing the second and the third trimester of pregnancy. As evidenced in past research, pregnancy imposes major changes in the lifestyles of women and requires important psychological resources for an adequate adaptation to these changes [1], which means that pregnancy can become a stressful period for women [49]. An interesting finding was that, according to our results, it is at the last stage during pregnancy when women experience greater limitations in their life areas (e.g., work activity, leisure, or social life). Based on our data, these increased difficulties in adaptation did not result in a proportional depressed mood, which suggests that a deterioration of adjustment with time might have been expected by the participants or was well tolerated at an emotional level. While acknowledging the aforementioned increase in adjustment challenges in the third trimester due to biological reasons, it is also true that preventive interventions focused on offering information about changes during pregnancy and guidelines to better adjust to such changes, such as maintaining social and leisure activities and physical activity, could help mitigate the degree of maladjustment in this period of pregnancy. As stated in previous research, ICTs can help to provide information-based interventions, physical exercise, or behavioral activation in perinatal women at reduced costs and high disseminability [37,50,51].

As noted in the previous lines, depressive symptomatology did not change during pregnancy in the present study, which contrasts with some past research [16]. These differences could be explained by several reasons, such as the sample sizes used in previous investigations, the country of origin of women participating in the studies, or their educational level, which was very high in the present study and this is known to be a protective factor for depression [52]. In addition, it is also possible that our participants have present protective factors for depression, such as an adequate evolution of pregnancy, an overall good health status, or adequate coping strategies.

Similar to depression, no changes were observed in perceived social support, which was high at both assessment times. This is an important finding considering that social support seems to have a buffering effect on women's health during the perinatal stage and, as some authors affirm, social support could contribute to reducing the impact of stress and depressive symptomatology [48]. Related to this, the fact that in the present study baseline support from family and friends was prospectively associated with reduced depressive symptomatology is consistent with the idea that social support facilitates the journey to motherhood [53].

Regarding the relationships between personality and outcomes, our results showed significant associations both at the cross-sectional and longitudinal level between personality traits and outcomes. Consistent with the literature, N and E showed the strongest associations with outcomes, and P was mostly associated with the social variables included in the study (i.e., social support) [16,17]. As expected, women who presented high N and low E scores reported more depressive symptoms, poorer adjustment, and less social support cross-sectionally. This adds to the existing literature showing that N is a risk factor for well-being and adaptation to challenges, such as those experienced during pregnancy, while E would be a protective factor in such situations [11,17,25].

Interestingly and one of the key contributions of the present study was the finding that the aforementioned contribution of personality, particularly in the case of N and P, was preserved in the multivariate analyses, including prospective data and controlling for the auto-regressions. This design allowed us to confirm that personality is not only associated with prenatal outcomes in a cross-sectional manner, but that N and P might be risk factors for the deterioration of many of these outcomes. It is important to note that personality explained an important percentage of the variance of prospective outcomes (13.3% for depressive symptoms, 11.2% for adjustment, and 10% for perceived social support), considering baseline scores in the outcomes were controlled for. While cross-sectional associations are indeed important and informative, the prospective relationships evidenced in the present investigation add to past research in suggesting that, if prevention or intervention programs are not provided to populations at risk (i.e., high N and P), they are likely to continue to worsen in the mental symptomatology, adaptation, and social satisfaction during pregnancy, which puts them at risk for their own well-being and that of the newborns [54].

Note that one of the present study goals was to investigate whether personality characteristics were indeed associated with social support during pregnancy. Our results support past research in showing that E is associated with satisfaction with social life, and N and P are inversely associated with this outcome [40]. Because social support was inversely associated with depressive symptoms and maladjustment, these results support the idea that intervention programs should be addressed to women at risk for poor perceived social support (i.e., those with a low E and high N and P profile). Again, ICT solutions might be useful tools to provide social support to women during pregnancy [55].

Contrary to our expectations, age did not show significant associations with any of the study variables. The literature is ambiguous when establishing a relationship between age and the risk of depression during pregnancy [11]. While some studies suggest that younger women are at greater risk of developing depressive symptoms [56], inconsistent findings have also been reported [57]. These discrepancies are probably due to differences in the mean age of women from the different studies. However, a review by Biaggi et al. [11] indicated no association between age and perinatal outcomes, which is consistent with our findings and suggests that older age might not be a key protective factor for well-being and adjustment in pregnant women.

A final contribution of the present study was the implementation of a web-based application for data collection. From our experience, the use of a web page for the longitudinal evaluation of risk factors and associated psychological variables during pregnancy has represented a simple, inexpensive, and confidential alternative that we believe helped overcome some of the current barriers for the longitudinal assessment of mental health problems in perinatal care, most notably the insufficient consultation time [34,58]. Additionally, research suggests that the application of ICT facilitates perinatal mental health screening due to the reduced stigma associated with non-face-to-face evaluations, the flexibility with which assessments can be completed (anywhere and anytime), and the reduced costs in terms of professional time [50,59].

While acknowledging the benefits of ICT for mental health screening, as noted by our low participation and retention rates, the implementation of online longitudinal assessments with very limited professional involvement is still challenging. One of the main barriers for participation, as informally reported by some of the participants, was associated with the time required to complete the evaluation protocol, which was perceived as being too extensive. As indicated by recent research conducting longitudinal and ecological momentary assessments, a reduction of items (e.g., validation of individual item measures against full traditional scales) and the selection of key questionnaires only is fundamental in design with technology and longitudinal designs [60]. The use of apps, which are more accessible and acceptable for perinatal women, might help as well in this direction [39]. Finally, the inclusion of gamification or treatment elements (i.e., tips to be used during pregnancy) might also facilitate engagement with longitudinal studies [61].

Limitations

This study has some limitations that should be taken into account. First, note that the sample is composed of a group of women with very similar sociodemographic characteristics, which limits the generalization of our findings. The small sample size (N = 85) also represents a problem. In this sense, it is important to consider the main obstacle associated with using the Internet in self-applied screening, prevention, or treatment programs, which is low adherence. In our case, as noted in the previous lines, the fact that this was a longitudinal study with a significant load in terms of the number of questionnaires to be completed might have negatively impacted on sample participation and retention. Note, however, that this is a frequent finding in the perinatal research using technology, even when treatment is provided [62]. As noted earlier, there are a number of initiatives that could be implemented to minimize this problem when conducting longitudinal assessments. Another limitation refers to the reliance on self-report measures only, which might have led to interpretation bias or social desirability. However, and in relation to social desirability, the anonymous and online nature of the evaluations should have encouraged honesty [63].

5. Conclusions

In sum, our results support the idea that certain personality characteristics (high N and P) might pose a risk to women for a deterioration of important well-being outcomes. This is important for prevention purposes and would suggest that women characterized by high N or high P should be monitored more frequently during pregnancy (e.g., using ICTs). Additionally, in order to promote changes in personality tendencies, self-applied programs, again using ICTs, could be the first solution in a stepped manner of care, which is more feasible than offering face-to-face individual treatments for all, considering the limited existing resources in public health settings in Spain [64].

It is important to note that an intervention program specifically aimed at reducing N and the negative consequences derived from this vulnerability factor currently exists [14]. This intervention, called the Unified Protocol, allows individuals to acquire a set of emotional regulation strategies that facilitate tolerance to discomfort derived from intense emotions, such as sadness or anxiety [65]. Future studies should test if the Unified Protocol effectively reduces N levels in a sample of pregnant women and whether, consequently, an improvement in outcomes (e.g., depressive symptoms, adaptation to pregnancy, and perceived social support) occurs. Again, and according to previous similar research, ICTs could be used to conduct and easily disseminate these interventions in women in the perinatal stage [60]. This opens fascinating avenues for future research in the field.

Author Contributions: Conceptualization J.O., C.S.-R., L.A.-P., and V.M.-B.; methodology, J.O. and C.S.-R.; formal analysis, C.S.-R.; investigation, L.A.-P.; resources, J.O., C.S.-R., L.A.-P., and V.M.-B.; data curation, J.O. and C.S.-R.; writing—original draft preparation, L.A.-P.; writing—review and editing, J.O., C.S.-R., and V.M.-B.; supervision, J.O.; project administration, J.O.; funding acquisition J.O. and V.M.-B. All authors have read and agreed to the published version of the manuscript.

Funding: This research was funded by the Universitat Jaume I, grant number Predoc/2018/43; the Gobierno de Aragon (Departamento de Innovacion, Investigación y Universidad) and Feder 2014–2020 "Construyendo Europa Desde Aragón", research group grant S31_20D; the Conselleria de Sanidad (Agencia Valenciana de Salud), grant number SMP 45/2011; the Fundación Universitaria Antonio Gargalo and the Obra Social Ibercaja, grant numbers 2013/B006 and 2014/B006.

Acknowledgments: The authors thank all the women who voluntarily participate in this study and all collaborating centers for their support in the dissemination campaigns.

Conflicts of Interest: The authors declare no conflict of interest.

References

1. Glazier, R.H.; Elgar, F.J.; Goel, V.; Holzapfel, S. Stress, social support, and emotional distress in a community sample of pregnant women. *J. Psychosom. Obstet. Gynecol.* **2005**, *25*, 247–255. [CrossRef] [PubMed]
2. Rubertsson, C.; Hellström, J.; Cross, M.; Sydsjö, G. Anxiety in early pregnancy: Prevalence and contributing factors. *Arch. Women's Ment. Heal.* **2014**, *17*, 221–228. [CrossRef] [PubMed]
3. Rallis, S.; Skouteris, H.; McCabe, M.P.; Milgrom, J. A prospective examination of depression, anxiety and stress throughout pregnancy. *Women Birth* **2014**, *27*, e36–e42. [CrossRef] [PubMed]
4. Accortt, E.E.; Cheadle, A.C.D.; Schetter, C.D. Prenatal depression and adverse birth outcomes: An updated systematic review. *Matern. Child Heal. J.* **2015**, *19*, 1306–1337. [CrossRef]
5. Rodriguez, M.D.L.F.; Le, H.-N.; La Cruz, I.V.-D.; Crespo, M.E.O.; Méndez, N.I. Feasibility of screening and prevalence of prenatal depression in an obstetric setting in Spain. *Eur. J. Obstet. Gynecol. Reprod. Boil.* **2017**, *215*, 101–105. [CrossRef]
6. Clinical Practice Guideline for Care in Pregnancy and Puerperium. Available online: https://portal.guiasalud.es/wp-content/uploads/2018/12/GPC_533_Embarazo_AETSA_compl_en.pdf (accessed on 6 May 2020).
7. The American College os Obstetricians and Gynecologist. ACOG Screening for perinatal depression. *Obstet. Gynecol.* **2018**, *132*, e208–e212. [CrossRef]
8. Antenatal and Postnatal Mental Health: Clinical Management and Service Guidance. Available online: https://www.nice.org.uk/guidance/cg192 (accessed on 6 May 2020).
9. Guia De Practica Clinica de atención en el embarazo y puerperio. Available online: https://portal.guiasalud.es/wp-content/uploads/2018/12/GPC_533_Embarazo_AETSA_compl.pdf (accessed on 6 May 2020).
10. Force, U.P.S.T.; Curry, S.J.; Krist, A.H.; Owens, U.K.; Barry, M.J.; Caughey, A.B.; Davidson, K.W.; Doubeni, C.A.; Epling, J.W.; Grossman, D.C.; et al. Interventions to Prevent Perinatal Depression: US Preventive Services Task Force Recommendation Statement. *JAMA* **2019**, *321*, 580–587. [CrossRef]
11. Biaggi, A.; Conroy, S.; Pawlby, S.; Pariante, C.M. Identifying the women at risk of antenatal anxiety and depression: A systematic review. *J. Affect. Disord.* **2015**, *191*, 62–77. [CrossRef]
12. Lancaster, C.A.; Gold, K.J.; Flynn, H.A.; Yoo, H.; Marcus, S.M.; Davis, M.M. Risk factors for depressive symptoms during pregnancy: A systematic review. *Am. J. Obstet. Gynecol.* **2010**, *202*, 5–14. [CrossRef]
13. Dennis, C.-L.; Boyce, P. Further psychometric testing of a brief personality scale to measure vulnerability to postpartum depression. *J. Psychosom. Obstet. Gynecol.* **2005**, *25*, 305–311. [CrossRef]
14. Barlow, D.H.; Sauer-Zavala, S.; Carl, J.R.; Bullis, J.R.; Ellard, K.K. The Nature, Diagnosis, and Treatment of Neuroticism. *Clin. Psychol. Sci.* **2013**, *2*, 344–365. [CrossRef]
15. Barlow, D.; Ellard, K.K.; Sauer-Zavala, S.; Bullis, J.R.; Carl, J.R. The Origins of Neuroticism. *Perspect. Psychol. Sci.* **2014**, *9*, 481–496. [CrossRef] [PubMed]

16. Bunevicius, R.; Kusminskas, L.; Bunevicius, A.; Nadisauskiene, R.J.; Jureniene, K.; Pop, V.J. Psychosocial risk factors for depression during pregnancy. *Acta Obstet. et Gynecol. Scand.* **2009**, *88*, 599–605. [CrossRef] [PubMed]
17. Podolska, M.Z.; Bidzan, M.; Majkowicz, M.; Podolski, J.; Sipak-Szmigiel, O.; Ronin-Walknowska, E. Personality traits assessed by the NEO Five-Factor Inventory (NEO-FFI) as part of the perinatal depression screening program. *Med Sci. Monit.* **2010**, *16*, 77–81.
18. Swickert, R. Personality and social support processes. In *The Cambridge Handbook of Personality Psychology*; Cambridge University Press: New York, NY, USA, 2012; pp. 524–540.
19. Johnston, R.; Brown, A. Maternal trait personality and childbirth: The role of extraversion and neuroticism. *Midwifery* **2013**, *29*, 1244–1250. [CrossRef]
20. Watson, D.; Clark, L.A. Extraversion and Its Positive Emotional Core. In *Handbook of Personality Psychology*, 1st ed.; Hogan, R., Johnson, J., Briggs, S., Eds.; Academic Press: Amsterdam, The Netherlands, 1997; pp. 767–793.
21. Yang, S.K.; Ha, Y. Predicting Posttraumatic Growth among Firefighters: The Role of Deliberate Rumination and Problem-Focused Coping. *Int. J. Environ. Res. Public Heal.* **2019**, *16*, 3879. [CrossRef]
22. Kotov, R.; Gamez, W.; Schmidt, F.; Watson, D. Linking "big" personality traits to anxiety, depressive, and substance use disorders: A meta-analysis. *Psychol. Bull.* **2010**, *136*, 768–821. [CrossRef]
23. Peñacoba-Puente, C.; Marín-Morales, D.; Carmona-Monge, F.J.; Furlong, L.V. Post-Partum Depression, Personality, and Cognitive-Emotional Factors: A Longitudinal Study on Spanish Pregnant Women. *Heal. Care Women Int.* **2015**, *37*, 1–21. [CrossRef]
24. Eysenck, H. The definition and measurement of psychoticism. *Pers. Individ. Differ.* **1992**, *13*, 757–785. [CrossRef]
25. Zeng, Y.; Cui, Y.; Li, J. Prevalence and predictors of antenatal depressive symptoms among Chinese women in their third trimester: A cross-sectional survey. *BMC Psychiatry* **2015**, *15*, 66. [CrossRef]
26. McCrae, R.R.; Costa, P.T., Jr. Comparison of EPI and psychoticism scales with measures of the five-factor model of personality. *Pers. Individ. Differ.* **1985**, *6*, 587–597. [CrossRef]
27. Peñacoba, C.; Rodriguez, L.; Carmona, J.; Marin, D. Agreeableness and pregnancy: Relations with coping and psychiatric symptoms, a longitudinal study on Spanish pregnant women. *Women Heal.* **2017**, *58*, 204–220. [CrossRef] [PubMed]
28. Martini, J.; Petzoldt, J.; Einsle, F.; Beesdo-Baum, K.; Höfler, M.; Wittchen, H.-U. Risk factors and course patterns of anxiety and depressive disorders during pregnancy and after delivery: A prospective-longitudinal study. *J. Affect. Disord.* **2015**, *175*, 385–395. [CrossRef] [PubMed]
29. Milgrom, J.; Hirshler, Y.; Reece, J.; Holt, C.; Gemmill, A.W. Social Support-A Protective Factor for Depressed Perinatal Women? *Int. J. Environ. Res. Public Heal.* **2019**, *16*, 1426. [CrossRef]
30. Bouvette-Turcot, A.-A.; Bernier, A.; Leblanc, E. Maternal Psychosocial Maladjustment and Child Internalizing Symptoms: Investigating the Modulating Role of Maternal Sensitivity. *J. Abnorm. Child Psychol.* **2016**, *45*, 157–170. [CrossRef]
31. Field, T. Prenatal depression effects on early development: A review. *Infant Behav. Dev.* **2011**, *34*, 1–14. [CrossRef]
32. Outomuro, D.; Actis, A. Estimación del tiempo de consulta ambulatoria en clínica médica. *Revista médica de Chile* **2013**, *141*, 361–366. [CrossRef]
33. McLoughlin, J. Stigma associated with postnatal depression: A literature review. *Br. J. Midwifery* **2013**, *21*, 784–791. [CrossRef]
34. Kingston, D.; Austin, M.-P.; Heaman, M.; McDonald, S.; Lasiuk, G.; Sword, W.A.; Giallo, R.; Hegadoren, K.; Vermeyden, L.; Van Zanten, S.V.; et al. Barriers and facilitators of mental health screening in pregnancy. *J. Affect. Disord.* **2015**, *186*, 350–357. [CrossRef]
35. Internet Use by Individuals. Available online: https://ec.europa.eu/eurostat/databrowser/view/tin00028/default/table?lang=en (accessed on 15 April 2020).
36. Osma, J.; Barrera, A.Z.; Ramphos, E. Are Pregnant and Postpartum Women Interested in Health-Related Apps? Implications for the Prevention of Perinatal Depression. *Cyberpsychol. Behav. Soc. Netw.* **2016**, *19*, 412–415. [CrossRef]

37. Lewis, B.A.; Gjerdingen, D.K.; Avery, M.D.; Guo, H.; Sirard, J.R.; Bonikowske, A.R.; Marcus, B.H. Examination of a telephone-based exercise intervention for the prevention of postpartum depression: Design, methodology, and baseline data from The Healthy Mom study. *Contemp. Clin. Trials* **2012**, *33*, 1150–1158. [CrossRef] [PubMed]
38. Belisario, J.M.; Gupta, A.K.; O'Donoghue, J.; Ramchandani, P.; Morrison, C.; Car, J. Implementation of depression screening in antenatal clinics through tablet computers: Results of a feasibility study. *BMC Med Inform. Decis. Mak.* **2017**, *17*, 59. [CrossRef]
39. Martínez-Borba, V.; Suso-Ribera, C.; Osma, J. The Use of Information and Communication Technologies in Perinatal Depression Screening: A Systematic Review. *Cyberpsychol. Behav. Soc. Netw.* **2018**, *21*, 741–752. [CrossRef] [PubMed]
40. Ozer, D.; Benet-Martinez, V. Personality and the Prediction of Consequential Outcomes. *Annu. Rev. Psychol.* **2006**, *57*, 401–421. [CrossRef] [PubMed]
41. Eysenck, S.; Eysenck, H.; Barrett, P. A revised version of the psychoticism scale. *Pers. Individ. Differ.* **1985**, *6*, 21–29. [CrossRef]
42. Eysenck, H.J.; Eysenck, S.B.G. *EPQ-R: Cuestionario Revisado de Personalidad de Eysenck: Versiones Completa (EPQ-R) y Abreviada (EPQ-RS): Manual*, 2nd ed.; Hodder & Stoughton: London, UK, 2001.
43. Vázquez, M.B.; Míguez, M.D.C. Validation of the Edinburgh postnatal depression scale as a screening tool for depression in Spanish pregnant women. *J. Affect. Disord.* **2019**, *246*, 515–521. [CrossRef]
44. Cox, J.L.; Holden, J.M.; Sagovsky, R. Detection of postnatal depression. Development of the 10-item Edinburgh Postnatal Depression Scale. *Br. J. Psychiatry* **1987**, *150*, 782–786. [CrossRef]
45. Echeburúa, E.; de Corral, P.; Fernandez-Montalvo, J. Escala de inadaptación (EI): Propiedades psicométricas en contextos clínicos. *Análisis y Modificación de Conducta* **2000**, *26*, 325–340.
46. Zimet, G.D.; Dahlem, N.W.; Zimet, S.G.; Farley, G.K. The Multidimensional Scale of Perceived Social Support. *J. Pers. Assess.* **1988**, *52*, 30–41. [CrossRef]
47. Landeta, O.; Calvete, E. Adaptación y validación de la escala multidimensional de apoyo social percibido. *Ansiedad y estrés* **2002**, *8*, 173–182.
48. Guedes, M.; Canavarro, M.C. Personal competencies, social resources, and psychosocial adjustment of primiparous women of advanced maternal age and their partners. *Child Adolesc. Soc. Work. J.* **2015**, *36*, 506–521. [CrossRef] [PubMed]
49. Rodriguez, A.; Bohlin, G.; Lindmark, G. Symptoms across pregnancy in relation to psychosocial and biomedical factors. *Acta Obstet. et Gynecol. Scand.* **2001**, *80*, 213–223. [CrossRef] [PubMed]
50. O'Mahen, H.; A Richards, D.; Woodford, J.; Wilkinson, E.; McGinley, J.; Taylor, R.S.; Warren, F.C. Netmums: A phase II randomized controlled trial of a guided Internet behavioural activation treatment for postpartum depression. *Psychol. Med.* **2013**, *44*, 1675–1689. [CrossRef] [PubMed]
51. Salonen, A.; Pridham, K.F.; Brown, R.L.; Kaunonen, M. Impact of an internet-based intervention on Finnish mothers' perceptions of parenting satisfaction, infant centrality and depressive symptoms during the postpartum year. *Midwifery* **2014**, *30*, 112–122. [CrossRef]
52. Bjelland, I.; Krokstad, S.; Mykletun, A.; Dahl, A.A.; Tell, G.S.; Tambs, K. Does a higher educational level protect against anxiety and depression? The HUNT study. *Soc. Sci. Med.* **2008**, *66*, 1334–1345. [CrossRef]
53. Warren, P.L. First-time mothers: Social support and confidence in infant care. *J. Adv. Nurs.* **2005**, *50*, 479–488. [CrossRef]
54. Gavin, N.I.; Gaynes, B.; Lohr, K.; Meltzer-Brody, S.; Gartlehner, G.; Swinson, T. Perinatal Depression: A Systematic Review of Prevalence and Incidence. *Obstet. Gynecol.* **2005**, *106*, 1071–1083. [CrossRef]
55. Caramlau, I.; Barlow, J.; Sembi, S.; McKenzie-McHarg, K.; McCabe, C. Mums 4 Mums: Structured telephone peer-support for women experiencing postnatal depression. Pilot and exploratory RCT of its clinical and cost effectiveness. *Trials* **2011**, *12*, 88. [CrossRef]
56. Siegel, R.S.; Brandon, A.R. Adolescents, Pregnancy, and Mental Health. *J. Pediatr. Adolesc. Gynecol.* **2014**, *27*, 138–150. [CrossRef]
57. Fellenzer, J.L.; Cibula, D.A. Intendedness of Pregnancy and Other Predictive Factors for Symptoms of Prenatal Depression in a Population-Based Study. *Matern. Child Heal. J.* **2014**, *18*, 2426–2436. [CrossRef]
58. Goodman, J.H. Women's Attitudes, Preferences, and Perceived Barriers to Treatment for Perinatal Depression. *Birth* **2009**, *36*, 60–69. [CrossRef] [PubMed]

59. Danaher, B.G.; Milgrom, J.; Seeley, J.R.; Stuart, S.; Schembri, C.; Tyler, M.S.; Ericksen, J.; Lester, W.; Gemmill, A.W.; Lewinsohn, P.; et al. Web-based Intervention for Postpartum Depression: Formative Research and Design of the MomMoodBooster Program. *JMIR Res. Protoc.* **2012**, *1*, e18. [CrossRef] [PubMed]
60. Suso-Ribera, C.; Castilla, D.; Zaragozá, I.; Ribera-Canudas, M.V.; Arbona, C.B.; Palacios, A.G. Validity, Reliability, Feasibility, and Usefulness of Pain Monitor, a Multidimensional Smartphone App for Daily Monitoring of Adults with Heterogeneous Chronic Pain. *Clin. J. Pain* **2018**, *34*, 900–908. [CrossRef] [PubMed]
61. Sardi, L.; Idri, A.; Fernández-Alemán, J.L. A systematic review of gamification in e-Health. *J. Biomed. Inform.* **2017**, *71*, 31–48. [CrossRef]
62. Barrera, A.Z.; Kelman, A.R.; Muñoz, R.F.; Donker, T.; Danaher, B. Keywords to Recruit Spanish- and English-Speaking Participants: Evidence From an Online Postpartum Depression Randomized Controlled Trial. *J. Med Internet Res.* **2014**, *16*, e6. [CrossRef]
63. Kingston, D.; Biringer, A.; Toosi, A.; Heaman, M.; Lasiuk, G.C.; McDonald, S.; Kingston, J.; Sword, W.A.; Jarema, K.; Austin, M.-P. Disclosure during prenatal mental health screening. *J. Affect. Disord.* **2015**, *186*, 90–94. [CrossRef]
64. Commissioning Stepped Care for People with Common Mental Health Disorders. Available online: http://www.swscn.org.uk/wp/wp-content/uploads/2015/03/non-guidance-commissioning-stepped-care-for-people-with-common-mental-health-disorders-pdf.pdf (accessed on 6 May 2020).
65. Barlow, D.; Farchione, T.J.; Bullis, J.R.; Gallagher, M.W.; Murray-Latin, H.; Sauer-Zavala, S.; Bentley, K.H.; Thompson-Hollands, J.; Conklin, L.R.; Boswell, J.F.; et al. The Unified Protocol for Transdiagnostic Treatment of Emotional Disorders Compared With Diagnosis-Specific Protocols for Anxiety Disorders: A Randomized Clinical Trial. *JAMA Psychiatry* **2017**, *74*, 875–884. [CrossRef]

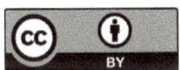

© 2020 by the authors. Licensee MDPI, Basel, Switzerland. This article is an open access article distributed under the terms and conditions of the Creative Commons Attribution (CC BY) license (http://creativecommons.org/licenses/by/4.0/).

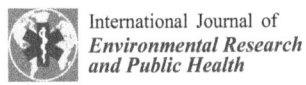

Review

How Are Information and Communication Technologies Supporting Routine Outcome Monitoring and Measurement-Based Care in Psychotherapy? A Systematic Review

Patricia Gual-Montolio [1], Verónica Martínez-Borba [1], Juana María Bretón-López [1], Jorge Osma [2] and Carlos Suso-Ribera [1,*]

[1] Department of Basic and Clinical Psychology and Psychobiology, Jaume I University, Avda. Vicent Sos Baynat s/n, 12071 Castellon de la Plana, Spain; al384421@uji.es (P.G.-M.); borba@uji.es (V.M.-B.); breton@uji.es (J.M.B.-L.)
[2] Department of Psychology and Sociology, Universidad de Zaragoza and Instituto de Investigación Sanitaria de Aragón, Ciudad Escolar s/n, 44003 Teruel, Spain; osma@unizar.es
* Correspondence: susor@uji.es

Received: 6 April 2020; Accepted: 29 April 2020; Published: 2 May 2020

Abstract: Psychotherapy has proven to be effective for a wide range of mental health problems. However, not all patients respond to the treatment as expected (not-on-track patients). Routine outcome monitoring (ROM) and measurement-based care (MBC), which consist of monitoring patients between appointments and using this data to guide the intervention, have been shown to be particularly useful for these not-on-track patients. Traditionally, though, ROM and MBC have been challenging, due to the difficulties associated with repeated monitoring of patients and providing real-time feedback to therapists. The use of information and communication technologies (ICTs) might help reduce these challenges. Therefore, we systematically reviewed evidence regarding the use of ICTs for ROM and MBC in face-to-face psychological interventions for mental health problems. The search included published and unpublished studies indexed in the electronic databases PubMed, PsycINFO, and SCOPUS. Main search terms were variations of the terms "psychological treatment", "progress monitoring or measurement-based care", and "technology". Eighteen studies met eligibility criteria. In these, ICTs were frequently handheld technologies, such as smartphone apps, tablets, or laptops, which were involved in the whole process (assessment and feedback). Overall, the use of technology for ROM and MBC during psychological interventions was feasible and acceptable. In addition, the use of ICTs was found to be effective, particularly for not-on-track patients, which is consistent with similar non-ICT research. Given the heterogeneity of reviewed studies, more research and replication is needed to obtain robust findings with different technological solutions and to facilitate the generalization of findings to different mental health populations.

Keywords: information and communication technologies; outcome monitoring; therapist feedback; measurement-based care; mental health

1. Introduction

The effectiveness of psychotherapy for the treatment of mental disorders has been supported by an impressive amount of evidence. However, some patients do not respond to treatment as expected, either because they do not show an improvement during the intervention or they discontinue it, or because they show a deterioration [1,2]. There might be several reasons explaining individual differences in response to psychological treatments, including unchallengeable patient characteristics (e.g., age), their personality and behavioral profiles, treatment characteristics and context, and patient physical health status and life context, to name some examples [3]. While acknowledging the previous, an increased number of studies have pointed to methodological deficits, namely, in how patients are monitored during treatments, as key factors influencing current treatment effectiveness [4,5].

Specifically, it has been proposed that a paradigm shift in the practice of psychotherapy towards an ecological momentary assessment (EMA) is necessary in order to monitor patients repeatedly and frequently in their natural environment [6,7]. However, simply monitoring the patient does not appear to be enough to improve the patient's outcomes [8,9]. In this sense, therapist (and patient) feedback has been argued to be a fundamental aspect if patient monitoring during therapy is to be effective [1,10].

The aforementioned procedure is known by different terms in the literature, such as routine outcome monitoring, with outcome or continuous feedback; progress monitoring; or, probably the most popular, measurement-based care (MBC) [9,11]. For simplicity and readability, the latter will be preferred throughout this text.

MBC is defined as a periodic and recurrent assessment of the patient's status over the course of an intervention using standardized measures. Importantly, the evaluation is followed by immediate, frequent, and systematic feedback of the patient's information to the therapist [12,13]. This procedure has been argued to help therapists to assess actual patient progress, suggest necessary adjustments to the treatment, and identify patient deterioration or improvement trajectories, thus enhancing the patient's response to the intervention [1,14–16]. According to the American Psychological Association's (APA) Division 28 Task Force on Empirically Supported Relationships, MBC may also lead to an improvement in the therapeutic alliance and may avoid premature treatment termination, because MBC encourages collaboration between patients and therapists, thus promoting engagement, dialogue and discussion of real-life, daily patient difficulties during sessions. Furthermore, giving feedback to patients raises awareness of their progress and makes them become more mindful of their symptoms, which may also enhance the quality of psychological interventions and the patient–therapist alliance [14].

Several studies have shown the efficacy of this systematic patient monitoring with progress feedback to the therapist in psychological interventions [10,17]. Research also indicates that feedback from outcome measures enhances treatment effectiveness, particularly in not-on-track patients (i.e., those who do not make the expected changes) or when it is provided both to clinicians and patients [8,10,13,14,17,18]. Specifically, providing the therapists with immediate feedback about the patient's symptoms appears to reduce the number of early dropouts and improve several treatment outcomes (depressive and anxiety symptoms, psychosocial functioning, psychosis, quality of life, therapeutic alliance, etc.) when compared against usual treatment [17,19]. Overall, medium effect sizes have been reported when using MBC [1,14].

What the existent literature suggests is that MBC is a promising methodology to enhance the effectiveness of psychological treatments. However, there are a number of flaws into the literature on MBC that might have limited the impact and dissemination of this procedure [20,21]. Traditionally, MBC has been conducted with self-report, paper-and-pencil questionnaires that patients complete before or after therapy sessions. Additionally, assessments are mostly retrospective and based on the patient's recalled experiences during the past week [11]. With this information, the therapist examines and discusses the results during the actual therapy session [22]. As noted earlier, while this practice has been shown to provide some relevant information, relying on paper-and-pencil retrospective reports only, where daily experiences are not reported, might result in recall bias, thus making it difficult to understand patient fluctuations over time [23,24]. Furthermore, focusing on self-reports exclusively is problematic, as more objective data (e.g., actual number of steps taken or time spent out of the home) is ignored or based on patient appraisal only.

Currently, the rapid growth of new technologies in our society has changed the way psychotherapy is conducted. For example, information and communication technologies (ICT) have been argued to allow therapists to evaluate and receive patient progress feedback in real time, thus minimizing patient recall bias [25]. Additionally, the use of ICT allows obtaining objective data of patient changes in natural settings, for example, using sensors (accelerometers, positioning system, or pedometers, among others) [22]. Therefore, the use of handheld ICT devices such as smartphones, tablets, or laptops might increase the effectiveness of MBC by facilitating EMA before, during, and after treatment, providing the information immediately to therapists and researchers, and making it easier to combine collection of objective and subjective patient data [11,21,25].

In order to investigate to what extent ICTs are being implemented to enhance psychological interventions and how their application is effectively improving outcomes, we have conducted a systematic review to explore how ICT is being used for MBC in face-to-face psychological treatments. In doing so, we have investigated: 1. what the different technologies and procedures used for MBC during psychological interventions are and 2. to what extent the use of ICT for MBC is feasible, acceptable, and effective.

2. Materials and Methods

2.1. Search Strategy

The search was conducted in accordance with the Preferred Reporting Items for Systematic Reviews and Meta-Analyses [26]. The search was conducted in February 2020 and included published and unpublished studies from the electronic databases PubMed, PsycINFO, and SCOPUS. In addition, reference mining was performed by searching through bibliographies of relevant articles. The selection of these databases was motivated by previous research showing that PsycINFO has high sensitivity and specificity when retrieving intervention studies and is especially suitable for psychology research, and that SCOPUS offers about 20% more coverage than other important databases such as Web of Science. Additionally, it has been argued that Google Scholar provides inaccurate results, and PubMed is one of the preferred tools for biomedical research [27,28].

The search strategy included variations of the terms "psychological treatment", "progress monitoring", and "technology" (See Appendix A for the complete list of search terms and combinations). Due to the diversity of terms, a broad search strategy of terms was used. Synonyms, abbreviations, and spelling variations were identified for the three concepts and combined in the search using the "OR" Boolean operator, with non-synonymous concepts combined using "AND". These terms were searched in titles and abstracts. The references of included studies and relevant systematic reviews were searched to identify studies that were missed during the literature search. There were no restrictions regarding language or publication period, but the search was only conducted in English.

2.2. Inclusion Criteria

Included studies were psychological treatments enhanced by MBC using technology systems. Specifically, included studies 1. were clinical trials (either feasibility, case studies, and both randomized or non-randomized investigations); 2. included the use of technology during MBC (both for monitoring and feedback provision) while undergoing a face-to-face psychological intervention; and 3. involved feedback to the therapist or to both therapists and patients based on standardized measures.

To be considered MBC, the intervention must satisfy the following components: 1. routine assessment of a symptom, an outcome, or a process measure; 2. therapist review of data; and 3. therapist use of data to inform clinical decisions. Therefore, the study population can include patients with any mental disorder from all ages who are routinely monitored via validated outcome measures using technologies over the course of a face-to-face psychological treatment.

2.3. Exclusion Criteria

Studies in which technology systems were not used in the whole MBC process, including the assessment and feedback parts, or where only patients but not therapists were provided with feedback, were excluded. In addition, studies were excluded if they did not include a face-to-face psychological intervention.

2.4. Search and Screening

Initially, 193 publications were identified from database searches and screening of reference lists (see Figure 1 for the study diagram flow). After excluding duplicates (*n* = 63), 130 publications were retained for screening. After initial screening of titles and abstracts, 84 of these documents were excluded due to eligibility reasons. For the remaining 46 publications, full texts were retrieved. After eligibility assessment of the full texts, 28 publications were excluded. The majority of publications were excluded because they did not meet the eligibility criteria, resulting in a final sample that comprised 18 publications.

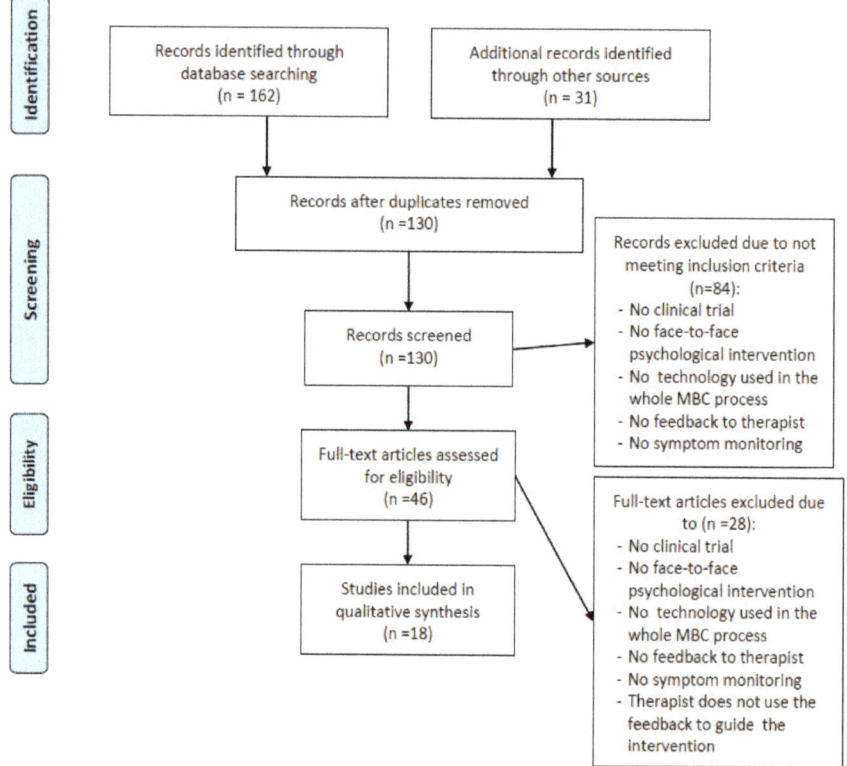

Figure 1. Flow diagram of study selection following PRISMA guidelines [26].

The search, screening process, and data extraction were conducted independently by the first two authors (PGM and VMB). When in doubt, study eligibility was discussed with a third author (CSR). After the phase of study eligibility assessment, inter-rater agreement was calculated (Cohen's kappa). This coefficient showed a substantial overall agreement, represented by a kappa of 0.908 (*SD* = 0.064; 95% CI, 0.781, 1.000).

2.5. Data Extraction

The following data were extracted from each included study, using a standardized data-extraction form developed a priori: authors, study setting (geographical setting and type of clinic), sample size, study design, study participants (demographics and type of mental disorder), type of psychological intervention, assessment characteristics (frequency and setting), primary outcomes, feedback characteristics (to whom, frequency, and setting), type of technology used, technology

2.6. Risk of Bias Assessment

All studies included in this review were independently rated for quality by two reviewers (PGM and VMB). If the rating differed, reviewers discussed the articles to reach consensus with a third reviewer (CSR). The Study Quality Assessment Tools from the National Heart Lung and Blood Institute [29] were used to assess study quality and risk of bias. This tool was preferred because it includes six types of studies and specific criteria according to the study design (i.e., controlled intervention studies; systematic reviews and meta-analyses; observational cohort and cross-sectional studies; case-control studies; before–after studies with no control group; and case series studies). This tool allows reviewers to rate studies as "good", "fair", or "poor". Total quality scores ranged from 9 to 14 points depending on the study design.

2.7. Synthesis of Results

Frequency tables were used to summarize the characteristics of individual studies. We conducted a systematic review and not a meta-analysis, because the emphasis was not on effect sizes, but on how MBC with technology was being conducted. Additionally, we anticipated that included studies would be very heterogeneous, because the review includes any form of psychological intervention, all types of technologies, several trial designs, and different types of mental disorders and outcomes. Thus, we performed a narrative synthesis only.

2.8. Additional Analyses

Factors affecting study heterogeneity included variations in the type of mental disorder (e.g., major depressive disorder or anxiety disorders), outcomes included, treatment characteristics (type, format, and duration), measures used (clinician-rated versus self-rated), study design, and differences in the means by which MBC was delivered. The description of the findings was sensitive about the aforementioned subgroups when possible.

3. Results

3.1. Characteristics of Included Studies

The characteristics of included studies are shown in Table 1. Of the 18 studies included in the systematic review, eight were published in the USA [30–37], with the remaining studies being published in Australia (n = 3 [38–40]), the United Kingdom (n = 3 [41–43]), Austria (n = 2 [44,45]), Greece (n = 1 [46]), and the Netherlands (n = 1 [47]). Most studies took place in outpatient settings (n = 15, 83.33%) such as mental health services (n = 3 [33,34,47]), specialist clinics (n = 4 [36,38,39,43]), hospital clinics (n = 7 [31,35,37,41,42,45,46]), and university clinics (n = 1 [32]); only three of them were conducted in inpatient settings [30,40,44]. In terms of design, six studies were feasibility pilot investigations (single group) [30,31,34,36,37,44]; four studies were case studies [32,39,45,46]; four studies were randomized controlled trials (RCTs) [35,38,42,47]; two of them were non-randomized controlled trials [33,40]; and two were pre–post investigations [41,43]. The sample sizes of the included investigations ranged from 1 to 2233 participants.

Table 1. Characteristics of the included studies.

Reference	Country	Setting	Psychological Disorder	Sample size	Study Design	Type of Psychological Intervention
[30]	California (USA)	Specialist inpatient treatment center	PTSD	27 Tx	SG (feasibility study)	Residential group psychotherapy (4-5 months)
[31]	Pittsburgh (USA)	Outpatient Psychiatric Institute and Clinic	Anxiety disorders (children from 9 to 14 years old)	9 Tx (3 received 16-sessions CBT, 6 received 8-sessions Brief CBT)	SG (feasibility pilot trial)	"Coping Cat": 16 CBT sessions"Brief Coping Cat": 8 CBT sessions
[32]	Evanston, Illinois (USA)	Outpatient clinic at the Family Institute at Northwestern University	Couple problems	1 Tx	Case study	Four Couple Multisystemic Psychotherapy sessions
[33]	California University: Berkeley (USA)	Outpatient behavioural health clinic	Depression	85 (40 cont. + 45 Tx)	nRCT (not blinded)	16 weeks of weekly group CBT therapy
[34]	California (USA)	4 Outpatient Early Psychosis clinics	Psychotic disorder	61 Tx	SG (feasibility study)	Early Psychosis Program (up to 5 months)
[35]	New York (USA)	Outpatient primary care	Substance use	240 (83 cont. + 77 Tx + 80 Tx HealthCall)	Three-arm RCT (1:1:1 allocation ratio)	Brief (25-30 min) individual (motivational interview) psychoeducation (3 sessions: every 30 days)
[36]	California University (USA)	Outpatient specialist clinic	Psychotic disorder (adolescent and young)	76 Tx	SG (feasibility pilot trial)	Early Psychosis Program (minimum 3 months)
[37]	Washington University (USA)	Outpatient primary care clinic affiliated with the Washington University	Depression and Anxiety	17 Tx	SG (feasibility and acceptability pilot study)	Collaborative care program (over 6 months)
[38]	Melbourne (Australia)	Outpatient Specialist Voices Clinic and clinical services	Schizophrenia	34 (17 cont. + 17 Tx)	A single-blind, parallel group, pilot RCT (1:1 allocation ratio)	Brief CBT (four in-person therapy sessions) + EMA + EMI
[39]	Melbourne (Australia)	Outpatient Specialist Voices clinic	Schizophrenia	1 Tx	Case study	Brief CBT (four in-person therapy sessions) + EMA+ EMI
[40]	Perth (Australia)	Private inpatients and day-patients psychiatric hospital	Mood and Anxiety	1308 (408 Tx Fb +, 439 nFb + 461 cont.)	nRCT	10 days of intensive CBT group

Table 1. *Cont.*

Reference	Country	Setting	Psychological Disorder	Sample size	Study Design	Type of Psychological Intervention
[41]	Leeds (England)	Outpatient clinic	Depression and Anxiety	594 (349 cont. + 245 Tx)	Quasi-experimental pre-post study	Low-intensity guided self-help CBT or High-intensity CBT, interpersonal psychotherapy and counselling
[42]	England	8 outpatient clinics	Depression and Anxiety	2233 (1057 cont. + 1176 Tx)	Multisite, open-label, cluster RCT	Low-intensity guided self-help CBT or High-intensity CBT, interpersonal psychotherapy and counselling
[43]	Oxford (UK)	Outpatient specialist mental health	Bipolar disorder	19 Tx	SG (pre-post)	five sessions of psychoeducational intervention (FIMM) + pharmacotherapy
[44]	Salzburg (Austria)	Inpatient and a day-treatment clinic	Mood disorders; Psychoactive substance use mental disorders; Schizophrenia, schizotypal, and delusional disorders; Neurotic, stress-related, and somatoform disorders; Personality disorders, and others	151 Tx	SG (feasibility pilot trial)	Psychotherapy (8 weeks in the day-treatment clinic and 12 weeks in the inpatient clinic)
[45]	Salzburg (Austria)	Outpatient clinic	Bulimia nervosa	1 Tx	Case study	six Rogerian person-centred psychotherapy sessions
[46]	Thessaloniki (Greece)	Alzheimer day care centre (at home)	Dementia	4 Tx	Case study	15 Individual psychotherapy sessions (psychosocial intervention, CBT, relaxation techniques, etc.)
[47]	The Netherlands	Outpatient mental health institutions or private practices	Mood disorder, Adjustment disorder, Anxiety disorder, Relational problems, Personality disorders, and others	475 (159 Tx FbT; 172 Tx FbTP; 144 cont. nFb)	RCT	Long and short psychotherapy (CBT, client-centered, psychodynamics)

Note: Cont., control group; Tx, treatment group; nRCT, non-randomized controlled trial; CBT, Cognitive-Behavioural Therapy; RCT, randomized controlled trial; EMA, ecological momentary assessment; EMI, ecological momentary intervention; FbT, feedback to the therapist; FbTP, feedback to the therapist and the patient; Fb, feedback; nFb, no-feedback; FIMM, Facilitated Integrated Mood Management; SG, single group design.

The included studies targeted very heterogeneous diagnoses. However, depression and anxiety disorders were the most frequent (n = 6, 33.33% of studies [31,33,37,40–42]). The remaining disorders were schizophrenia spectrum disorders (n = 4, 22.22% of studies [34,36,38,39]), bulimia nervosa (n = 1, 5.6% of studies [45]), substance use (n = 1, 5.6% of studies [35]), dementia (n = 1, 5.6% of studies [46]), post-traumatic stress (n = 1, 5.6% of studies [30]), bipolar disorder (n = 1, 5.6% of studies [43]), couple problems (n = 1, 5.6% of studies [32]), and combinations of heterogeneous disorders together (n = 2, 11.11% of studies [44,47]). The majority of treatments were addressed to adult populations (n = 16) and only two investigations (n = 2 [34,36]) aimed at treating mental health problems in younger populations (i.e., adolescents and young adults).

Regarding the treatments offered in the included studies, different face-to-face interventions were provided across studies. However, cognitive behavioral therapy (CBT) was the most frequent (n = 13). Other therapeutic options were client-centered psychotherapy (n = 1 [45]), collaborative care (n = 1 [37]), an early psychosis program (n = 2 [34,36]), and couple multisystemic psychotherapy (n = 1 [32]). The format of the intervention was mainly individual (n = 15), but some studies included group treatments (n = 3 [30,33,40]). Finally, the intensity (i.e., frequency) of the intervention also differed across investigations. Some studies implemented a low-intensity treatment plan (i.e., less than eight sessions; n = 6 [32,35,38,39,43,45]), while others applied a higher-intensity intervention (i.e., more than eight sessions; n = [30,33,34,36,37,40,44,46]) or both a low- and a high-intensity treatment (n = 4 [31,41,42,47]).

3.2. MBC Characteristics

3.2.1. Assessment Procedure Used to Track the Patient's Status

The characteristics of studies included in the review are described in Table 2. Most studies (n = 9 [30,31,33,35,38–40,44,46]) monitored their patients daily. The remaining studies monitored their patients weekly (n = 4 [32,41,42,47]), before every therapy session, or both daily and weekly (n = 5 [34,36,37,43,45]). In the latter studies conducting assessments both daily and weekly, daily assessments usually included shorter questionnaires that evaluated therapeutic process outcomes, mood, or medication adherence, while longer outcome scales (i.e., measures of depressive or anxiety symptoms) were administered weekly. Treatment effectiveness was assessed most commonly with the primary outcome measures of interest for the investigation, which most often were the Patient Health Questionnaire-9 for depressive symptoms and the Generalised Anxiety Disorder-7 for anxiety symptoms (n = 4 [33,37,41,42]). Other outcomes included the frequency and amount of drug use (n = 1 [35]); the Subjective Experiences of Psychosis Scale, the Auditory Hallucinations subscale of the Psychotic Symptom Rating Scales for psychotic symptoms, and the Depression Anxiety Stress Scale for negative emotional symptoms (n = 2 [38,39]); the Outcome Questionnaire-45 (n= 1 [47]); the Therapy Process Questionnaire (n = 1 [44]); the World Health Organization's Wellbeing Index (n = 1 [40]) for well-being; the Symptom Checklist-90 for bulimia symptoms and the Intersession Experience Questionnaire for the psychotherapy process (n = 1 [45]); the Altman Self-Rating Mania scale and the 16-item Quick Inventory of Depressive Symptoms-Self Report scale (n = 1 [43]); and other clinical measures related to sleep, mood, medication use, or daily functioning (n = 6 [30–32,34,36,46]).

Table 2. Measurement-based care characteristics.

Reference	Assessment Frequency and Setting	Primary Outcome Measures	Feedback to	Feedback Frequency and Setting	Type of Technology Used
[30]	Daily at a random time	Adapted questionnaire from Symptom Checklist-6, the BriefCOPE and Beck Depression Inventory-II	T and P	P: T regularly shared P progress in order to incorporate strategies in therapy sessions and treatment plan. T: They got patient information several times a week in a graph format to discuss with them during sessions, to encourage them and monitor them.	EMA and Text messages
[31]	Daily questions about recent emotional events (e.g., emotions, scenario, somatic symptoms, automatic thoughts) + answers on demand by the participant	Skills entries and satisfaction with the treatment.	P and T	P: They received personalized feedback from therapists. T: Information and graphs from the portal about patients' progress were discussed in weekly CBT sessions with the patients.	Smartphone app: SmartCAT app + SmartCAT therapist portal.
[32]	Online before every session	STIC: set of questionnaires	T and clinicians stakeholders	T: On-demand graphs of patient progress were provided to the therapist through STIC	STIC online
[33]	Once daily mood monitoring messages at random between 8 a.m. and 8 p.m.	Attendance to therapy, duration of therapy and PHQ-9	P and T	P: They received feedback about their mood responses T: T reviewed information from an online dashboard were patient progress is shown. T can periodically review the graphs, identify key aspects and address any important event during or between sessions.	Automated text messages and Web-based platform (HealthySMS)
[34]	Daily and weekly surveys (between 5 p.m. and 10:30 p.m.)	Mood, medication use, socialization and conflict	P and T	P: They discussed their feedback with the T at every session. T: They reviewed and discussed patient information (plots of symptoms over time, etc.) on the dashboard with P during sessions and between sessions.	Smartphone app: RealLife Exp + web-based platform
[35]	Once daily call (HealthCall) for self-monitoring	Primary drug use (frequency and amount), use of other drugs, medication adherence, and mood	P and T	P: They received the feedback at 30 and 60 days, where their information was discussed with the T. T: At 30 and 60 days, T discussed with P the generated graphs based on HealthCall about their drug use, moods and health behaviors.	Phone IVR system
[36]	Daily surveys (at 5 p.m. until 11:55 p.m.), weekly surveys (Sundays at 10 a.m. until Monday 11:55) and monthly in-person psychosocial assessments with research staff	Daily surveys assessing mood, medication adherence, and social interaction, weekly surveys assessing symptoms, sleep, and medication adherence	T	T: They received alerts from the dashboard when P scores were clinically significant and took the proper decisions according to the patient demand.	Ginger.io (software) = Smartphone app + Clinician dashboard
[37]	3/4 times daily, weekly; 8/12 weeks	PHQ-9 and GAD-7	P and T	P: P received notifications about their progress in the app, becoming more aware of their symptoms. T: T reviewed patient-reported information via an online dashboard and visualized patient progress graphs.	Smartphone app + online platform
[38]	Session 1 and 2: 10 daily evening EMA for 6 days. Session 3 and 4: 8 evening daily EMA (monitor changes in voices and coping strategies)	SEPS, PSYRATS-AH, and DASS-21	P and T	P: In session 2, P received a summary sheet with their EMA progress. T: In session 2, EMA feedback was discussed with the P in order to guarantee understanding, detect predictors and avoid causation.	Smartphone app: MovisensXS + web-based platform

Table 2. *Cont.*

Reference	Assessment Frequency and Setting	Primary Outcome Measures	Feedback to	Feedback Frequency and Setting	Type of Technology Used
[39]	Session 1 and 2: 10 daily evening EMA for 6 days. Session 3 and 4: 8 evening daily EMA (monitor changes in voices and coping strategies)	SEPS, PSYRATS-AH, and DASS-21	P and T	P: In session 2, P received a summary sheet with their EMA progress. T: In session 2, EMA feedback was discussed with the P in order to guarantee understanding, detect predictors and avoid causation.	Smartphone app: RealLife Exp + web-based platform
[40]	Daily self-reported measures of well-being	Well-being (WHO-5)	P and T	P: They received routinely individualized information about their progress in group discussion with the therapist. T: T received daily automatic plots of each patient's outcomes within trajectories.	Touch-screen technology in therapy rooms
[41]	Weekly (session-by-session)	PHQ-9 and GAD-7	P and T	P: They received their feedback in session with the therapist, where the information was reviewed, discussed and used to guide the treatment plan. T: They had access to patient progress graphs and response curves from the monitoring system, and they were warned automatically when a P was not-on-track.	Computer PCMIS
[42]	Weekly (session-by-session)	PHQ-9 and GAD-7	P and T	P: They received their feedback in session with the therapist, where the information was reviewed, discussed and used to guide the treatment plan. T: They had access to patient progress graphs and response curves from the monitoring system, and they were warned automatically when a P was not-on-track.	Computer PCMIS
[43]	Twice a day (only during psychoeducation sessions) and once a week	Daily: mood and sleep Weekly: QIDS, ASRM and mood management strategies questionnaire	P and T	P: P received their feedback at every session with the T. T: T reviewed patient progress from daily mood rating and weekly scales from the previous week and discussed with the P the relationship between his/her mood changes and stressors.	Phone text messages or e-mails (True Colours mood monitoring system)
[44]	Daily process monitoring (during evenings).	TPQ	T	T: On demand. Feedback was used for individualizing therapeutic decisions.	SNS
[45]	Daily measures of psychotherapy process. Weekly measure of therapy outcome.	IEQ daily, weekly SCL-90 (Bulimia)	P, T and researchers	P: They viewed their progress and estimated their moods and symptoms during the past day. T: They had access to P data from the system in order to adapt the intervention delivered.	Smartphone: DynAMo web app
[46]	Daily monitoring	Sleep patterns, physical activity, and activities of daily living	P, T and caregivers	P and caregiver: They could see a proportionate share of the information adapted to their needs. T: Information collected was available at all times in order to design personalized interventions.	Tablet app (assistive technology: wearable, sleep, movement, presence sensors)
[47]	Once a week just before therapy session (at waiting room)	OQ-45	P and T, or only T	P: P can access the feedback via email or into their portal system. T: T could access the feedback via email or in their portal system and could discuss the feedback information (progress charts and a message) with the P based on the OQ-45 patient's scores.	Computer: Web-based monitoring app

Note: PHQ-9, Patient Health Questionnaire-9; P, patient; T, therapist; GAD-7, Generalised Anxiety Disorder-7; EMA, Ecological Momentary Assessment; SEPS, Subjective Experiences of Psychosis Scale; PSYRATS-AH, Auditory Hallucinations subscale of the Psychotic Symptom Rating Scales; DASS-21, Depression Anxiety Stress Scale; OQ-45, Outcome Questionnaire; IEQ, Intersession Experience Questionnaire; SCL-90, Symptom Checklist-90; QIDS, Quick Inventory of Depressive Symptomatology; ASRM, Altman Self Rating Mania Scale; WHO-5, World Health Organization's Wellbeing Index; STIC, Systemic Therapy Inventory of Change System; CBT, Cognitive Behavioral Therapy; TPQ, Therapy Process Questionnaire; IVR, interactive voice response; App, mobile application; STIC, Systemic Therapy Inventory of Change System; SNS, Synergetic Navigation System; PCMIS, Patient Case Management Information System.

3.2.2. Feedback Procedure

The majority of studies provided feedback to both therapists and patients (n = 15). The remaining studies gave feedback to therapists only (n = 3 [32,36,44]). Most studies used feedback to track the patients' progress focusing on key aspects during treatment and to monitor responses in-between sessions. Even when the feedback was not directly provided to the patient, this information was used to discuss patient progress during treatment sessions or to take clinical decisions (e.g., emphasize a specific content during session).

Feedback included information about treatment evolution in progress charts, summary sheets, graphs of scores and curves, and plots of scores within trajectories. Feedback information was either sent periodically to the therapist in response to patient assessments or on-demand (weekly or daily). In some studies, feedback to the therapist appeared when the patients' responses were considered clinically significant according to pre-established criteria.

3.3. Technology Characteristics

The technology characteristics of included studies are presented in Table 2. Most studies included handheld technology, such as smartphone apps (n = 7 [31,34,36–39,45]), touch-screen technologies (n = 2 [40,46]), or laptops (n = 5 [32,41,42,44,47]), together with a web-based platform for the therapist. The remaining studies used phone text messages (n = 2 [30,33]), e-mail (n = 1 [43]), or a phone interactive voice response system (n = 1 [35]). For example, in one study, automated text messages and a web-based platform (e.g., HealthySMS) were used [33]. In other investigations, authors implemented an Internet-based system, such as the Patient Case Management Information System (PCMIS), or an electronic clinical record system which includes outcome-monitoring graphs that chart depression and anxiety scores at every session [41,42]. A similar example was the Synergetic Navigation System, an Internet-based device for data collection (with web-compatible devices such as PCs, tablets, or smartphones) and data analysis that allows for the implementation of questionnaires at any chosen interval [44]. Another Internet-based system was the DynAMo web app, a piece of software that combines algorithm-based treatment planning, process monitoring, and outcome monitoring, which can be used by both researchers and clinicians to plan treatments and monitor psychotherapeutic processes [45]. One investigation used the Systemic Therapy Inventory of Change System, an online system that assesses and tracks changes in the patients' interpersonal system, as well as in the therapeutic alliance, and also feeds these data back to the therapists on demand [32]. A final example of an Internet-based system used in one of the included investigations was Ginger.io, an mHealth software program comprising a therapist dashboard and an app which can collect data from self-report surveys sent to the participant in addition to "passive" data from the participant's phone, such as number of calls and SMS messages, and movement patterns based on Global Positioning System data [36].

3.3.1. Technology Feasibility

Because of the large differences in sample sizes across investigations (Table 3), case studies with one to four participants [32,39,45,46] have been described in previous sections but will not be considered in the feasibility and effectiveness summaries. The remaining studies included at least 17 participants, and therefore will be discussed in detail here and in Table 3. Overall, the results demonstrated that enhancing MBC in psychological therapy with technology was generally feasible and acceptable (Table 3). This statement is supported by the high average response rate for daily (mean = 63.3%, range = 40%–81% [34,36,43]), weekly (mean = 73.0%, range = 39%–88% [34,36,37,43]), and monthly (92.7% [30]) symptom monitoring across studies, low average missing data rates amongst patients (13% [44]), and high completion rates (mean = 77.8%; range = 64.1%–90% [31,35,38,40,44]). In addition, several studies reported satisfaction with the technology used to improve MBC in the intervention delivered, and most of them revealed that patients and therapists would recommend the technology used as part of the treatment [31,34,38].

Table 3. Usability, acceptability, and effectiveness of technology-supported measurement-based care.

Reference	Sample Size	Feasibility of Technology	Clinical Effectiveness
[30]	27 Tx	Monthly: 92.7%.	NA
[31]	9 Tx	Completion rate was 82.8%. Patients reported the app being easy to use. All parents report treatment satisfaction and would recommend the program.	NA
[33]	85 (40 cont. + 45 Tx)	NA	Technology-supported MBC significantly increased treatment adherence (median of 13.5 weeks before dropping out) compared to traditional CBT (median of 3 weeks before dropping out). Effect sizes of technology-supported MBC CBT on depressive symptoms' severity ($z = -5.80$) were larger than for traditional CBT ($z = -3.12$), but differences were not significant
[34]	61 Tx	Moderate survey completion (daily = 40%; weekly = 39%). In general, both T (66%) and P (85%) reported they would continue using the app as part of the treatment.	NA
[35]	240 (83 cont. + 77 Tx + 80 Tx)	HealthCall shows a great retention rate and response rate (64.1%), supporting feasibility, patient acceptability and generalizability.	At 12-month follow-up, reductions in non-injection drug use were comparable in traditional and technology-supported MBC motivational interviewing and superior than in the control condition. In the subset of patients with drug dependence, drug use was significantly lower in the technology-supported MBC condition at 12 months post-treatment. At 60 days, treatment retention in the technology-supported MBC group (88.8%) was superior than in the motivational intervention only condition (81.8%) and the control condition (78.3%)
[36]	76 Tx	Feasibility and acceptability of the smartphone app as an adjunct treatment tool is supported by the high response rate sate (weekly surveys: 77%; daily surveys: 69%)	NA
[37]	17 Tx	The feasibility and acceptability of the mobile platform is supported by the high early response rate (weekly = 88%).	NA
[38]	34 (17 cont. + 17 Tx)	High completion rates (74%) of EMA questionnaires and good satisfaction of participants support the feasibility and acceptability of the study, respectively.	Compared with the usual treatment, the technology-supported MBC treatment resulted in large improvements in confidence in coping with voices (Hedges $g = 1.45$) and medium improvements in understanding of voices (Hedges $g = 0.61$) and in psychotic symptoms (Hedges $g = 0.51$). Both groups showed similar changes in the impact of psychosis.
[40]	1308 (408 Tx Fb +, 439 nFb + 461 cont.)	High rates of touch-screen questionnaire completion (over 90%).	Technology-supported MBC for NOT patients was more effective than traditional CBT or monitoring without feedback in reducing depressive symptoms and the impact of emotions on functioning, as well as on increasing vitality. By contrast, changes in well-being, anxiety, and stress were comparable across conditions.
[41]	594 (349 cont. + 245 Tx)	MBC technology was generally acceptable and feasible to integrate in routine practice.	Technology-supported MBC achieved comparable reductions in depression and anxiety compared to controls, but with significantly less time (adjusted mean = 10.25, SE = 0.45 vs. adjusted mean = 6.59, SE = 0.51) and cost (between £65.88 and £129.20 cost reductions per treatment). Cases in the control condition were twice as likely to become not-on-track patients compared to those in the technology-supported MBC.

Table 3. Cont.

Reference	Sample Size	Feasibility of Technology	Clinical Effectiveness
[42]	2233 (1057 cont. + 1176 Tx)	NA	NOT patients in the technology-enhanced MBC condition obtained significantly larger reductions in depressive ($d = 0.23$) and anxiety symptom severity ($d = 0.19$), as well as improved work and social adjustment ($d = 0.19$) compared with active controls (traditional CBT).
[43]	19 Tx	High response rate (daily = 81%, weekly = 88%)	NA
[44]	151 Tx	High average compliance rates (78.3%) and low average missing data rates (13%) amongst the inpatients support the feasibility.	NA
[47]	475 (159 Tx FbT; 172 Tx FbTP; 144 cont. nFb)	NA	In short-term interventions (less than 35 weeks), receiving feedback was protective of negative outcomes in NOT cases ($d = 1.28$). No significant differences between conditions were found for on-track patients, but there was a trend for the technology-supported MBC group to be more effective ($d = 0.24$ at 35 weeks and $d = 0.29$ at 78 weeks) and to have lower deterioration rates ($z = 1.3$), especially when feedback was provided to both patient and therapist.

Note: Cont., Control Group; Tx, Treatment Group; FbT, Feedback to The Therapist; FbTP, Feedback to The Therapist and The Patient; Fb, Feedback; nFb, No Feedback; NA, Not Applicable/Not Specified; IVR, Interactive Voice Response; App, Mobile Application; EMA, Ecological Momentary Assessment; MBC, Measurement-Based Care; NOT, Not-on-Track patients; T, Therapist; P, Patient. The feasibility and effectiveness reports are not provided for case studies due to the reduced number of patients ($n \leq 4$).

3.3.2. Clinical Effectiveness

As summarized in Table 3, data about clinical effectiveness was described in seven studies, including four RCTs [35,38,42,47], two nRCTs [33,40], and a quasi-experimental pre–post investigation [41]. All RCTs included active controls (i.e., traditional face-to-face psychological treatment) without MBC. According to these investigations, the use of technology-supported MBC appears to significantly reduce symptom severity, and changes are sometimes larger than with traditional interventions [38], especially in patients at risk of poor response to treatment (i.e., not-on-track cases) [35,40,42,47], which is consistent with previous research [42,46]. Furthermore, one study showed that although traditional CBT and technology-enhanced MBC CBT were comparable in terms of treatment effectiveness, the latter significantly reduced therapy duration and cost of treatment [41]. Also in favor of technology-assisted MBC, another investigation revealed that patients stayed in therapy longer (i.e., higher adherence) in the experimental condition, that is, when MBC was supported by technology (group CBT with a text messaging adjunct) as opposed to traditional MBC without technology (group CBT without the text messaging adjunct) [33]. In sum, most studies suggest that technology-supported MBC has the potential to improve the efficacy and cost-effectiveness of psychotherapy, especially for not-on-track individuals.

3.4. Risk of Bias Assessment

As observed in Tables 4–7, studies included in this review could be placed in four of the categories proposed by the National Heart Lung and Blood Institute [29], namely, case studies, before-after studies; observational cohort and cross-sectional studies; and controlled intervention studies. Overall, the four studies classified as case studies had a "good" quality, with total scores ranging from 5 to 7 points out of a maximum of 9 points [32,39,45,46]. Even so, none of them had follow-up sessions, or these were not reported, and two studies did not include a complete case definition [32,45]. Secondly, the two before–after studies could also be rated as "good" quality investigations, as both obtained 9 points of a maximum of 12 [41,43]. The main issue with one of the studies was related to sample size, although this concern was justified, as this was a pilot study and authors reported the previous in the limitation section [43]. The six studies classified as observational, cohort and cross-sectional studies correspond to feasibility and acceptability studies, and some quality criteria, such as numbers 7, 8, 12, and 14, were not applicable [30,31,34,36,37,44]. Overall, feasibility and acceptability studies did not meet most criteria required in observational and cross-sectional studies (they met only seven or eight criteria of a maximum of 14), so their quality could only be rated as "fair". It is important to note that just two studies maintained 80% of the sample [30,31] and four studies did not meet the participation rate of 50% from eligible participant criteria [30,31,37,44]. Finally, two of the controlled intervention studies [33,40] were rated as "poor" quality as they were non-randomized and did not follow most of the criteria for controlled studies (i.e., randomization, blind allocation, or assessment). These two studies met, respectively, only two [40] and eight [33] criteria of a maximum of 14. The remaining four controlled intervention studies [35,38,42,47] were "good" quality investigations despite the lack of blinded allocation and assessment [35,42,47] and relatively high drop-out rates [42,47].

Table 4. Quality assessment of case studies.

	[32]	[39]	[45]	[46]
1. Was the study question or objective clearly stated?	Yes	Yes	Yes	Yes
2. Was the study population clearly and fully described, including a case definition?	No	Yes	No	Yes
3. Were the cases consecutive?	NA	NA	NA	No
4. Were the subjects comparable?	NA	NA	No	Yes
5. Was the intervention clearly described?	Yes	Yes	Yes	Yes
6. Were the outcome measures clearly defined, valid, reliable, and implemented consistently across all study participants?	Yes	Yes	Yes	Yes
7. Was the length of follow-up adequate?	NR	No	No	NR
8. Were the statistical methods well-described?	Yes	Yes	Yes	Yes
9. Were the results well-described?	Yes	Yes	Yes	Yes
Total score (maximum 9 points)	5	6	5	7

Note: CD, Cannot Determine; NA, Not Applicable; NR, Not Reported.

Table 5. Quality assessment of before–after studies.

	[41]	[43]
1. Was the study question or objective clearly stated?	Yes	Yes
2. Were eligibility/selection criteria for the study population prespecified and clearly described?	Yes	Yes
3. Were the participants in the study representative of those who would be eligible for the test/service/intervention in the general or clinical population of interest?	NR	Yes
4. Were all eligible participants that met the prespecified entry criteria enrolled?	NR	No
5. Was the sample size sufficiently large to provide confidence in the findings?	Yes	No
6. Was the test/service/intervention clearly described and delivered consistently across the study population?	Yes	Yes
7. Were the outcome measures prespecified, clearly defined, valid, reliable, and assessed consistently across all study participants?	Yes	Yes
8. Were the people assessing the outcomes blinded to the participants' exposures/interventions?	No	NA
9. Was the loss to follow-up after baseline 20% or less? Were those lost to follow-up accounted for in the analysis?	Yes/Yes	Yes/Yes
10. Did the statistical methods examine changes in outcome measures from before to after the intervention? Were statistical tests done that provided p values for the pre-to-post changes?	Yes	Yes
11. Were outcome measures of interest taken multiple times before the intervention and multiple times after the intervention (i.e., did they use an interrupted time-series design)?	Yes	Yes
12. If the intervention was conducted at a group level (e.g., a whole hospital, a community, etc.) did the statistical analysis take into account the use of individual-level data to determine effects at the group level?	Yes	Yes
Total score (maximum 12 points)	9	9

Note: CD, Cannot Determine; NA, Not Applicable; NR, Not Reported.

Table 6. Quality assessment of observational cohort and cross-sectional studies.

	[30]	[31]	[34]	[36]	[37]	[44]
1. Was the research question or objective in this paper clearly stated?	Yes	Yes	Yes	Yes	Yes	Yes
2. Was the study population clearly specified and defined?	Yes	Yes	Yes	Yes	Yes	Yes
3. Was the participation rate of eligible persons at least 50%?	NR	NR	Yes	Yes	No	NR
4. Were all the subjects selected or recruited from the same or similar populations? Were inclusion and exclusion criteria for being in the study prespecified and applied uniformly to all participants?	Yes	Yes	Yes	Yes	Yes	Yes
5. Was a sample size justification, power description, or variance and effect estimates provided?	NR	NR	NR	NR	NR	NR
6. For the analyses in this paper, were the exposure(s) of interest measured prior to the outcome(s) being measured?	Yes	Yes	Yes	NA	Yes	Yes
7. Was the timeframe sufficient so that one could reasonably expect to see an association between exposure and outcome if it existed?	NA	NA	NA	NA	NA	NA
8. For exposures that can vary in amount or level, did the study examine different levels of the exposure as related to the outcome (e.g., categories of exposure, or exposure measured as continuous variable)?	NA	NA	NA	NA	NA	NA
9. Were the exposure measures clearly defined, valid, reliable, and implemented consistently across all study participants?	Yes	Yes	Yes	Yes	Yes	Yes
10. Was the exposure(s) assessed more than once over time?	Yes	Yes	Yes	Yes	Yes	Yes
11. Were the outcome measures clearly defined, valid, reliable, and implemented consistently across all study participants?	Yes	Yes	Yes	Yes	Yes	Yes
12. Were the outcome assessors blinded to the exposure status of participants?	NA	NA	NA	NA	NA	NA
13. Was loss to follow-up after baseline 20% or less?	Yes	Yes	No	No	No	No
14. Were key potential confounding variables measured for their impact on the relationship between exposure(s) and outcome(s)?	NA	NA	NA	NA	NA	NA
Total score (maximum 14 points)	8	8	8	7	7	7

Note: CD, Cannot Determine; NA, Not Applicable; NR, Not Reported.

Table 7. Quality assessment of controlled intervention studies.

	[33]	[35]	[38]	[40]	[42]	[47]
1. Was the study described as randomized, a randomized trial, a randomized clinical trial, or an RCT?	No	Yes	Yes	No	Yes	Yes
2. Was the method of randomization adequate (i.e., use of randomly generated assignment)?	NA	Yes	Yes	NA	Yes	Yes
3. Was the treatment allocation concealed (so that assignments could not be predicted)?	NA	Yes	Yes	NA	Yes	Yes
4. Were study participants and providers blinded to treatment group assignment?	No	No	No	No	No	No
5. Were the people assessing the outcomes blinded to the participants' group assignments?	No	NA	Yes	No	No	NA
6. Were the groups similar at baseline on important characteristics that could affect outcomes (e.g., demographics, risk factors, co-morbid conditions)?	Yes	Yes	Yes	Yes	Yes	No
7. Was the overall drop-out rate from the study at endpoint 20% or lower of the number allocated to treatment?	Yes	Yes	Yes	NR	No	No
8. Was the differential drop-out rate (between treatment groups) at endpoint 15 percentage points or lower?	Yes	Yes	Yes	NR	Yes	Yes
9. Was there high adherence to the intervention protocols for each treatment group?	Yes	Yes	Yes	NR	Yes	Yes
10. Were other interventions avoided or similar in the groups (e.g., similar background treatments)?	Yes	NR	Yes	NR	Yes	NR
11. Were outcomes assessed using valid and reliable measures, implemented consistently across all study participants?	Yes	Yes	Yes	No	Yes	Yes
12. Did the authors report that the sample size was sufficiently large to be able to detect a difference in the main outcome between groups with at least 80% power?	No	Yes	No	NR	Yes	Yes
13. Were outcomes reported or subgroups analyzed prespecified (i.e., identified before analyses were conducted)?	Yes	Yes	Yes	Yes	Yes	Yes
14. Were all randomized participants analyzed in the group to which they were originally assigned, i.e., did they use an intention-to-treat analysis?	Yes	No	Yes	NR	Yes	Yes
Total score (maximum 14 points)	8	10	12	2	11	9

Note: CD, Cannot Determine; NA, Not Applicable; NR, Not Reported.

4. Discussion

The aim of the present study was to systematically review evidence on how ICT is being used for MBC in psychological treatments. To the best of our knowledge, this is the first attempt to systematically examine the different technologies that have been used so far for MBC during psychological interventions and to explore to what extent the use of ICT for MBC is feasible, acceptable, and effective.

One important finding was that only 18 studies met our inclusion criteria, which suggests that this is a field that requires more research. Additionally, the included studies varied greatly in terms of study design, diagnoses, MBC characteristics, and technology used, which again suggests that more investigation and replication will be needed to obtain robust findings about different technological solutions for MBC and to facilitate the generalization of the results to different populations. Future research should also examine the implication of technology systems for MBC in specific populations (e.g., children and adolescents, who are more familiar with technology systems). Furthermore, most of the included studies focused on mood and anxiety disorders, so it would be interesting to investigate the effects of technology used for MBC in other mental disorders.

As noted in the results section, the included technologies to support MBC were frequently handheld ICTs, such as smartphone apps, tablets, or laptops, which were involved both in the patient monitoring process and in the feedback to the therapists. In this sense, while tablets and laptops might be more difficult to use for EMA, it is encouraging that smartphone apps, which might facilitate EMA to a greater extent than other technologies, are also being used as supporting technologies for MBC.

An important finding regarding technology was that, overall, the use of technology for MBC during psychological interventions appears to be feasible and acceptable. In addition, technology in MBC was found to be effective [38] and cost-effective [41], particularly for not-on-track patients [35,40,42,47], as revealed in previous studies using MBC without technology [1]. Importantly, treatment engagement (i.e., time until dropout) was also enhanced with technology-supported MBC [33]. While these findings should be interpreted with caution, due to the limited number of existing investigations and the reduced number of controlled trials comparing technology-supported and non-supported MBC, the results suggest that the use of ICT to support MBC should continue to be tested in the future.

It is important to acknowledge that technology-supported EMA for MBC is different to a similar concept, which is ecological momentary intervention (EMI). Specifically, while in EMI a given intervention is provided in response to EMA in a timely manner (e.g., providing therapeutic skills with an app based on patient responses), in MBC EMA is only used to enhance face-to-face psychological interventions.

It is also important to note that some studies were excluded from this systematic review for several reasons which should be mentioned here. For instance, in some investigations, the monitoring process was not used to guide therapeutic decisions, even though technology was used for monitoring (thus, this would not be considered MBC). Conversely, in other studies, the technology was only used in one part of the MBC process, most frequently during the feedback part, but not for EMA (e.g., assessments were made in a paper-and-pencil approach, but then the information was introduced in a computer and presented in graphs or charts to the therapists and/or patients) [16,48–50].

4.1. Limitations

Some limitations should also be considered when interpreting the results of the present systematic review. As in previous similar reviews [13,18], the heterogeneity of studies with respect to sample size, measures used, and methodology, to name some examples, made it difficult to piece together the results and restricted the implementation of a meta-analysis which affects the generalizability and robustness of findings. Moreover, the majority of included studies were feasibility pilot studies, case studies, or non-RCTs. Although these designs can yield valuable information, RCTs, which have been rarer, are considered superior because of their higher internal validity and, therefore, higher robustness of the evidence indicating a (causal) relationship. Additionally, some factors might have biased the present systematic review findings, including the fact that only three databases were used for the search, and the possibility that studies where ICT was not feasible or did not add any value have not been published. Finally, it is important to note that this systematic review is limited to the interpretations of the authors who conducted the systematic review.

4.2. Conclusions

To conclude, this systematic review found preliminary support for the use of technology in MBC during psychological interventions. The use of ICTs in MBC has brought some encouraging contributions to the evolution of psychotherapy and its inclusion in routine care might significantly change the way psychotherapists work. Particularly, the provision of real-time information on symptom progress over the course of psychological interventions might help therapists detect and rapidly react to problems that might occur during treatment (e.g., exacerbation in symptomatology or low adherence to recommended practices). This would make current interventions more flexible and personalized [22] and should favor the psychotherapeutic relationship during face-to-face interventions. Additionally, this might increase the patients' awareness of their own progress.

In addition, technology was generally found to be a feasible and acceptable add-on tool for the MBC process. Therefore, the use of technology for improving the MBC process is mostly supported, as it might facilitate EMA and offer some potential for improving psychotherapy thanks to the real-time connection between patient assessment and therapist and patient feedback [32]. While the presented results are, overall, encouraging, especially for not-on-track patients, more research is required in this field, especially RCTs comparing technology-supported MBC with traditional MBC without technology.

Author Contributions: Conceptualization, P.G.-M., V.M.-B., J.M.B.-L., J.O., and C.S.-R.; Methodology, P.G.-M., V.M.-B., J.M.B.-L., J.O., C.S.-R.; Validation, J.M.B.-L. and C.S.-R.; Formal Analysis, P.G.-M. and V.M.-B.; Investigation, P.G.-M. and V.M.-B.; Resources, J.M.B.-L. and C.S.-R.; Data Curation, P.G.-M., V.M.-B., and C.S.-R.; Writing Original Draft Preparation, P.G.-M., V.M.-B., and C.S.-R.; Writing Review & Editing, P.G.-M., V.M.-B., J.M.B.-L., J.O., and C.S.-R.; Visualization, P.G.-M., V.M.-B., and C.S.-R.; Supervision, J.M.B.-L., J.O., and C.S.-R.; Project Administration, J.M.B.-L., J.O., and C.S.-R. All authors have read and agreed to the published version of the manuscript.

Funding: This research received no external funding.

Conflicts of Interest: The authors declare no conflict of interest

Appendix A. Complete List of Search Terms and Combinations

The first set of search terms were related to psychological treatment: "psychotherapy" OR "psychological treatment" OR "psychological intervention" OR "CBT" OR "cognitive-behavioral therapy" OR "cognitive behavioral therapy" OR "cognitive-behavioural therapy" OR "cognitive behavioural therapy". The second set of search terms were related to progress monitoring: "outcome feedback" OR "ecological momentary", OR "outcome monitoring" OR "enhanced treatment" OR "enhanced assessment" OR "enhanced monitoring". The last set of search terms were related to the use of technology through diverse devices: "mHealth" OR "eHealth" OR "technology" OR "app" OR "smartphone" OR "phone". These sets of search terms were linked with the Boolean operator AND.

References

1. Shimokawa, K.; Lambert, M.J.; Smart, D.W. Enhancing treatment outcome of patients at risk of treatment failure: Meta-analytic and mega-analytic review of a psychotherapy quality assurance system. *J. Consult. Clin. Psychol.* **2010**, *78*, 298–311. [CrossRef] [PubMed]
2. Lambert, M.J.; Hansen, N.B.; Finch, A.E. Patient-focused research: Using patient outcome data to enhance treatment effects. *J. Consult. Clin. Psychol.* **2001**, *69*, 159–172. [CrossRef] [PubMed]
3. Kaplan, S.H.; Billimek, J.; Sorkin, D.H.; Ngo-Metzger, Q.; Greenfield, S. Who can respond to treatment? *Med. Care* **2010**, *48*, S9–S16. [CrossRef] [PubMed]
4. McDevitt-Murphy, M.E.; Luciano, M.T.; Zakarian, R.J. Use of ecological momentary assessment and intervention in treatment with adults. *Focus (Madison)* **2018**, *16*, 370–375. [CrossRef]
5. Suso-Ribera, C.; Mesas, Á.; Medel, J.; Server, A.; Márquez, E.; Castilla, D.; Zaragozá, I.; García-Palacios, A.; Mesas, A.; Medel, J.; et al. Improving pain treatment with a smartphone app: Study protocol for a randomized controlled trial. *Trials* **2018**, *19*, 145. [CrossRef]
6. Colombo, D.; Fernández-Álvarez, J.; Suso-Ribera, C.; Cipresso, P.; Valev, H.; Leufkens, T.; Sas, C.; Garcia-Palacios, A.; Riva, G.; Botella, C. The need for change: Understanding emotion regulation antecedents and consequences using ecological momentary assessment. *Emotion* **2020**, *20*, 30–36. [CrossRef]
7. Beute, F.; De Kort, Y.; Ijsselsteijn, W. Restoration in its natural context: How ecological momentary assessment can advance restoration research. *Int. J. Environ. Res. Public Health* **2016**, *13*, 420. [CrossRef]
8. Kendrick, T.; Moore, M.; Gilbody, S.; Churchill, R.; Stuart, B.; El-Gohary, M. Routine use of patient reported outcome measures (PROMs) for improving treatment of common mental health disorders in adults. *Cochrane Database Syst. Rev.* **2014**, *2014*. [CrossRef]
9. Canadian Psychological Association. *Outcomes and Progress Monitoring in Psychotherapy*; A Report of the Canadian Psychological Association, Prepared by the Task Force on Outcomes and Progress Monitoring in Psychotherapy; Canadian Psychological Association: Ottawa, ON, Canada, 2018.
10. Knaup, C.; Koesters, M.; Schoefer, D.; Becker, T.; Puschner, B. Effect of feedback of treatment outcome in specialist mental healthcare: Meta-analysis. *Br. J. Psychiatry* **2009**, *195*, 15–22. [CrossRef]

11. Scott, K.; Lewis, C.C. Using measurement-based care to enhance any treatment. *Cogn. Behav. Pract.* **2015**, *22*, 49–59. [CrossRef]
12. Lambert, M.J.; Whipple, J.L.; Smart, D.W.; Vermeersch, D.A.; Nielsen, S.L.; Hawkins, E.J. The effects of providing therapists with feedback on patient progress during psychotherapy: Are outcomes enhanced? *Psychother. Res.* **2001**, *11*, 49–68. [CrossRef] [PubMed]
13. Goldberg, S.B.; Buck, B.; Raphaely, S.; Fortney, J.C. Measuring psychiatric symptoms remotely: A systematic review of remote measurement-based care. *Curr. Psychiatry Rep.* **2018**, *20*, 81. [CrossRef] [PubMed]
14. Reese, R.J.; Norsworthy, L.A.; Rowlands, S.R. Does a continuous feedback system improve psychotherapy outcome? *Psychotherapy* **2009**, *46*, 418–431. [CrossRef] [PubMed]
15. Lambert, M.J.; Harmon, C.; Slade, K.; Whipple, J.L.; Hawkins, E.J. Providing feedback to psychotherapists on their patients' progress: Clinical results and practice sugges tions. *J. Clin. Psychol.* **2005**, *61*, 165–174. [CrossRef] [PubMed]
16. Bickman, L.; Kelley, S.D.; Breda, C.; De Andrade, A.R.; Riemer, M. Effects of routine feedback to clinicians on mental health outcomes of youths: Results of a randomized trial. *Psychiatr. Serv.* **2011**, *62*, 1423–1429. [CrossRef]
17. Carlier, I.V.E.; Meuldijk, D.; Van Vliet, I.M.; Van Fenema, E.; Van Der Wee, N.J.A.; Zitman, F.G. Routine outcome monitoring and feedback on physical or mental health status: Evidence and theory. *J. Eval. Clin. Pract.* **2012**, *18*, 104–110. [CrossRef]
18. Gondek, D.; Edbrooke-Childs, J.; Fink, E.; Deighton, J.; Wolpert, M. Feedback from outcome measures and treatment effectiveness, treatment efficiency, and collaborative practice: A systematic review. *Adm. Policy Ment. Health Ment. Health Serv. Res.* **2016**, *43*, 325–343. [CrossRef]
19. Imel, Z.E.; Caperton, D.D.; Tanana, M.; Atkins, D.C. Technology-enhanced human interaction in psychotherapy. *J. Couns. Psychol.* **2017**, *64*, 385–393. [CrossRef]
20. Aboraya, A.; Nasrallah, H.A.; Elswick, D.E.; Elshazly, A.; Estephan, N.; Aboraya, D.; Berzingi, S.; Chumbers, J.; Berzingi, S.; Justice, J.; et al. Measurement-based care in psychiatry—Past, present, and future. *Innov. Clin. Neurosci.* **2018**, *15*, 13–26.
21. Hallgren, K.A.; Bauer, A.M.; Atkins, D.C. Digital technology and clinical decision making in depression treatment: Current findings and future opportunities. *Depress. Anxiety* **2017**, *34*, 494–501. [CrossRef]
22. Bauer, S.; Moessner, M. Technology-enhanced monitoring in psychotherapy and e-mental health. *J. Ment. Health* **2012**, *21*, 355–363. [CrossRef] [PubMed]
23. Silk, J.S.; Forbes, E.E.; Whalen, D.J.; Jakubcak, J.L.; Thompson, W.K.; Ryan, N.D.; Axelson, D.A.; Birmaher, B.; Dahl, R.E. Daily emotional dynamics in depressed youth: A cell phone ecological momentary assessment study. *J. Exp. Child Psychol.* **2011**, *110*, 241–257. [CrossRef] [PubMed]
24. Suso-Ribera, C.; Castilla, D.; Zaragozá, I.; Ribera-Canudas, M.V.; Botella, C.; García-Palacios, A. Validity, reliability, feasibility, and usefulness of Pain Monitor. A multidimensional smartphone app for daily monitoring of adults with heterogeneous chronic pain. *Clin. J. Pain* **2018**, *34*, 900–908. [CrossRef] [PubMed]
25. Hegland, P.A.; Aasprang, A.; Hjelle Øygard, S.; Nordberg, S.; Kolotkin, R.; Moltu, C.; Tell, G.S.; Andersen, J.R. A review of systematic reviews on the effects of patient-reported outcome monitoring with clinical feedback systems on health-related quality of life-implications for a novel technology in obesity treatment. *Clin. Obes.* **2018**, *8*, 452–464. [CrossRef]
26. Moher, D.; Liberati, A.; Tetzlaff, J.; Altman, D.G.; Altman, D.G.; Antes, G.; Atkins, D.; Barbour, V.; Barrowman, N.; Berlin, J.A.; et al. Preferred reporting items for systematic reviews and meta-analyses: The PRISMA statement (Chinese edition). *J. Chin. Integr. Med.* **2009**, *7*, 889–896. [CrossRef]
27. Falagas, M.E.; Pitsouni, E.I.; Malietzis, G.A.; Pappas, G. Comparison of PubMed, Scopus, Web of Science, and Google Scholar: Strengths and weaknesses. *FASEB J.* **2008**, *22*, 338–342. [CrossRef]
28. Eady, A.M.; Wilczynski, N.L.; Haynes, R.B. PsycINFO search strategies identified methodologically sound therapy studies and review articles for use by clinicians and researchers. *J. Clin. Epidemiol.* **2008**, *61*, 34–40. [CrossRef]
29. National Heart Lung and Blood Institute (NHLBI). Study Quality Assessment Tools. Available online: https://www.nhlbi.nih.gov/health-topics/study-quality-assessment-tools (accessed on 1 May 2020).
30. Smith, B.; Harms, W.D.; Burres, S.; Korda, H.; Rosen, H.; Davis, J. Enhancing behavioral health treatment and crisis management through mobile ecological momentary assessment and SMS messaging. *Health Inform. J.* **2012**, *18*, 294–308. [CrossRef]

31. Pramana, G.; Parmanto, B.; Kendall, P.C.; Silk, J.S. The SmartCAT: An m-health platform for ecological momentary intervention in child anxiety treatment. *Telemed. e-Health* **2014**, *20*, 419–427. [CrossRef]
32. Pinsof, W.M.; Goldsmith, J.Z.; Latta, T.A. Information technology and feedback research can bridge the scientist–practitioner gap: A couple therapy example. *Couple Fam. Psychol. Res. Pract.* **2012**, *1*, 253–273. [CrossRef]
33. Aguilera, A.; Bruehlman-Senecal, E.; Demasi, O.; Avila, P. Automated Text messaging as an adjunct to cognitive behavioral therapy for depression: A clinical trial. *J. Med. Internet Res.* **2017**, *19*, e148. [CrossRef] [PubMed]
34. Kumar, D.; Tully, L.M.; Iosif, A.-M.; Zaskorn, L.N.; Nye, K.E.; Zia, A.; Niendam, T.A. A mobile health platform for clinical monitoring in early psychosis: Implementation in community-based outpatient early psychosis care. *JMIR Ment. Health* **2018**, *5*, e15. [CrossRef] [PubMed]
35. Aharonovich, E.; Sarvet, A.; Stohl, M.; DesJarlais, D.; Tross, S.; Hurst, T.; Urbina, A.; Hasin, D. Reducing non-injection drug use in HIV primary care: A randomized trial of brief motivational interviewing, with and without HealthCall, a technology-based enhancement. *J. Subst. Abuse Treat.* **2017**, *74*, 71–79. [CrossRef] [PubMed]
36. Niendam, T.A.; Tully, L.M.; Iosif, A.M.; Kumar, D.; Nye, K.E.; Denton, J.C.; Zakskorn, L.N.; Fedechko, T.L.; Pierce, K.M. Enhancing early psychosis treatment using smartphone technology: A longitudinal feasibility and validity study. *J. Psychiatr. Res.* **2018**, *96*, 239–246. [CrossRef]
37. Bauer, A.M.; Iles-Shih, M.; Ghomi, R.H.; Rue, T.; Grover, T.; Kincler, N.; Miller, M.; Katon, W.J. Acceptability of mHealth augmentation of Collaborative Care: A mixed methods pilot study. *Gen. Hosp. Psychiatry* **2018**, *51*, 22–29. [CrossRef]
38. Bell, I.H.; Rossell, S.L.; Farhall, J.; Hayward, M.; Lim, M.H.; Fielding-Smith, S.F.; Thomas, N. Pilot randomised controlled trial of a brief coping-focused intervention for hearing voices blended with smartphone-based ecological momentary assessment and intervention (SAVVy): Feasibility, acceptability and preliminary clinical outcomes. *Schizophr. Res.* **2019**. [CrossRef]
39. Bell, I.H.; Fielding-Smith, S.F.; Hayward, M.; Rossell, S.L.; Lim, M.H.; Farhall, J.; Thomas, N. Smartphone-based ecological momentary assessment and intervention in a blended coping-focused therapy for distressing voices: Development and case illustration. *Internet Interv.* **2018**, *14*, 18–25. [CrossRef]
40. Newnham, E.A.; Hooke, G.R.; Page, A.C. Progress monitoring and feedback in psychiatric care reduces depressive symptoms. *J. Affect. Disord.* **2010**, *127*, 139–146. [CrossRef]
41. Delgadillo, J.; Overend, K.; Lucock, M.; Groom, M.; Kirby, N.; McMillan, D.; Gilbody, S.; Lutz, W.; Rubel, J.A.; De Jong, K. Improving the efficiency of psychological treatment using outcome feedback technology. *Behav. Res. Ther.* **2017**, *99*, 89–97. [CrossRef]
42. Delgadillo, J.; De Jong, K.; Lucock, M.; Lutz, W.; Rubel, J.; Gilbody, S.; Ali, S.; Aguirre, E.; Appleton, M.; Nevin, J.; et al. Feedback-informed treatment versus usual psychological treatment for depression and anxiety: A multisite, open-label, cluster randomised controlled trial. *Lancet Psychiatry* **2018**, *5*, 564–572. [CrossRef]
43. Miklowitz, D.J.; Price, J.; Holmes, E.A.; Rendell, J.; Bell, S.; Budge, K.; Christensen, J.; Wallace, J.; Simon, J.; Armstrong, N.M.; et al. Facilitated Integrated Mood Management for adults with bipolar disorder. *Bipolar Disord.* **2012**, *14*, 185–197. [CrossRef] [PubMed]
44. Schiepek, G.; Aichhorn, W.; Gruber, M.; Strunk, G.; Bachler, E.; Aas, B. Real-time monitoring of psychotherapeutic processes: Concept and compliance. *Front. Psychol.* **2016**, *7*, 604. [CrossRef] [PubMed]
45. Kaiser, T.; Laireiter, A.R. DynAMo: A modular platform for monitoring process, outcome, and algorithm-based treatment planning in psychotherapy. *JMIR Med. Inform.* **2017**, *5*, e20. [CrossRef] [PubMed]
46. Lazarou, I.; Karakostas, A.; Stavropoulos, T.G.; Tsompanidis, T.; Meditskos, G.; Kompatsiaris, I.; Tsolaki, M. A novel and intelligent home monitoring system for care support of elders with cognitive impairment. *J. Alzheimer's Dis.* **2016**, *54*, 1561–1591. [CrossRef] [PubMed]
47. De Jong, K.; Timman, R.; Hakkaart-Van Roijen, L.; Vermeulen, P.; Kooiman, K.; Passchier, J.; Van Busschbach, J. The effect of outcome monitoring feedback to clinicians and patients in short and long-term psychotherapy: A randomized controlled trial. *Psychother. Res.* **2014**, *24*, 629–639. [CrossRef]

48. Amble, I.; Gude, T.; Stubdal, S.; Andersen, B.J.; Wampold, B.E. The effect of implementing the Outcome Questionnaire-45.2 feedback system in Norway: A multisite randomized clinical trial in a naturalistic setting. *Psychother. Res.* **2015**, *25*, 669–677. [CrossRef]
49. Janse, P.D.; De Jong, K.; Van Dijk, M.K.; Hutschemaekers, G.J.M.; Verbraak, M.J.P.M. Improving the efficiency of cognitive-behavioural therapy by using formal client feedback. *Psychother. Res.* **2017**, *27*, 525–538. [CrossRef]
50. Lucock, M.; Halstead, J.; Leach, C.; Barkham, M.; Tucker, S.; Randal, C.; Middleton, J.; Khan, W.; Catlow, H.; Waters, E.; et al. A mixed-method investigation of patient monitoring and enhanced feedback in routine practice: Barriers and facilitators. *Psychother. Res.* **2015**, *25*, 633–646. [CrossRef]

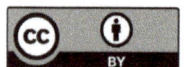 © 2020 by the authors. Licensee MDPI, Basel, Switzerland. This article is an open access article distributed under the terms and conditions of the Creative Commons Attribution (CC BY) license (http://creativecommons.org/licenses/by/4.0/).

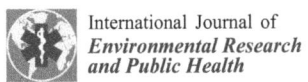

Article

Working Alliance Inventory for Online Interventions-Short Form (WAI-TECH-SF): The Role of the Therapeutic Alliance between Patient and Online Program in Therapeutic Outcomes

Rocío Herrero [1,2], Mª Dolores Vara [1,2], Marta Miragall [2,3,*], Cristina Botella [2,3], Azucena García-Palacios [2,3], Heleen Riper [4,5], Annet Kleiboer [4] and Rosa Mª Baños [1,2,6]

1. Polibienestar Research Institute, University of Valencia, 46022 Valencia, Spain; ro.herrero.09@gmail.com (R.H.); m.dolores.vara@uv.es (M.D.V.); banos@uv.es (R.M.B.)
2. CIBERObn Physiopathology of Obesity and Nutrition, Instituto de Salud Carlos III, 28029 Madrid, Spain; botella@uji.es (C.B.); azucena@uji.es (A.G.-P.)
3. Department of Basic and Clinical Psychology and Psychobiology, Faculty of Health Sciences, Jaume I University, 12071 Castellon de la Plana, Spain
4. Department of Clinical, Neuro and Developmental Psychology, Vrije Universiteit, 1081-BT Amsterdam, The Netherlands; h.riper@vu.nl (H.R.); a.m.kleiboer@vu.nl (A.K.)
5. Department of Research and Innovation GGZ InGeest, Amsterdam University Medical Center, 1081-HJ Amsterdam, The Netherlands
6. Department of Personality, Evaluation and Psychological Treatment, Faculty of Psychology, University of Valencia, 46010 Valencia, Spain
* Correspondence: miragall@uji.es

Received: 17 July 2020; Accepted: 19 August 2020; Published: 25 August 2020

Abstract: Background: Therapeutic alliance (TA) between the patient and therapist has been related to positive therapeutic outcomes. Because Internet-based interventions are increasingly being implemented, a tool is needed to measure the TA with Internet-based self-guided programs. The Working Alliance Inventory for online interventions (WAI-TECH-SF) was adapted based on the WAI Short Form (Hatcher & Gillaspy, 2006). The objectives of this study were: (1) to analyse the psychometric properties of the WAI-TECH-SF; (2) to explore the differences in the WAI-TECH-SF scores according to different categories of the sample; and (3) to analyse whether the WAI-TECH-SF can predict therapeutic outcomes and satisfaction with the treatment. Methods: 193 patients diagnosed with depression were included and received blended Cognitive-Behavioural Therapy. Measures of preferences, satisfaction, and credibility about the treatment, TA with the online program, depressive symptoms, and satisfaction with the treatment were administered. Results: An exploratory factor analysis revealed a one-dimensional structure with adequate internal consistency. Linear regression analyses showed that the WAI-TECH-SF predicted changes in depressive symptoms and satisfaction with the treatment. Conclusions: WAI-TECH-SF is a reliable questionnaire to assess the TA between the patient and the online program, which is associated with positive therapeutic outcomes and satisfaction with the treatment.

Keywords: therapeutic alliance; online interventions; therapeutic outcomes; satisfaction with the treatment

1. Introduction

Evidence shows that the therapeutic alliance (TA) (also called the working alliance) has a relevant influence on therapeutic outcomes [1]. Several meta-analyses have found that TA is moderately associated with better treatment outcomes in face-to-face therapy [1,2], regardless of the therapeutic framework or patient characteristics, among other aspects [3]. One of the most widely used definitions of TA was proposed by Bordin [4], who considered the alliance to be a general factor with three interrelated components: (a) the degree of mutual trust, collaboration, and acceptance between the therapist and the patient (i.e., the bonds); (b) the agreement between patient and therapist about specific tasks or activities (i.e., the tasks); and (c) the agreement about the therapeutic objectives (i.e., the goals).

Currently, the ways of delivering therapeutic interventions are changing. The need for psychological support is growing, and the dominant model of psychotherapy from past centuries—individual, face-to-face, and long-lasting—is not likely to fulfil this need [5]. New forms of treatment delivery are emerging to face the challenge of providing well-established interventions that can reach a wider population. This situation has promoted the development of interventions that require less therapist involvement, such as Internet-based Interventions (IBIs) [6], either self-guided or hybrid therapeutic approaches (blended treatments) where face-to-face sessions are combined with online therapy [7]. Well-established evidence shows that interventions fully or partially delivered through the Internet (especially those based on Cognitive Behavioural Therapy (CBT)) are effective in treating different psychological disorders [8–10] and can be as effective as face-to-face therapy [11,12]. Therefore, IBIs are attractive and useful strategies to be applied by healthcare professionals in clinical settings [13]. Nevertheless, different questions have arisen about the therapeutic process, such as what happens to the TA when there is no direct contact with a therapist or when this contact is scarce [14].

The research triggered by this question has focused on the development and validation of measures that make it possible to assess the TA in IBIs and study of the role of the TA in predicting the therapeutic outcomes. To measure the TA in therapies supported by technological tools, most studies have used an adapted version of the Working Alliance Inventory (WAI) [15], or its short form (WAI-SF) [16,17]. In general, evidence supports the relevance of the TA in IBIs, because similar TA scores have been found for face-to-face therapy and IBIs [3,14,18–20], as well as similar moderate effect sizes for the relationship between TA and therapeutic outcomes [3,21]. In this regard, Clarke et al. [22] conducted a qualitative and quantitative study to examine the TA in the context of a self-guided intervention, and they found that TA is high even when the intervention does not involve human support. In addition, the study highlighted that a positive TA, in terms of feeling a meaningful connection and working collaboratively, is relevant for engaging with the intervention. In this study, they did not find a relationship between TA and therapeutic outcomes. Nonetheless, a systematic review showed an effect of TA on anxiety and depressive outcomes, pointing out that higher levels of TA were related to better clinical outcomes [23]. Recently, Gómez-Penedo et al. [24] explored the reliability and validity of the WAI-SF in guided IBIs, taking into account the relational aspects involved in this type of intervention (e.g., therapist support, online program). In this validation, the bond subscale was adapted to refer to the acceptance and trust between the patient and the therapist who supported him/her in the online program. Results of the WAI for guided Internet interventions (i.e., WAI-I) showed a two-factor solution ("tasks-goals" and "bonds") with adequate internal consistency and external validity in a sample of patients with mild to moderate depression. Moreover, patients with higher scores on TA were more satisfied with the intervention after the treatment.

The approach used to carry out the adaptation of the WAI questionnaire in previous studies consisted of following Bordin's classic conceptualization [4], considering the three dimensions of TA (bond, tasks, and goals) and making slight modifications in the statements [25,26]. This approach has been questioned by some authors, who suggest that the definition of TA is grounded in the specific characteristics of face-to-face therapy and, therefore, is not necessarily the same in other formats [27,28]. In fact, in the WAI adapted to measure the TA between the patients and the virtual environment, where the word "therapist" was replaced by "virtual environment", the three dimensions proposed by Bordin [4] did not arise in the exploratory factor analysis, and only one general dimension was found [25]. By contrast, Kiluk et al. [29] conducted an adaptation of the 36-item original version of the WAI called WAI-Tech, which was designed to measure the TA between cocaine-dependent patients and the online program, and it showed similar psychometric properties to the original scale (i.e., the WAI). In this adaptation, items were slightly adapted by replacing "therapist" with "online program", and items corresponding to the bond subscale were reworded to preserve comprehension. Results showed lower scores on the bond subscale, and the total scores on WAI-Tech were not associated with the change in therapeutic outcomes. However, findings are limited due to the small sample size and the absence of factor analysis to analyse the psychometric properties in this study.

Thus, the TA developed by the patients in IBIs and, specifically, in blended Cognitive-Behavioural Therapy (CBT) (i.e., combining individual face-to-face sessions with online intervention modules) has not been completely understood. The present study was conducted in the context of a European project called "e-Compared", in which previous findings found that only therapist-rated TA (but not patient-rated TA) was predictive of changes in depression scores during a blended treatment in a sample of 73 patients [30]. Thus, it seems that technology is a third factor in the relationship between patient and therapist, which adds more complexity to this relationship. Hence, the need to measure not only the relationship between the patient and the therapist, but also between the patient and the technology, is undeniably relevant due to the growing emergence of IBIs.

Previous studies have found that individuals have the ability to form a bond and be open with an online application [28]. However, it is still important to develop a reliable questionnaire and explore whether the three-dimensional structure proposed originally for face-to-face therapy is also maintained in the TA with the online program in self-guided IBIs where there is hardly any interaction with a therapist or person supporting the intervention. To do so, an adaptation of the WAI-SF to measure the TA with the online program was carried out. An exploratory factor analysis was conducted in order to avoid determining the psychometric structure a priori, given the controversial structure of TA when technologies are involved (e.g., the structure was uni-dimensional in Miragall et al. [25]; or bi-dimensional in Gómez-Penedo et al. [24]). In addition, other potential variables influencing the TA with the online program were explored, as well as the capacity of the TA with the online program to predict therapeutic outcomes and satisfaction with the treatment. The study was conducted in a sample of depressive patients who were receiving a self-guided IBI in the context of the National Health Systems of different European countries.

Hence, the aims of this study were: (1) to analyse the psychometric structure of the WAI-TECH-SF, a questionnaire designed to assess the TA between the patient and the online program in a self-guided IBI; (2) to explore whether there are differences in WAI-TECH-SF scores based on sex, age-range, level of education, initial severity of depression, preference for any of the treatments offered, and expectations about and credibility of the treatment; and (3) to explore whether higher WAI-TECH-SF scores predict the therapeutic outcomes (i.e., change in depressive symptom scores) and satisfaction with the treatment.

2. Materials and Methods

2.1. Participants

One-hundred and ninety-three patients took part in this study (ages ranging from 19 to 69 years old: $M = 40.44$ years old; $SD = 12.79$; 64.2% women). Patients were recruited as part of the clinical trial conducted in the e-Compared Project (EU-HEALTH.2013 N.603098). The sample was composed of European citizens diagnosed with depression in either primary or specialized care. Regarding their nationalities, 38.2% of the sample were from Germany, 16.2% from Sweden, 12.0% from Spain, 9.8% from France, 8.4% from the Netherlands, 6.3% from the UK, and 2.1% from Switzerland. Patients were excluded if they were under 18 years old, had serious psychiatric comorbidity, or did not have access to a computer or the Internet. All the patients were diagnosed with depression using the MINI. In terms of their symptoms, 10.9% of the sample showed mild symptoms of depression, 33.2% showed moderate symptoms, 36.8% showed moderate–severe symptoms, and 19.2% showed severe depressive symptomatology. In addition, 50.8% of the sample had some suicidal risk, and 61.1% of the sample had a comorbid diagnosis, such as panic disorder, agoraphobia, or social phobia. Regarding their educational level, 56.0% of the sample had a high educational level, 31.6% had a medium educational level, and 12.4% had a low educational level. All participants were informed about the study and gave their informed consent before the beginning of the trial, in accordance with the Declaration of Helsinki. The study was approved by the corresponding ethical committee in each country: (a) France: Comité de protection des personnes, Ile de France V (15033-n° 2015-A00565-44); (b) Germany: Ethik Kommison DGPsychologie, Universitat Trier (MB 102014); (c) The Netherlands: METC VUMC (2015.078); (d) Poland: Komisja ds. Etyki Badan Naukowych (10/2014); (e) Spain: Comision Deontologica/Comite Ético de Investigacion en Humanos de la Universidad de Valencia (H1414775276823); (f) Sweden: Regionala etikprovningsnamnden (2014/428-31); (g) Switzerland: Kantonale Ethikkomission Bern (001/2015); (h) UK: NRES Committee London-Camden and King's Cross (15/LO/0511). All participants received a blended CBT (bCBT) for depression.

2.2. Intervention

All the e-Compared project interventions combined individual CBT delivered through face-to-face sessions and online sessions [31]. The interventions received by patients had some variations across the countries, but followed common guidelines [31]. In this regard, the ratio between the number of face-to-face sessions and the number of online modules varied across countries, but at least 1/3 of the sessions were face-to-face (i.e., between 3 and 10 sessions), and at least 1/3 were online (i.e., between 6 and 10 sessions). As a minimum, the bCBT included modules of psychoeducation, cognitive restructuring, behavioural activation, and relapse prevention. In addition, each country site was able to include additional components, such as mindfulness, coping skills training, or problem solving, but these additional components could not make up more than a quarter of the total intervention. Face-to-face sessions were provided by: (1) licensed CBT therapists in mental health care; (2) CBT therapists in training under the supervision of an experienced licensed CBT therapist in mental health care; (3) a licensed psychologist with a CBT orientation in primary care; or (4) psychologists in training under the supervision of a licensed psychologist with a CBT orientation in primary care. All of them were trained in how to deliver the blended treatment. Each face-to-face session lasted around 20–60 min (i.e., 45–60 min in specialized care and 20–45 min in primary care), while the online session lasted for as long as the patients took to read each session. A summary of the intervention components and the online vs. face-to face ratio are shown in Table 1.

Table 1. Overview of blended treatment applied in each country.

Country	Platform	Duration	Online/Face-to-Face Sessions	Session Sequence	Mandatory Modules				Additional Modules		
					PE	CR	BA	RP	Problem Solving	Physical Exercise	Other
Netherlands	Moodbuster	20 weeks	10/10	Alternate	X	X	X	X	X	X	
France	Moodbuster	16 weeks	8/8	Alternate	X	X	X	X	X	X	
Poland	Moodbuster	6–10 weeks	6/6	Alternate	X	X	X	X	X	X	
United Kingdom	Moodbuster	11 weeks	5/6	Alternate	X	X	X	X	X	X	
Switzerland	Deprexis	18 weeks	9/9	Alternate	X	X	X	X	X	X	X
Sweden	Itherapi	12 weeks	8/4	Alternate	X	X	X	X			
Spain	Smiling is fun	10 weeks	8/3	1-4-1-4-1	X	X	X	X			X
Germany	Moodbuster	10–13 weeks	10/5	Alternate	X	X	X	X	X	X	

Notes. PE = Psychoeducation; CR = Cognitive restructuring; BA = Behavioral activation; RP = Relapse prevention.

2.3. Measures

Working Alliance Inventory applied to Internet (WAI-TECH-SF) is an adaptation of the WAI-SF [16] elaborated by the authors. It is a 12-item self-report questionnaire designed to assess the TA with the online program in a self-guided IBI, with responses rated on a seven-point Likert scale, ranging from 1 (never) to 7 (always). The questionnaire was designed to cover the same structure as the original scale, with three dimensions: (1) therapeutic goals (items 1, 2, 8, 10), (2) tasks (items 4, 6, 10, 11), and (3) bonds (items 3, 5, 7, 9). The total score ranges from 12 to 84. The mean and standard deviation for this sample were $M = 57.84$ and $SD = 16.39$. Details about its adaptation appear in the "Procedure" section. The questionnaire was administered at post-assessment.

Patient Health Questionnaire-9 (PHQ-9; [32]) is a nine-item mood module that can be used to screen and diagnose patients with depressive disorders. It is based directly on the criteria for major depressive disorder in the Diagnostic and Statistical Manual of Mental Disorders (4th ed.) [33] and its accuracy for screening to detect major depression has been demonstrated [34]. The nine items are each scored on a 0–3 scale, with the total score ranging from 0–27 and higher scores indicating more severe depression. The means and standard deviations for this sample were $M = 15.50$ and $SD = 4.63$ (pre-assessment), and $M = 9.05$ and $SD = 5.35$ (post-assessment). The PHQ-9 has been shown to have good psychometric properties [35]. The questionnaire was administered at pre- and post-assessment. In this study, Cronbach's alphas ranged from 0.73 to 0.87.

International Neuropsychiatric Interview (MINI 5.0; [36]) is a structured diagnostic interview based on the Diagnostic and Statistical Manual of Mental Disorders (DSM-IV) and on International Classification of Diseases (ICD-10) criteria. The MINI has been translated into 65 languages and is used for both clinical and research practices. The full MINI. 5.0, with the exception of Anorexia Nervosa, Bulimia Nervosa, and Antisocial Personality Disorder, was used to provide a diagnosis at pre-assessment.

Preference for Treatment Questionnaire (ad-hoc instrument) was used to assess participants' treatment preference from the options of bCBT, TAU, or no preference. Specifically, the following question was asked: "If you had the chance to choose your depression treatment, which one would you prefer to receive?"

Credibility and Expectancy Questionnaire (CEQ; [37]) was used to assess the prior predisposition of patients to the proposed intervention. The scale consists of six items divided into two factors: expectancy (with three questions rated on a 10-point scale, ranging from 1 to 9) and credibility (with one question rated on a 10-point scale and two questions rated on a 1–100% scale). The means and standard deviations for this sample were $M = 17.59$ and $SD = 4.92$ (in a scale ranging from 3 to 27) and $M = 19.32$ and $SD = 5.15$ (on a scale ranging from 3 to 27) for expectancy and credibility, respectively. In this study, Cronbach's alphas were 0.86 for expectancy and 0.72 for credibility.

Client Satisfaction Questionnaire (CSQ-8; [38]) was used to assess patients' satisfaction with the treatment. This questionnaire has been translated into multiple languages, and it is used to measure global patient satisfaction. The questionnaire consists of eight items rated on a four-point scale, with total scores ranging from 8 to 32. The mean and standard deviation for this sample were $M = 25.39$ and $SD = 5.00$. The questionnaire was administered at post-assessment. In this study, Cronbach's alpha was 0.92.

2.4. Procedure

An adaptation of the patient version of the WAI-SF [16] was carried out following the recommendations of Hambleton and Patsula [39]. Thus, the purpose of the WAI-TECH-SF is to measure agreement about goals, tasks, sense of trust, comfort, and bonding between the patient and the "online program". To this end, the sentences on the current scale were kept as similar as possible to the originals, but "my therapist" or therapy was replaced with "online program". Items are displayed in Table 2.

Table 2. Psychometric properties of the WAI-TECH: Descriptive statistics and factorial loadings with a one-factor structure using Maximum Likelihood.

	Skewness Index	Kurtosis Index	M (SD)	λ	h^2
Item 1. As a result of these sessions using the program____ I am clearer as to how I might be able to change.	−0.72	0.19	5.11 (1.40)	0.76	0.58
Item 2. What I am doing with the program____ gives me new ways of looking at my problem.	−0.56	−0.40	4.89 (1.48)	0.88	0.77
Item 3. I believe that I am a good candidate for the program____.	−0.50	−0.36	4.84 (1.46)	0.86	0.74
Item 4. The program____ and I collaborate on setting goals for my therapy.	−0.47	−0.58	4.72 (1.72)	0.87	0.75
Item 5. The program____ and I respect each other.	−0.57	−0.28	4.94 (1.58)	0.84	0.70
Item 6. The program____ and I are working towards mutually agreed upon goals.	−0.64	−0.05	5.04 (1.48)	0.85	0.72
Item 7. I feel that the program____ appreciates me.	−0.35	−0.75	4.44 (1.74)	0.81	0.67
Item 8. The program____ and I agree on what is important for me to work on.	−0.62	−0.25	4.84 (1.61)	0.85	0.73
Item 9. I feel the program____ cares about me even when I do things that he/she does not approve of.	−0.61	−0.13	4.91 (1.62)	0.89	0.78
Item 10. I feel that the things I do with the program____ will help me to accomplish the changes that I want.	−0.48	−0.34	4.56 (1.54)	0.87	0.76
Item 11. The program____ and I have established a good understanding of the kind of changes that would be good for me.	−0.66	−0.07	4.93 (1.55)	0.91	0.83
Item 12. I believe the way that the program____ and I are working with my problem is correct.	−0.52	−0.43	4.62 (1.65)	0.89	0.79

Notes. λ = Factor loading; h^2 = Communalities.

Once the WAI-TECH-SF had been adapted, it was applied in the context of the e-Compared European project to the participants receiving the bCBT. All the patients in the project were recruited in the National Health Systems of the countries involved, in either primary or specialised care. Their status was assessed with the MINI interview, performed by a clinical psychologist. If patients met the inclusion criteria, they were allocated to one of two conditions: bCBT or Treatment as Usual (TAU) (for more details about the trial, see Kleiboer et al. [31]). All participants filled out the PHQ-9 questionnaire to assess the severity of their depressive symptoms and their preference for the intervention ("blended", "TAU", or "no preference"), and the CEQ scale was used to assess the patients' expectations and credibility with regard to the intervention offered. For the purposes of the current study, only participants allocated to the bCBT condition were taken into account, given that those in the TAU condition did not receive any therapeutic support online. Once patients had finished the intervention, they were assessed again on their depressive symptoms, their satisfaction with the treatment through the CSQ scale, and their TA with the self-guided IBIs using the WAI-TECH-SF.

2.5. Data Analyses

All statistical analyses were performed using the SPSS v.26 (IBM Corp, Armonk, NY, USA). The percentage of missing values in the WAI-TECH-SF, PHQ-9, and CEQ scores ranged from 0% to 1.6%. After testing that the values were missing at random using Little's MCAR test ($p > 0.05$), they were imputed using the Expectation–Maximization Algorithm method [40]. Then, several analyses were carried out. First, to analyse the psychometric properties of the WAI-TECH-SF, skewness and kurtosis were analysed to check the normality of the data [41]. Kaiser-Meyer-Olkin (KMO), and Barlett's Test of Sphericity was used to ensure the suitability of the data for performing an Exploratory Factor Analysis (EFA). Parallel Analysis [42] was applied using a macro for SPSS [43] to determine the number of factors retained in the EFA. Then, to explore the factor structure of the WAI-TECH-SF, an EFA was conducted using a Maximum Likelihood estimation extraction method because the data were normally distributed [41]. Internal consistency of the total score was assessed using Cronbach's alpha coefficient [44].

Second, preliminary analyses were conducted to ensure that relevant assumptions of t-tests, ANOVAs, and simple/multiple regression (i.e., normality, linearity, homoscedasticity, and absence of multicollinearity) were met. Third, independent-samples t-tests and one-way ANOVAs were performed to find out whether there were significant differences in the WAI-TECH-SF scores based on sex, age range (18–34 vs. 35–49 vs. > 50), level of education (low vs. medium vs. high), initial severity on PHQ scores (mild vs. moderate vs. moderate–severe vs. severe), preference for any of the treatments offered (no preference vs. blended vs. TAU), and expectations and credibility towards the treatment. Expectations and credibility scores were categorized as low (Mean−1 Standard deviation), medium (Mean), and high (Mean + 1 Standard deviation). *T*-values are reported as absolute values.

Fourth, two simple linear regression analyses (using the enter method) were carried out to study whether the WAI-TECH-SF scores predicted the changes in PHQ scores and satisfaction with the treatment. PHQ scores were calculated using the differences between post- and pre-assessment scores (Post−Pre). Thus, positive values indicated an increase in depression symptoms, whereas negative values indicated a decrease in depression symptoms.

Finally, a power analysis was conducted to determine whether the present study was adequately powered with our sample size ($N = 193$) (the sample size of this study was initially calculated for testing the hypothesis that bCBT was not inferior to the TAU condition on the primary clinical outcome (i.e., symptoms of depression at 3 months after baseline) (see Kleiboer et al. [31]), but not for the secondary outcomes and analyses). Using G*power v. 3.1.9.743 (Heinrich-Heine-Universität, Düsseldorf, Germany), we calculated power for: (1) an omnibus *F*-test "Fixed effects, one-way"; (2) a *t*-test "Differences between two independent means"; and (3) an omnibus *F*-test "Lineal multiple regression: fixed model, R^2 deviation from zero". An effect size of $f = 0.20$ or $f^2 = 0.12$ was used because there is still limited data in this field and $d = 0.40$ is a standard in Psychology, according to Brysbaert [45]. Results indicated that the current study had 69.38% and 62.68% power for one-way ANOVAs with three and four groups, respectively, 75.49% for the *t*-test, and 99.77% for the regression analyses with one predictor to detect a medium effect size at $p < 0.05$.

3. Results

3.1. Psychometric Properties of WAI-TECH-SF

A random percentage of missing values was found, with Little's MCAR test, $\chi^2(33) = 14.27$, $p = 0.998$, ranging from 0 to 1.6% per item. Consequently, items' missing values were imputed using the Expectation–Maximization Algorithm method [38]. The sample's normality was assumed because skewness values were <|2|, and kurtosis values were <|7| [46,47] (see Table 2). The KMO value was (0.96), and the Barlett's Test of Sphericity value, $\chi^2(66) = 2587.26$, $p < 0.001$, showed that it was appropriate to perform a factor analysis. Regarding the number of factors to extract, Parallel Analysis [40] showed that one factor had to be retained because only one factor had an eigenvalue (raw data eigenvalue = 9.08) greater than the eigenvalue at the 95th percentile for randomly generated data (95th percentile eigenvalue = 1.53) [48]. Factorial rotation with one dimension was performed using the Maximum Likelihood extraction method, which showed that one dimension explained 73.49% of the total variance. The factorial solution showed that all the items had minimum factor loadings and communalities above ≥0.30 (see Table 2). Cronbach's alpha coefficient for the WAI-TECH-SF was high for the overall scale ($\alpha = 0.97$). We analysed the item–total correlation, and the exclusion of any item increased the alpha value for the overall scale.

3.2. Differences in WAI-TECH-SF Scores According to Socio-Demographic Variables, Initial Severity on PHQ Scores, Preference for the Treatment Offered, and Expectations and Credibility towards the Treatment

Table 3 shows the means and standard deviations of the WAI-TECH-SF scores according to sex, age-range, level of education, initial severity on PHQ scores, preference for any of the treatments offered, and expectations and credibility towards the treatment.

Table 3. Descriptive statistics of WAI-TECH scores in each category.

	Independent-Sample *t*-Tests/ One-Way ANOVAs	N	M	SD
Total sample		193	57.84	16.39
Sex	$t(191) = 0.49, p = 0.627$, Cohen's $d = 0.07$			
Men		69	57.07	15.03
Women		124	58.27	17.14
Age-range	$F(2,190) = 1.75, p = 0.177, \eta^2_p = 0.02$			
18–34		70	55.84	17.09
35–49		66	57.12	17.89
>50		57	61.13	13.14
Level of education	$F(2,190) = 3.21, p = 0.043, \eta^2_p = 0.03$			
Low		24	50.01	15.06
Medium		61	58.72	15.52
High		108	59.08	16.80
Initial severity of depression	$F(3,189) = 0.91, p = 0.436, \eta^2_p = 0.01$			
Mild		21	59.86	16.16
Moderate		64	56.50	16.38
Moderate-Severe		71	56.66	17.03
Severe		37	61.27	15.27
Preference for any of the treatments offered	$F(2,190) = 1.66, p = 0.194, \eta^2_p = 0.02$			
No preference		54	57.78	16.09
Blended		107	56.48	16.09
Treatment as usual		32	62.47	17.53
Expectations towards the treatment	$F(2,182) = 1.34, p = 0.265, \eta^2_p = 0.02$			
Low		34	59.84	15.41
Medium		119	57.92	16.82
High		32	53.47	16.18
Credibility towards the treatment	$F(2,183) = 0.57, p = 0.567, \eta^2_p = 0.01$			
Low		28	56.38	17.19
Medium		126	57.13	15.65
High		32	60.34	19.13

Independent-sample *t*-tests and one-way ANOVAs showed that there were no significant differences in the WAI-TECH-SF scores based on sex, age-range, initial severity of depression, preferences for any of the treatments offered, expectations about the treatment, and credibility of the treatment. However, there were significant differences in the WAI-TECH-SF scores based on the level of education. Patients with high (vs. low) education levels achieved higher scores on the WAI-TECH-SF, $p = 0.042$.

An Exploratory Multiple Regression Analysis: Socio-Demographic Variables, Initial Severity on PHQ Scores, Preference for the Treatment Offered, and Expectations and Credibility towards the Treatment as Predictors of WAI-TECH-SF Scores

Given the number of potential predictor variables of the WAI-TECH-SF, we also carried out a stepwise linear regression in order to analyse the explained variance by each variable. To do so, age, expectations, and credibility towards the treatment were maintained as continuous variables. Categorical predictor variables (i.e., level of education, initial severity of depression, and preference for any of the treatments offered) were transformed into dummy-coded variables. The reference category was "low" (vs. "medium and high") for level of education, "mild" (vs. moderate, moderate-severe and severe) for initial severity of depression, and "no preference" (vs. blended and treatment as usual) for preference for any of the treatments offered.

Results of this regression analysis showed that two models were significant. The first model included level of education ($\beta = 0.180$, $t = 2.462$, $p = 0.015$) as a positive significant predictor of the WAI-TECH-SF scores. This model was significant, $F(1,181) = 6.059$, $p = 0.015$, explaining 2.7% of the variance.

The second model included level of education ($\beta = 0.205$, $t = 2.798$, $p = 0.006$) and age ($\beta = 0.167$, $t = 2.279$, $p = 0.024$) as positive significant predictors of the WAI-TECH-SF scores. This model was significant, $F(2,181) = 5.696$, $p = 0.004$, explaining 4.9% of the variance.

3.3. Predictive Models: Are Changes in PHQ Scores and Satisfaction with the Treatment Predicted by WAI-TECH-SF Scores?

The model where changes in PHQ pre-post intervention scores were predicted by WAI-TECH-SF scores was statistically significant, $F(1,188) = 14.42$, $p < 0.001$, explaining 6.7% of the variance. Higher scores on the WAI-TECH-SF predicted a greater decrease in depression symptoms.

Similarly, the model in which satisfaction with the treatment was predicted by the WAI-TECH-SF scores was statistically significant, $F(1,187) = 185.53$, $p < 0.001$, explaining 49.7% of the variance. Higher scores on the WAI-TECH-SF predicted higher scores on satisfaction with the treatment (see Table 4).

Table 4. Simple linear regressions of change in PHQ scores and satisfaction with the treatment.

	R	R²	B	SE	β	t
Change in PHQ scores						
Constant			0.186	1.829		
WAI-TECH	0.268	0.072	−0.115	0.030	−0.268	3.797 ***
Satisfaction with the treatment						
Constant			12.929	0.951		13.601 ***
WAI-TECH	0.707	0.497	0.214	0.016	0.707	13.621 ***

Note. Statistical significance: *** $p < 0.001$. PHQ-9 = Patient Health Questionnaire-9; WAI-TECH-SF = Working Alliance Inventory applied to Internet–Short Form. R = Multiple Correlation Coefficient; R² = Coefficient of determination; R² Change = Coefficient of determination Change; B = Unstandardized coefficient; SE = Standard Error; β = Beta coefficient; t = t statistic (estimated coefficient divided by its own SE).

4. Discussion

The objectives of this study were: (1) to explore the psychometric structure of a questionnaire (i.e., the WAI-TECH-SF) designed to assess the TA with an online program in a self-guided IBI and CBT program in a sample of depressive patients in the context of the National Health Systems of different European countries; (2) to analyse whether there were differences in the WAI-TECH-SF scores based on several socio-demographic variables, initial symptoms of depression, preference for any of the treatments offered, and expectations and credibility towards the treatment; and (3) to study the capacity of the WAI-TECH-SF scores to predict the therapeutic outcomes (i.e., changes in depressive symptoms) and satisfaction with the treatment.

With regard to the psychometric properties of the WAI-TECH-SF, a unidimensional structure emerged in the EFA that accounted for 73.49% of the explained variance. All the factors had high factor loadings, and the overall scale had excellent internal consistency. This unidimensionality is in line with the structure found in the validation of the WAI applied to virtual and augmented reality (WAI-VAR, [25]). However, this structure is inconsistent with the three-dimensional structure of Bordin's [4] theory and the original validation of the WAI-SF carried out by Hatcher and Gallispy [16] to measure TA in the face-to-face context, distinguishing three separate factors: tasks, goals, and bonds. Nevertheless, the structure of this questionnaire is controversial because a bi-factorial structure has also been found in other validations of the WAI, such as in Gómez-Penedo et al. [24], who found that in the TA with the therapist in IBIs, "goals and tasks" loaded in the same factor, whereas "bond" loaded in a separate factor. According to our findings, a three-dimensional structure cannot be assumed a priori in the context of IBIs. More specifically, in the case of the TA with an online program during a self-guided IBI, the theoretical distinction between task, goals, and bond with the online program was not psychometrically significant, and a single factor could explain the majority of the explained variance of the TA between the patient and the online program. However, these results should be interpreted with caution because IBIs are continuously evolving, and a more personalized treatment that uses algorithms to provide personalized feedback or set individualized goals or tasks depending on the emotional state or unique needs of each patient throughout the treatment could generate a more differentiated factorial structure of the WAI-TECH-SF.

Another possible explanation for the structure of the WAI-TECH-SF is related to the fact that the TA with the online programs is highly complex, and merely replacing the words is not sufficient to capture the subtle differences in these different kinds of TA. In other words, perhaps the dimensions of the questionnaire should be completely reframed [28]. In this regard, Henson, Peck, and Torous [49] developed the Digital-WAI (D-WAI), a six-item self-report questionnaire based on Bordin's three dimensions, but aligned with the purpose of smartphone-based interventions (e.g., "bond" is aimed at measuring the capacity of the app to offer support and guide them through challenges). More recently, Miloff et al. [50] adopted this approach of developing novel items and validated the Virtual Therapist Alliance Scale (VTAS), which assesses the three components of the TA with virtual therapists in an automated exposure treatment format for patients with fear of spiders. Two factors emerged in the exploratory factor analysis ("task, goal, and copresence" and "bond and empathy") that had small and non-significant correlations with therapeutic outcomes at post-treatment, but moderate and significant correlations at follow-up.

Regarding the differences in the WAI-TECH-SF scores according to different characteristics of the sample, overall, no differences were found. That is, the TA with the self-guided IBI was achieved by the patients independently of their sex, their age, the severity of their depression before starting the intervention, their preferences for doing the intervention in the assigned condition, or the expectations and credibility towards the treatment. The average score on the WAI-TECH-SF was around 58 (on a scale ranging from 12 to 84). Nevertheless, patients with a higher level of education scored higher on TA with the online program than patients with a low level of education. This finding was also corroborated by the exploratory multiple regression analysis, in which all the different characteristics of the sample were introduced as potential predictors of the WAI-TECH-SF scores. Results showed that level of education, but also the age, were positive significant predictors of the TA with the self-guided IBI, explaining 4.9% of the variance. Regarding level of education, this higher TA could be related to the fact that more positive therapeutic outcomes in IBIs are also predicted by having a higher level of education [51]. Moreover, these findings may be associated with the lower preferences for IBIs expressed by people with a lower level of education [52], or the related barriers to the use of a less-known technology (e.g., low trust and lack of confidence in the capacity of IBIs to actually help).

The lower preference for technology adoption has also been related to age (e.g., because of their lower proficiency). Moret-Tatay et al. [53] found that older adults showed lower scores in mobile device and computer proficiency than younger adults. Consequently, adapted computer systems for older people have been designed to reduce the barriers that this population encounter. Mitzer et al. [54] found that the use of an adapted computer system for older people at the mid- and long-term was predicted by the earlier use of the system, the higher cognitive abilities (i.e., executive functioning), and computer efficacy. Hence, future studies should assess technology proficiency and cognitive abilities before starting a self-guided IBI in order to avoid the problems associated with the level of education and age, such as the adherence to the therapy. Nevertheless, older patients achieved higher TA in our study. One possible explanation for this finding is that the lower technology proficiency typically found in the population could have been compensated by the greater involvement in the therapy.

Regarding the capacity of the TA with the self-guided IBI to predict therapeutic outcomes, the findings highlight the importance of considering the WAI-TECH-SF scores to predict the change in depressive symptoms and satisfaction with the intervention. The TA with the online program explained 6.7% of the change in depressive symptoms, and 49.7% of the satisfaction with the treatment. Consequently, the relationship between "patient-online program TA" and therapeutic outcomes is also in line with the positive relationship found between the "patient-therapist TA" and the therapeutic outcomes in face-to-face therapy [1,2] and IBIs [3,21]. However, to our knowledge, this is the first study to confirm the relationship between "patient and online program TA" and therapeutic outcomes. By contrast, Kiluk et al. [29] did not find that the total scores on the long form of the WAI-Tech were associated with the change in therapeutic outcomes. Hence, so far, only the present study and Miragall et al. [25] found a significant relationship between the TA with the technology (i.e., the TA between the patient and virtual and augmented reality) and therapeutic outcomes. Therefore, this finding supports the need to work directly on the TA when it is poor because it has important consequences for therapeutic outcomes. Future studies should include algorithms to detect low TA scores after each session, in order to adjust the goals, tasks, and bond between the patient and the online program during an IBI.

This study has some limitations. First, the WAI-TECH-SF was only administered at the end of the treatment, which did not allow us to explore whether the "patient and online program TA" preceded the symptoms and satisfaction throughout the therapeutic sessions. Thus, having these measures during the treatment would allow us to establish the causal effect of TA on the therapeutic outcomes. Future studies should administer the WAI-TECH-SF in earlier therapeutic sessions (e.g., third session) in order to examine the TA through the therapy. Second, the study sample was only composed of depressive patients. Therefore, future studies should replicate this study in a sample of patients with several diagnoses (e.g., anxiety, post-traumatic stress disorder) in order to confirm whether the same psychometric structure is found, and to detect its capacity to predict therapeutic changes in other mental disorders. Third, the adherence or number of sessions performed by the patients was not registered. Thus, future studies should analyse whether the TA affects adherence and, in turn, the therapeutic outcomes. Fourth, the statistical analyses of TA were only conducted with the patients that accepted to fill in the questionnaire after the self-guided IBI was finished. However, the normal distribution (e.g., skewness = -0.56; kurtosis = -0.83) and the wide range of variability of the WAI-TECH-SF scores (i.e., from 12 to 84) allowed us to draw reliable conclusions. The importance shown by the TA with the technology points out the question regarding the impact of TA at early stages of the treatment, and the role that it can play in predicting efficacy and preventing dropouts.

Finally, the importance of having self-guided IBI that promotes an adequate TA between the patient and the online program should be noted, especially when resources are scarce. Several situations, such as the COVID-19 pandemic, could prevent individuals from accessing the traditional face-to-face therapy. Consequently, CBT delivered through telehealth services are undeniably crucial in order to provide timely psychological support, especially in vulnerable populations [55].

5. Conclusions

In conclusion, this study reveals that patients with major depression can develop TA with an online program during a self-guided IBI in the context of primary care. Thus, patients can feel that the program is "taking care" of them, in terms of allowing them to achieve therapeutic goals, proposing appropriate tasks to achieve these goals, and making them feel "embraced" and "cared for" by the program. According to our exploratory factor analysis, the WAI-TECH-SF is a reliable questionnaire to measure this construct, but it would be advisable to calculate an overall score for the total scale, rather than using the traditional theoretical three-dimensional "task-goals-bonds" structure of TA. Moreover, it would be beneficial to explore the IBI preferences of the patients with lower education levels before starting the intervention, in order to ensure that their level of education does not interfere with their capacity to develop TA with the online program. Finally, this study highlights the importance of considering the "patient and online program TA" because the WAI-TECH-SF score was a significant predictor variable of both the change in depressive symptoms and satisfaction at the end of the treatment. Further research is needed to more deeply understand the TA achieved in the "patient-technology-therapist" triangulation in blended treatments.

Author Contributions: Conceptualization, R.H., C.B., A.G.-P., H.R., A.K., and R.M.B.; methodology, R.H. and A.K.; software, R.H. and A.K.; formal analysis, R.H., M.D.V. and M.M.; resources, C.B., A.G.-P., H.R., and R.M.B.; data curation, R.H., M.D.V. and M.M.; writing—original draft preparation, R.H., M.D.V. and M.M.; writing—review and editing, all authors; supervision, C.B., A.G.-P., H.R., A.K. and R.M.B.; funding acquisition, C.B., A.G.-P., H.R., A.K. and R.M.B. All authors have read and agreed to the published version of the manuscript.

Funding: This research was funded by European Commission (grant number FP7-Health-2013-Innovation-N603098) and Excellence Research Program PROMETEO ("INTERSABIAS" project—PROMETEO/2018/110/ Conselleria d'Educació, Investigació, Cultura I Esport, Generalitat Valenciana).

Acknowledgments: We would like to thank CIBERObn, an initiative of ISCIII (ISC III CB06 03/0052).

Conflicts of Interest: The authors declare no conflict of interest.

References

1. Cameron, S.K.; Rodgers, J.; Dagnan, D. The relationship between the therapeutic alliance and clinical outcomes in cognitive behaviour therapy for adults with depression: A meta-analytic review. *Clin. Psychol. Psychother.* **2018**, *25*, 446–456. [CrossRef] [PubMed]
2. Horvath, A.O.; Del Re, A.C.; Flückiger, C.; Symonds, D. Alliance in individual psychotherapy. *Psychotherapy* **2011**, *48*, 9–16. [CrossRef] [PubMed]
3. Flückiger, C.; Del Re, A.C.; Wampold, B.E.; Horvath, A.O. The alliance in adult psychotherapy: A meta-analytic synthesis. *Psychotherapy* **2018**, *55*, 316–340. [CrossRef] [PubMed]
4. Bordin, E.S. The generalizability of the psychoanalytic concept of the working alliance. *Psychol. Psychother.* **1979**, *16*, 252–260. [CrossRef]
5. Kazdin, A.E.; Blase, S.L. Rebooting Psychotherapy Research and Practice to Reduce the Burden of Mental Illness. *Perspect. Psychol. Sci.* **2011**, *6*, 21–37. [CrossRef] [PubMed]
6. Mohr, D.C.; Tomasino, K.N.; Lattie, E.G.; Palac, H.L.; Kwasny, M.J.; Weingardt, K.; Karr, C.J.; Kaiser, S.M.; Rossom, R.C.; Bardsley, L.R.; et al. IntelliCare: An eclectic, skills-based app suite for the treatment of depression and anxiety. *J. Med. Internet Res.* **2017**, *19*, e10. [CrossRef]
7. Erbe, D.; Eichert, H.C.; Riper, H.; Ebert, D.D. Blending face-to-face and Internet-based interventions for the treatment of mental disorders in adults: Systematic review. *J. Med. Internet Res.* **2017**, *19*, e306. [CrossRef]
8. Richards, D.; Richardson, T. Computer-based psychological treatments for depression: A systematic review and meta-analysis. *Clin. Psychol. Rev.* **2012**, *32*, 329–342. [CrossRef]
9. Schröder, J.; Berger, T.; Westermann, S.; Klein, J.P.; Moritz, S. Internet interventions for depression: New developments. *Dialogues Clin. Neurosci.* **2016**, *18*, 203–212.
10. Sztein, D.; Koransky, C.; Fegan, L.; Himelhoch, S. Efficacy of cognitive behavioural therapy delivered over the Internet for depressive symptoms: A systematic review and meta-analysis. *J. Telemed. Telecare* **2018**, *24*, 527–539. [CrossRef]
11. Andersson, G.; Cuijpers, P.; Carlbring, P.; Riper, H.; Hedman, E. Guided internet-based vs. face-to-face cognitive behavior therapy for psychiatric and somatic disorders: A systematic review and meta-analysis. *World Psychiatry* **2014**, *13*, 288–295. [CrossRef] [PubMed]

12. Wagner, B.; Horn, A.B.; Maercker, A. Internet-based versus face-to-face cognitive-behavioral intervention for depression: A randomized controlled non-inferiority trial. *J. Affect. Disord.* **2014**, *152–154*, 113–121. [CrossRef] [PubMed]
13. Topooco, N.; Riper, H.; Araya, R.; Berking, M.; Brunne, M.; Chevreul, K.; Cieslak, R.; Ebert, D.D.; Etchemendy, E.; Herrero, R.; et al. On behalf of the E-COMPARED consortium. Attitudes towards digital treatment for depression: A European stakeholder survey. *Internet Interv.* **2017**, *8*, 1–9. [CrossRef] [PubMed]
14. Kooistra, L.; Ruwaard, J.; Wiersma, J.; van Oppen, P.; Riper, H. Working alliance in blended versus face-to-face cognitive behavioral treatment for patients with depression in specialized mental health care. *J. Clin. Med.* **2020**, *9*, 347. [CrossRef]
15. Horvath, A.O.; Greenberg, L.S. Development and validation of the Working Alliance Inventory. *J. Couns. Psychol.* **1989**, *36*, 223–233. [CrossRef]
16. Hatcher, R.L.; Gillaspy, J.A. Development and validation of a revised short version of the working alliance inventory. *Psychother. Res.* **2007**, *16*, 12–25. [CrossRef]
17. Tracey, T.J.; Kokotovic, A.M. Factor structure of the Working Alliance Inventory. *Psychol. Assess.* **1989**, *1*, 207–210. [CrossRef]
18. Jasper, K.; Weise, C.; Conrad, I.; Andersson, G.; Hiller, W.; Kleinstauber, M. The working alliance in a randomized controlled trial comparing internet-based self-help and face-to-face cognitive behavior therapy for chronic tinnitus. *Internet Interv.* **2014**, *1*, 49–57. [CrossRef]
19. Knaevelsrud, C.; Maercker, A. Internet-based treatment for PTSD reduces distress and facilitates the development of a strong therapeutic alliance: A randomized controlled clinical trial. *BMC Psychiatry* **2007**, *7*, 13. [CrossRef]
20. Preschl, B.; Maercker, A.; Wagner, B. The working alliance in a randomized controlled trial comparing online with face-to-face cognitive-behavioral therapy for depression. *BMC Psychiatry* **2011**, *11*, 189. [CrossRef]
21. Probst, G.H.; Berger, T.; Flückiger, C. The alliance-outcome relation in internet-based interventions for psychological disorders: A correlational meta-analysis. *Verhaltenstherapie* **2019**, 1–12. [CrossRef]
22. Clarke, J.; Proudfoot, J.; Whitton, A.; Birch, M.R.; Boyd, M.; Parker, G.; Manicavasagar, V.; Hadzi-Pavlovic, D.; Fogarty, A. Therapeutic alliance with a fully automated mobile phone and web-based intervention: Secondary analysis of a randomized controlled trial. *JMIR Ment. Health* **2016**, *3*, e10. [CrossRef] [PubMed]
23. Pihlaja, S.; Stenberg, J.H.; Joutsenniemi, K.; Mehik, H.; Ritola, V.; Joffe, G. Therapeutic alliance in guided internet therapy programs for depression and anxiety disorders–a systematic review. *Internet Interv.* **2018**, *11*, 1–10. [CrossRef] [PubMed]
24. Gómez-Penedo, J.M.; Babl, A.M.; Holtforth, M.G.; Hohagen, F.; Krieger, T.; Lutz, W.; Meyer, B.; Moritz, S.; Klein, J.P.; Berger, T. The association of therapeutic alliance with long-term outcome in a guided Internet Intervention for depression: Secondary analysis from a randomized control trial. *J. Med. Internet Res.* **2020**, *22*, e15824. [CrossRef] [PubMed]
25. Miragall, M.; Baños, R.M.; Cebolla, A.; Botella, C. Working alliance inventory applied to virtual and augmented reality (WAI-VAR): Psychometrics and therapeutic outcomes. *Front Psychol.* **2015**, *6*, 1531. [CrossRef]
26. Heim, E.; Roetger, A.; Lorenz, N.; Maercker, A. Working alliance with an avatar: How far can we go with internet interventions? *Internet Interv.* **2018**, *11*, 41–46. [CrossRef]
27. Berger, T.; Boettcher, J.; Caspar, F. Internet-based guided self-help for several anxiety disorders: A randomized controlled trial comparing a tailored with a standardized disorder-specific approach. *Psychotherapy* **2014**, *51*, 207–219. [CrossRef]
28. Berry, K.; Salter, A.; Morris, R.; James, S.; Bucci, S. Assessing therapeutic alliance in the context of mHealth interventions for mental health problems: Development of the mobile Agnew relationship measure (mARM) questionnaire. *J. Med. Internet Res.* **2018**, *20*, e90. [CrossRef]
29. Kiluk, B.D.; Serafini, K.; Frankforter, T.; Nich, C.; Carroll, K.M. Only connect: The working alliance in computer-based cognitive behavioral therapy. *Behav. Res.* **2014**, *63*, 139–146. [CrossRef]
30. Vernmark, K.; Hesser, H.; Topooco, N.; Berger, T.; Riper, H.; Luuk, L.; Backlund, L.; Carlbring, P.; Andersson, G. Working alliance as a predictor of change in depression during blended cognitive behaviour therapy. *Cogn. Behav.* **2019**, *48*, 285–299. [CrossRef]

31. Kleiboer, A.; Smit, J.; Bosmans, J.; Ruwaard, J.; Andersson, G.; Topooco, N.; Berger, T.; Krieger, T.; Botella, C.; Baños, R.; et al. European COMPARative Effectiveness research on blended Depression treatment versus treatment-as-usual (E-COMPARED): Study protocol for a randomized controlled, non-inferiority trial in eight European countries. *Trials* **2016**, *17*, 387. [CrossRef] [PubMed]
32. Kroenke, K.; Spitzer, R.L.; Williams, J.B. The PHQ-9: Validity of a brief depression severity measure. *J. Gen. Intern. Med.* **2001**, *16*, 606–613. [CrossRef] [PubMed]
33. American Psychiatric Association. *Diagnostic and Statistical Manual of Mental Disorders*, DSM IV-4th ed.; American Psychiatric Association: Washington, DC, USA, 1994.
34. Levis, B.; Benedetti, A.; Thombs, B.D. Accuracy of Patient Health Questionnaire-9 (PHQ-9) for screening to detect major depression: Individual participant data meta-analysis. *BMJ* **2019**, *365*. [CrossRef]
35. Wittkampf, K.A.; Naeije, L.; Schene, A.H.; Huyser, J.; van Weert, H.C. Diagnostic accuracy of the mood module of the Patient Health Questionnaire: A systematic review. *Gen. Hosp. Psychiatry* **2007**, *29*, 388–395. [CrossRef] [PubMed]
36. Sheehan, D.V.; Lecrubier, Y.; Sheehan, K.H.; Amorim, P.; Janavs, J.; Weiller, E.; Dunbar, G.C. The Mini-International Neuropsychiatric Interview (M.I.N.I.): The development and validation of a structured diagnostic psychiatric interview for DSM-IV and ICD-10. *J. Clin. Psychiatry* **1998**, *59*, 22–33.
37. Devilly, G.J.; Borkovec, T.D. Psychometric properties of the credibility/expectancy questionnaire. *J. Behav. Exp. Psychiatry* **2000**, *31*, 73–86. [CrossRef]
38. Nguyen, T.D.; Attkisson, C.C.; Stegner, B.L. Assessment of patient satisfaction: Development and refinement of a service evaluation questionnaire. *Eval. Program Plan.* **1983**, *6*, 299–314. [CrossRef]
39. Hambleton, R.K.; Patsula, L. Increasing the validity of adapted tests: Myths to be avoided and guidelines for improving test adaptation practices. *J. Appl. Test. Technol.* **1999**, *1*, 1–12.
40. Schafer, J.L. Analysis of Incomplete Multivariate Data. In *Monographs on Statistics and Applied Probability*; Chapman & Hall: London, UK, 1997; Volume 72.
41. Fabrigar, L.R.; Wegener, D.T.; MacCallum, R.C.; Strahan, E.J. Evaluating the use of exploratory factor analysis in psychological research. *Psychol. Methods* **1999**, *4*, 272–299. [CrossRef]
42. Horn, J.L. A rationale and test for the number of factors in factor analysis. *Psychometrika* **1965**, *30*, 179–185. [CrossRef]
43. O'Connor, B.P. SPSS and SAS programs for determining the number of components using parallel analysis and Velicer's MAP test. *Behav. Res. Methods Instrum. Comput.* **2000**, *32*, 396–402. [CrossRef] [PubMed]
44. Cronbach, L.J. Coefficient alpha and the internal structure of tests. *Psychometrika* **1951**, *16*, 297–334. [CrossRef]
45. Brysbaert, M. How many participants do we have to include in properly powered experiments? A tutorial of power analysis with reference tables. *J. Cogn.* **2019**, *2*, 1–38. [CrossRef] [PubMed]
46. West, S.G.; Finch, J.F.; Curran, P.J. Structural Equation Models with Non Normal Variables: Problems and Remedies. In *Structural Equation Modeling: Concepts, Issues, and Applications*, 1st ed.; Hoyle, R.H., Ed.; Sage Publications: Thousand Oaks, CA, USA, 1995; pp. 56–75.
47. Russell, D.W. In search of underlying dimensions: The use (and abuse) of factor analysis in Personality and Social Psychology Bulletin. *Pers. Soc. Psychol. Bull.* **2002**, *28*, 1629–1646. [CrossRef]
48. Fabrigar, L.R.; Wegener, D.T. *Exploratory Factor Analysis*; Oxford University Press: New York, NY, USA, 2012.
49. Henson, P.; Peck, P.; Torous, J. Considering the therapeutic alliance in digital mental health interventions. *Harv. Rev. Psychiatry* **2019**, *27*, 268–273. [CrossRef] [PubMed]
50. Miloff, A.; Carlbring, P.; Hamilton, W.; Andersson, G.; Reuterskiöld, L.; Lindner, P. Measuring alliance toward embodied virtual therapists in the era of automated treatments with the virtual therapist alliance scale (VTAS): Development and psychometric evaluation. *J. Med. Internet Res.* **2020**, *22*, e16660. [CrossRef]
51. Warmerdam, L.; Van Straten, A.; Twisk, J.; Cuijpers, P. Predicting outcome of Internet-based treatment for depressive symptoms. *Psychother. Res.* **2013**, *23*, 559–567. [CrossRef]
52. Batterham, P.J.; Calear, A.L. Preferences for internet-based mental health interventions in an adult online sample: Findings from an online community survey. *JMIR Ment. Health* **2017**, *4*, e26. [CrossRef]
53. Moret-Tatay, C.; Beneyto-Arrojo, M.J.; Gutierrez, E.; Boot, W.R.; Charness, N. A spanish adaptation of the computer and mobile device proficiency questionnaires (CPQ and MDPQ) for older adults. *Front Psychol.* **2019**, *10*, 1165. [CrossRef]

54. Mitzner, T.L.; Savla, J.; Boot, W.R.; Sharit, J.; Charness, N.; Czaja, S.J.; Rogers, W.A. Technology adoption by older adults: Findings from the PRISM trial. *Gerontologist* **2019**, *59*, 34–44. [CrossRef]
55. Ng, Q.X.; Chee, K.T.; De Deyn, M.L.Z.Q.; Chua, Z. Staying connected during the COVID-19 pandemic. *Int. J. Soc. Psychiatry* **2020**, *66*, 519–520. [CrossRef] [PubMed]

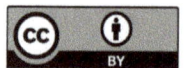

© 2020 by the authors. Licensee MDPI, Basel, Switzerland. This article is an open access article distributed under the terms and conditions of the Creative Commons Attribution (CC BY) license (http://creativecommons.org/licenses/by/4.0/).

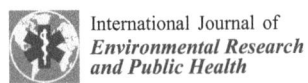

Article

Designing ICTs for Users with Mild Cognitive Impairment: A Usability Study

Diana Castilla [1,2,*], Carlos Suso-Ribera [3], Irene Zaragoza [2], Azucena Garcia-Palacios [3] and Cristina Botella [3]

1. Department of Personality, Evaluation and Psychological Treatment, University of Valencia, 46010 Valencia, Spain
2. CIBER of Physiopathology of Obesity and Nutrition (CIBEROBN), ISCIII CB06/03/0052 Instituto Salud Carlos III, 28029 Madrid, Spain; izaragoz@uji.es
3. Department of Basic Psychology, Clinical Psychology and Psychobiology, Universitat Jaume I, 12071 Castellón, Spain; susor@uji.es (C.S.-R.); azucena@uji.es (A.G.-P.); botella@uji.es (C.B.)
* Correspondence: Diana.Castilla@uv.es; Tel.: +34-9-6386-4394

Received: 14 June 2020; Accepted: 14 July 2020; Published: 17 July 2020

Abstract: Background: Research has supported the cost-effectiveness of cognitive training tools enhanced by information and communication technologies (ICT) in several populations, including individuals with mild cognitive impairment (MCI) and age-related cognitive decline. The implementation of ICTs in this population, however, is sometimes challenging to their cognitive and age characteristics. Ultimately, this might compromise the effectiveness of ICT-enhanced therapies in this population. The aim of this study is to test the usability and acceptability of a European project prototype for elderly care, in an attempt to explore the ICT design needs of users with MCI. Methods: Participants were 28 individuals aged 58–95 years and with a diagnosis of MCI. Results: The results showed a low perception of peripheral elements and the need to place main interaction elements in the centre of the screen. The correlation between the general level of autonomy (daily life activities) and the ICT autonomy level was significant and positive. The speed of audio help had a significant impact on performance. Conclusion: The present work contributes to the literature on ICT usability needs of users with MCI. Some usability recommendations for designing interfaces for this type of user are provided in the text.

Keywords: usability; speech interfaces; cognitive impairment; ICT; elderly; cognitive decline

1. Introduction

1.1. Demographic Changes and Mild Cognitive Impairment

The age profile is expected to change globally in the coming decades. According to the U.S. Census Bureau's latest ageing report, the population will be much older in 2050. Specifically, in the next 35 years it is expected that the increase in the number of older individuals will be considerably greater than that of the younger population [1]. Consequently, with the ageing of the population, the possibility of an increase in the number of cognitively impaired individuals will also rise.

According to a World Health Organization report dementia and cognitive impairment lead the list of chronic diseases contributing to disability and dependence among older people worldwide. Forty-seven million people suffered from dementia in the world in 2015, and due to the ageing of the population globally, this number is expected to be tripled by 2050. These demographic changes not only have a strong impact on the daily lives of patients and their relatives, but also they have substantial consequences for public finances. Specifically, the estimated global cost of dementia care in 2010 was US$604 billion, and it is projected that its worldwide cost in 2030 could be US$1.2 trillion or more [2].

In the previous paragraph, we have presented the global impact of dementia, which is often characterized by an important cognitive impairment. However, dementia and its associated cognitive impairment do not start abruptly. Conversely, dementia is a dimensional construct that begins with small changes in the brain and symptomatology. In this sense, mild cognitive impairment (MCI) is the clinical syndrome that describes the transitional zone between normal cognitive status and dementia and it is estimated that approximately 10% to 15% of individuals with MCI will develop dementia [3]. Therefore, an important societal goal is to delay the transition between MCI and dementia or at least to reduce the speed of the cognitive decline in patients with MCI. Cognitive training is the most frequently reported form of cognition-focused intervention. It contains sessions involving practice on tasks that target aspects of cognition such as attention, memory, and language [4]. There is now sufficient support for the effectiveness of such training in individuals with MCI [5,6]. However, traditional face-to-face interventions may not always be accessible to the older individuals on a large scale because of accessibility reasons (e.g., having to travel long distances to specialized treatment centres) and limited public economic resources. For this reason, interest in the development of technological applications for the cognitive treatment in older adults is increasing [7]. Several studies have provided evidence about the efficiency of cognitive training tools based on information and communication technologies (ICT) when applied as an adjunct therapy for recovering or improving performance on cognitive skills and self-confidence, as well as for an early intervention in individuals with MCI and age-related cognitive decline [8–12].

In particular, reminiscence therapy appears to be an important therapy in MCI and Alzheimer's disease. Reminiscence therapy is a non-pharmacological intervention used to prompt past memories with music and old photographs, which also facilitates social interactions and increases self-esteem. The use of ICT seems to be particularly appropriate in this kind of intervention. For example, some studies demonstrate the feasibility of using readily available technology (digital video, images, and music) to produce personalized multimedia biographies that hold special meaning for individuals with Alzheimer's disease and MCI and their families [13–16].

1.2. Information and Communication Technologies (ICTs) and Cognitive Decline

Rapid technological advances offer an excellent opportunity to face the challenge of promoting independence, strengthening social connectedness, and preventing isolation in older individuals [17,18]. Furthermore, a recent meta-analysis that using computers for leisure produced an overall significant reduction in the risk of dementia [19].

In addition to its recreational role, a systematic review of technology-supported reminiscence therapy also supported the benefits of using technology in the elderly, this time for therapeutic purposes [20]. Some of these benefits include access to rich and engaging multimedia reminiscence materials, opportunities for people with dementia to participate in social interactions and take ownership of conversations, and a reduction in barriers due to motor deficits during interactions with media. Reminiscence therapy interventions based on ICT have also showed their efficacy in depression treatment in the elderly [21]. This is important because several studies have pointed out that depression, social isolation, and loneliness can negatively impact cognitive impairment [22–26]. In a similar line of supporting the benefits of using technology in the elderly, another study suggested that interventions with tailored social networks and social contacts are also needed to increase social contact in the elderly and to help them to delay and cope with cognitive impairment [23].

Cognitive decline in capabilities, such as memory, attention, perceptual speed, or spatial abilities, is part of normal ageing [27], and for this reason, the new age demography brings new challenges related to the way to improve the independence and quality of life of elderly people and, especially, promote their well-being in different ways [28]. New technologies can help to face these challenges, but their utilization in the elderly and specifically in persons with MCI might have some associated challenges. Although technology is increasingly present in everyday life, the elderly usually face usability problems related to the unsuitable design of central features, such as the graphic user interface design and input device choices, to name some examples. On usability tests, elderly users face a greater number of usability problems than young users [29–31], and their ICT experience differs not only in terms of their success rate, but also in terms of emotional factors that should be included as an important part of their experience [32–35]. Often these negative experiences of older users are consolidated into what has been called a technophobia, that is a computer avoidance due to fear or phobia of interacting with computers [36].

Indeed, research has shown that the majority of non-ICT seniors feel "intimidated" and "anxious" about using technology and anticipate that the Internet is difficult to use and to understand [37,38]. In this scenario, a few studies have explored the possible benefits of improving usability by using embodied conversational agents as a form of assistive technology for users with cognitive impairment and the results so far are promising [39]. Nowadays, the technological barrier for elderly users goes far beyond the application design or the individual's fear of technologies. In this sense, usability for this type of user has to be conceptualized as a more complex problem in which related but different constructs such as web usability and web accessibility should be taken into consideration altogether when designing technological solutions.

Tim Berners-Lee, inventor of the World Wide Web and Director of the World Wide Web Consortium (W3C) states that *"the power of the Web is in its universality. Access by everyone regardless of disability is an essential aspect"* [40]. In this sense, the European Commission defines web accessibility as a policy of e-inclusion that aims *"to allow everyone, including people with disabilities, to perceive, understand, navigate and interact with the Internet"* [41]. In fact, the European Commission went a step further with the development of the Directive (EU) 2016/2102, an important document whose purpose is to ensure digital inclusion and web accessibility by indicating specific standards in the design of websites and mobile apps [42].

Other important contribution that aimed to make webs more accessible to people with disabilities was the Web Content Accessibility Guideline developed by the World Wide Web Consortium (W3C) [43]. The Accessibility Fundamentals summarized by the W3C revealed four relevant issues for older users, namely hearing loss, vision decline, physical decline, and cognitive decline. This important document highlighted that the cognitive decline can affect navigation, comprehension, and task completion due to difficulties with concentration and coping with information overload, distraction from movement or irrelevant material, and short-term memory limitations [44]. In 2019, the W3C developed a more specific section with accessibility standards for users with cognitive or learning disabilities. These include, to name some examples, the need to present content in different ways, make texts easily readable, and provide enough time to read and use content [45].

One key aspect of technology is its connectivity through the Internet. However, the technological characteristics of the Internet (mainly its undefined structure) can be barrier for accessibility and usability of technologies in the elderly. For instance, a meta analysis [41] revealed negative age effects on spatial abilities, so that time is likely to play an important role in ICT usability. This problem has an important impact when using technologies because the use of the Internet requires spatial abilities due to hypertext characteristics where the user must build the structure of the information or tasks during navigation (e.g., Where was I before? Where should I go now? In which order should I do the required steps?). As a consequence of the previous and the lack of ICT experience, elderly users show better performance on systems with linear navigation [32,46,47]. Another aspect that adds up to the complexity of usability in the elderly lies in the fact that the characteristics of elderly users are not static and vary over time because there are changes due to age-related decline [48].

The aforementioned barriers refer to the elderly in general. Not surprisingly, cognitive impairment in this population makes it even more difficult to use technology. For example, users with cognitive impairment make more mistakes and need more time to use web platforms due to their difficulties in orientation [49]. Thus, it has been suggested that people with mild to moderate cognitive impairment should be offered with simple technologies [50]. In addition to this, visual attention and control of visual short-term memory decline as a result of neurodegenerative processes that occur with ageing, MCI, and AD [51–53], which reduces the individual's ability to respond on a visually dynamic real-world task [54]. Ultimately, this means that, when interacting with computers, users do not behave the way the designers planned [55]. A popular related concept is change blindness, which is defined as the inability to detect changes in visual scenes, in the sense that users focus their attention on an image using visual short-term memory to store relevant information [53]. Because of this decrease in visual attention and control of visual short-term memory, change blindness may be much greater in people with cognitive impairment. Program designers, especially those of young ages, are not likely to be familiar with these characteristics and needs of elderly users. This poses important limitations in the design of technology for this population because taking into account the mental model of individuals with MCI is crucial for the adequate design and testing of user-friendly ICT-based applications and services [56].

Considering the previous, this study aims to analyse the ICT usability needs of users with MCI. Specifically, the purpose of the study is to provide some usability recommendations to design technologies for these users. To carry out this investigation we have used an application named the ehcoBUTLER project, a ground-breaking and comprehensive service solution designed to improve the quality of life of older people by promoting a healthy lifestyle and active ageing through the use of tools that enhance positive emotions and cognitive training [57]. This project has been developed with the support of the European Union's Horizon 2020 research and innovation programme [58]. The system has been developed following the guidelines of a software that has proven its usability with elderly users using linear navigation [32,46,59]. The study was performed in four iterative cycles to obtain more robust usability recommendations for ICT developments in MCI users.

2. Materials and Methods

2.1. Design

The study consisted of a classic usability test [60], where the first prototype of the ehcoButler system was used in a controlled environment. The assessment method used was a task analysis [61], applied individually, where the user performed several predefined tasks in order to obtain quantitative data. To carry out this study, only one group was defined. This included users with a diagnosis of cognitive impairment (mild and moderate) made by a physician (neurologist or geriatrician).

The study included performance measures during the test and measurements at pre-test and post-test. The main task consisted of writing an email to a specific recipient and attaching a picture facilitated by the experimenter. As a secondary task, qualitative information was collected about user preferences, iconography, appearance of the avatar, and reality judgments about the synthetic avatar voice.

2.2. Participants

The inclusion criteria were: age around 60 years old or more, MCI diagnosed by a geriatrician or neurologist, as well as conserving enough cognitive ability to have a conversation, sufficient hearing capacity, and sufficient visual and motor abilities to interact with the system or with the professional.

The Spanish health care system is universal (all citizens are covered), free of charge, and organized in 17 autonomous communities that apply the General Health Act [62]. The Spanish Ministry of Health, Social Services, and Equality approved the country's first National Health System strategy for Neurodegenerative Diseases in 2016. It includes early diagnosis strategies and a personalized social and health care plan for each patient [63]. Nursing homes have protocols for cognitive impairment assessment and interventions that are aligned with this national strategy. The users were assessed on cognitive functions (executive functions, episodic memory, visuospatial ability, naming ability, and verbal fluency), functionality (impairment in daily activities), neuropsychiatric symptoms, and biomarkers, by a neurologist or geriatrician, following the guidelines of the "Mild cognitive impairment in the elderly Consensus document" [64].

The final sample consisted of 28 participants with a MCI diagnosis from two nursing homes: 50% men and 50% women, aged between 58 and 95 years, with an average of 76.98 years ($SD = 9.56$).

The literacy level was mostly very basic because 84.6% of the sample only went to school up to the age of 14 (see Table A1). The average age when the sample left school was 11.27 ($SD = 5.07$), with a mean of 5.92 years of school attendance ($SD = 3.67$). Three participants never attended school, even though they could all read and write because they learned at home. Two participants did not recall going to school. This educational level (low or none) is representative of people from 65 to 85 years of age in small cities or towns in rural areas, given that the country had great economic difficulties during the 1940s and 1950s as a result of the Spanish civil war (1936 to 1939). At that moment, most of them left school and went to work at an early age to help their families.

Regarding their previous experience using ICTs, 82.1% had never used a personal computer or a tablet before this study, and only 7.1% of them had used a personal computer or a tablet more than 10 times.

The participants were randomly divided into four groups of seven participants each in order to test the system in four iterations.

Apart from the end-users, three professional caregivers (working at the recruitment centres) took part in the experiment as observers.

2.3. Materials

2.3.1. Main Software

The first ehcoBUTLER [58] functional prototype was the main software used for the study. The prototype was developed following all the usability characteristics of the BUTLER system, an emotional and social platform designed for elderly people with low digital literacy skills that has proven its usability and acceptability with elderly people without cognitive impairment [21,46,59,65].

The most important design feature of ehcoBUTLER is the navigation system, which follows a linear structure (i.e., like a step-by-step system) [46]. First, in the main menu, the user selects the application to use. Then, on each step, a human-looking avatar explains where they are and what they can do next. The avatar is "the butler" and its goal is to help them to decide what to do in every step of the system. The avatar is represented graphically as a young man and provides the help through audio (a synthetic voice) and text. The buttons have different colors depending on the type of action they allow: green is for buttons whose actions allow the user to continue with a task; red allows to interrupt a task (i.e., delete data or undo a concluded step); and orange represents secondary actions. Because all the system applications follow the same design principles, the email application was selected for the usability test. A complete description of the email task will be facilitated in the procedure section.

2.3.2. Variables and Measuring Instruments

As we described in more detail below, the assessment protocol consisted of three parts, namely user information (collected before the task), an evaluation of task-related information (performance and user's opinion), and effectiveness of the task as reported by professional caregivers.

User Profile

The user profile data were collected before the usability test. It included demographic data such as sex and educational level. In addition, we evaluated the user's experience with computers and the Internet, as well as whether the user had an e-mail account and had taken any computer training courses previously.

The level of autonomy in daily life activities was measured based on the professional's clinical judgement after an interview with the participant. The following item was then responded: "The user can perform his/her daily routines entirely unassisted" with a 5-point Likert scale with response labels: (0) strongly disagree, (1) somewhat disagree, (2) neither disagree nor agree, (3) somewhat agree, and (4) strongly agree.

Measures Based on User Performance

Success rate. The success rate was determined in absolute values: 0 (did not successfully perform the task); 1 (successfully performed the task).

Assistance received. The experimenter was not allowed to help the user solve the task. However, participants could be reminded that they could review the avatar's help, which counted as a new attempt. They could also be reminded about the name of the email recipient or on how to find a letter on the keyboard. Any help was annotated.

Number of attempts. The number of attempts was recorded, based on the number of times the experimenter had to show the user how to review the avatar instructions to find out how to continue.

Instruments Measuring the User's Opinion

Post-test questionnaire for the user: face scales [66] can help to evaluate the mood state in patients with cognitive impairment [67,68]. This questionnaire assesses the user's opinion of the system, with all the items using a 5-point face scale, rated from left to right with the following labels: strongly disagree, disagree, neither agree nor disagree, agree, and strongly agree. The variables measured were perceived ease of use, learnability and controllability, self-efficacy, flexibility, clear and easy to understand, usefulness, and intention to use.

Finally, a single item using a 5-point face scale to explore the feelings during the test was rated from left to right with the following labels: very bad, bad, neither bad nor good, good, very good.

All the items were obtained from a previous usability study with elderly users (see [32]).

Measures Regarding Professional's Judgment

The NASA Task Load Index–TLX [69] was filled in by the professional caregivers to evaluate the perceived workload. This is done to obtain a measure of the effectiveness of a task. This questionnaire provides an overall workload score based on six subscales: mental demand, physical demand, temporal demand, performance, effort, and frustration. Each scale is divided into 21 degrees from very low to very high. The experimenter trained the professional caregivers before the user test on how to fill in the NASA-TLX properly.

2.3.3. Hardware

Two set-ups were tested for this study. First, a 10"tablet (*Samsung Galaxy tablet Tab2*) was used because this was originally expected to be a suitable set-up due to its portability and affordable price. However, this was ruled out at the beginning of the study due to additional usability difficulties resulting from the use of the logical keyboard of the device, which hides half the screen during typing processes (see Figure A1). The second set-up which was finally used in the study, was a personal computer with a touch screen and physical keyboard, big keys in ABC order, and a normal keyboard with QWERTY order (*all in one MSI Model AE222-274 G3250 4GB 1TB W10 21.5* inches). A videocamera with a tripod was used to record the sessions.

In addition to the experimenter, the professional caregivers also assessed indicators of performance on the task (whether the user completed the task or not, the number of attempts, the degree of assistance needed during the test, and the technology used). They also reported their clinical judgment about the difficulty of the task, feelings observed in the user, together with suggestions and recommended improvements in the system. Finally, the professional assessed the ability of the user to use the system in an autonomous way (i.e., without any kind of support), using a 5-point Likert scale with response labels 0 = strongly disagree, 1 = somewhat disagree, 2 = neither disagree nor agree, 3 = somewhat agree, and 4 = strongly agree.

2.3.4. Statistical Software

For data analysis, IBM SPSS 22.0 (IBM Corp., Armonk, NY, USA) was used. Descriptive statistics were performed to explore the frequency and percentage of responses for all the variables and a Spearman correlation analysis was conducted to explore the relationship between the user's level of general autonomy and the number of attempts, as well as the relationship between the user's level of general autonomy and the extent to which the user could use the system autonomously in the future. A contingency table was created to explore the relationship between the user's performance and feelings during the task. This was done to explore whether the user's feelings were related to performance. To investigate whether the non-verbal language displayed by the users matched with their reported feelings, we asked the professionals to rate the observed user's feelings. Then both ratings were correlated by Spearman analysis. Then, results were graphically represented with Microsoft Excel (Microsoft Corporation, Redmond, WA, USA).

2.4. Procedure

To carry out this study, several nursing homes and socio-health organizations dedicated to elderly care in the region of Valencia (Spain) were contacted. We debriefed the managers of the organizations about the objective of the project and the need to test the system with people with MCI diagnosed by a physician (neurologist or geriatrician).

Two collaboration agreements were finally signed between the Jaume I University and two nursing homes from the Health Department of the Valencian Community (Spain). It took two months for the study to be conducted, including the development phases.

The medical staff of both nursing homes selected users with MCI as candidates for the study. Due to the candidates' cognitive state, the nursing homes contacted their families to obtain their informed consent to participate and permission to video-tape the sessions. For users under the tutelage of the local government (Health Counsel of the Valencian Community), an additional permit was required to carry out the study. The research was conducted following the American Psychological Association's ethical principles and code of conduct [70]. The study was approved by the Ethics Committee of the Gestión Sociosanitaria del Mediterráneo (GESMED, Socio-Sanitary Management of the Mediterranean; REC number: CD643566/2017). The participants' data confidentiality and anonymity were ensured. Forty-six users were asked to participate in this study voluntarily. Of these, 33 agreed to participate and 28 met the inclusion criteria and signed the data and recording confidentiality agreement. The experimental session consisted of a usability test [60], where a task analysis was carried out [61]. The experimenter took all the necessary hardware to be used in the study to the nursing homes. The rooms used in the centres were big enough to place the equipment and facilitate the movement of people with reduced mobility.

The centre's psychologists (the professional caregiver) accompanied the participants while the expert in usability (the experimenter) conducted the tests. Next, the experimenter presented the task and administered the pre-test assessment protocol (demographic data and previous experience with computers and the Internet). Once the questionnaires were completed, the experimenter explained the task to the user, gave them the instructions for the task on paper, and asked if they would prefer to use a physical or a logical keyboard.

The main task involved writing an email to a specific contact already registered in the address book and attaching a specific picture using the ehcoBUTLER system. The user had the instructions on paper, with the name of the contact in red, the text of the email, and the image to be attached, so that they could follow the instructions as easily as possible and could effectively perform the task. Therefore, the user did not have to memorize the instructions. The secondary task required the evaluation of the avatar and the help voice from a qualitative point of view. We also asked the participants to explain the reasons for their preferences. In order to obtain reliable data on task performance, the sessions were video-taped. A usability expert reviewed the sessions.

The role of the experimenter was to encourage the users to perform the task autonomously, without providing additional instructions. If the users required assistance, the experimenter encouraged them to interact with the avatar. Success meant that the user could complete the task without the help of the experimenter. If any kind of help was needed to complete the task, this was noted as failure. The number of attempts was recorded according to the number of times the experimenter had to show the user how to review the avatar instructions to find out how to continue. The experimenter stood next to the users throughout the usability test (see Figure A2).

In accordance with the Iterative User Interface Design [60], the study was divided into four iterative cycles. This began with the first functional prototype of the system and included seven new users in every iteration. Usability issues were found in each iteration and the proposals for improvement were implemented by the development team. In each iteration the usability issues found were fixed, and after tested again, until arriving to iteration 4, where no usability problems were found. Finally, a re-test was carried out with the users from iteration 1 (see Figure A3). Finally, after finalizing the test, the post-test questionnaires were answered by the users with the experimenter's support (their opinion about the system and how they felt during the test). The professional's clinical judgment was also recorded at this stage. As noted earlier, this included whether the user completed the task, the number of attempts, the assistance received, the opinion about the system and the technology used, the workload experienced, and suggestions and recommended changes.

3. Results

3.1. Main Usability Findings

3.1.1. Solved through Behavior Program Changes

An important problem was related to the way in which users pressed on the screen. The users performed very long pulsations (an average of 3–4 s pressing), which led to the following problems: instead of clicking on the main button (e.g., continue), the secondary button (e.g., copy) was activated. Thus, the text label button was copied, as shown in Figure 1, as opposed to following to the next action.

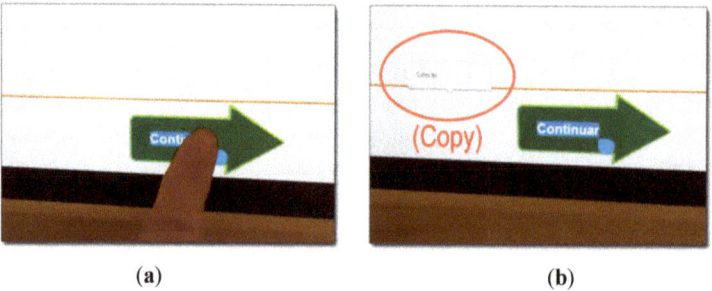

Figure 1. Troubles found due to very long pulsations. (**a**) Text label button selected due to very long pulsation. (**b**) Secondary button activated (copy) instead clicking on the main action button (the green arrow).

This problem was solved by writing a piece of code that overrides the behaviour in the web browsers related to the right-click mouse events by converting these events to left-click mouse events.

Another usability issue observed was the user's need to see what they are pressing while interacting with the touch screen. As a result of this, they clicked outside buttons. To solve this problem, we programmed an interaction area higher than the visual button only, thus preventing missclicking for this reason.

Regarding the help audio facilitated by the avatar voice (a synthetic voice), we found problems with standard speech speed (around 3 words per second). Some participants had problems following the instructions because these were too fast for them. The speed was changed to 2 words per second, adding 8 spaces (2 s) between sentences in order to clearly separate the concepts in the instructions. For example: "You are now viewing your letter (2 s of silence). If you like it (2 s of silence), press the green button that says: Send letter". After changing the voice speed, 92% of the users informed that they liked the voice and that it was easy to understand.

3.1.2. Solved through Graphical Changes

The main usability finding we encountered related to the cognitive state and mental model of this type of user had to do with their attentional capacity. A large number of users did not see the interaction buttons during the first usability iteration. Our first hypothesis was that maybe they suffer some cognitive blindness to bottom elements, which might be caused by the dark grey colour of the graphic user interface (GUI). This is shown in Figure 2a. Because we anticipated that some users might perceive that the dark grey band was an external element, the graphic user interface was redesigned and the dark grey colour was replaced by an orange line, following the upper design as in Figure 2b.

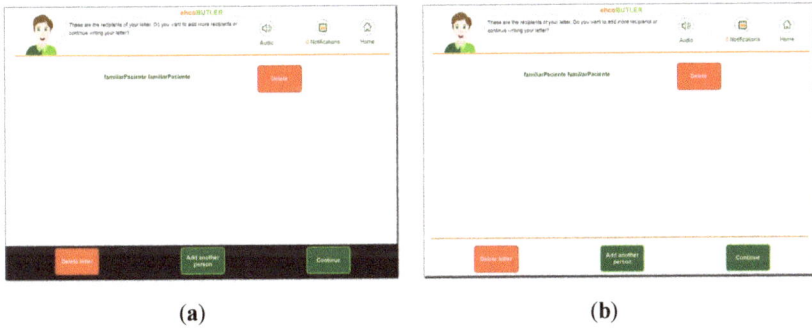

Figure 2. Graphic user interface (GUI) colour change in bottom interaction area. (**a**) Original design. (**b**) Modified design.

Despite this change, users still did not see the elements at the bottom. The study of the sessions revealed that the less autonomous users presented a very acute attentional focus towards the centre of the screen, to the detriment of the interaction elements placed at the bottom or sides of the screen. In order to solve this problem, the graphic user interface was redesigned again, placing the main interaction elements in the central area, that is, within the attentional focus of these users (see Figure 3). With this change, the interaction issues were fully resolved.

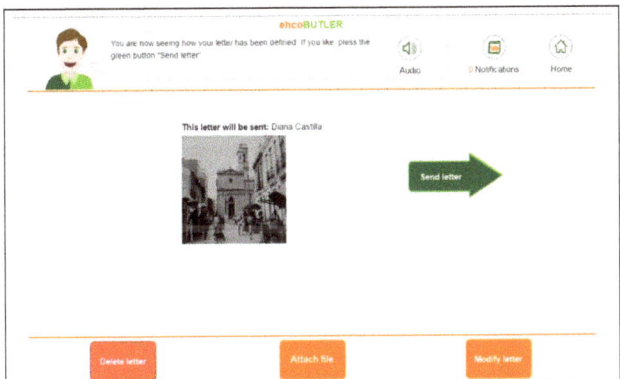

Figure 3. Final graphic user interface.

3.2. Quantitative Results

3.2.1. Task Performance

Good results were obtained on task performance. Specifically, 89% of the participants successfully completed the task (even though the majority of them had no previous ICT experience).

3.2.2. Number of Attempts

The number of attempts to complete the task varied across participants (range 1 to 6). However, 50% of the users managed to complete it in just 1 or 2 attempts (median = 2.50, SD = 1.59). Comparing the sum of attempts during the study, we observed that there was a higher number of attempts at the beginning of the study due to usability problems related to the touch interaction (long pulsations that activate selecting text or the contextual menu). We conducted a Spearman correlation analysis between the user's general level of autonomy, rated by the professional caregivers, and the number of attempts. The correlation was not significant (r_s = 0.17, p = 0.396).

3.2.3. Workload NASA Task Work Load Index)

The workload during the task was low or very low on all subscales (see Figure 4), achieving a general mean of 4.55 (SD = 5.65) and means on all scales below the central point of 11 (range 0 to 21, Very low demand = 0; Very high demand = 21).

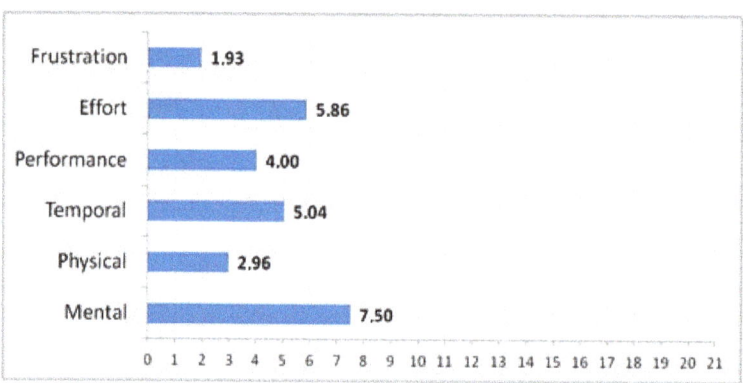

Figure 4. NASA task work load index results.

3.3. Quantitative Results

3.3.1. Usability Variables and User Opinion

In general, the users' opinion was good, as all the usability variables were scored on the positive side of the scale exceeding the midpoint (i.e., exceeding 2 points on a scale ranging from 0 to 4). Specifically, the users found the system easy to use and useful for their lives, they felt confident while using it, felt that they had control over the system, found the button size large enough to see it and interact with it, and reported that they would like to use the system in the future (see Figure 5).

The variable with the highest average score was ease of use, with 3.07 (SD = 0.98), followed by useful with 3.00 (SD = 1.19).

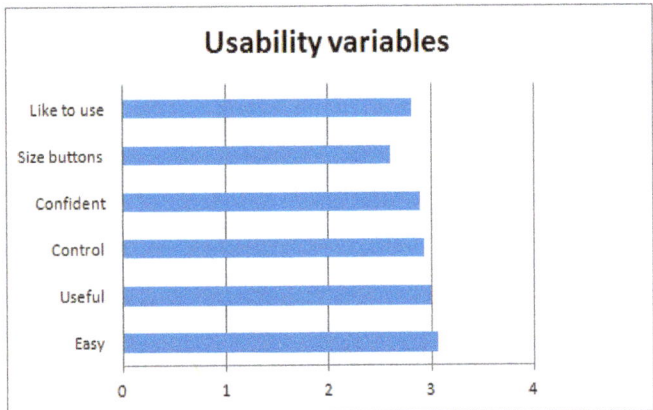

Figure 5. Average of usability variables.

Regarding their feelings during the test, 79% of the users felt from normal to very good. A contingency table was created to explore the relationship between user performance and feelings during the task (see Table 1).

Table 1. User performance vs. feelings during the task: contingency table.

		Task Performance		Total
		Fail	Success	
User Felt	Very bad	0	0	0
	Bad	2	1	3
	Neutral	1	4	5
	Good	0	15	15
	Very good	0	5	5
Total		3	25	28

Only three users (10%) referred to feeling bad during the experiment. They indicated that they felt nervous because of the test conditions (people looking at them and assessing what they were doing). The number of users who felt bad or failed the task were too low to perform a Chi-square analysis.

3.3.2. Intention to Use

Regarding the intention to use the system in the future, 82% of the users expressed that they would like to use it often in the future (21% strongly agree; 61% somewhat agree; 7% neither disagree nor agree; 0% somewhat disagree, 11% strongly disagree).

3.3.3. Preferences about Avatar Appearance and Voice

From a graphic point of view, users indicated that they liked the age of the avatar (young), estimating that it was about 30 years old. Regarding the voice, none of the participants perceived that it was a synthetic voice. Adjectives such as "nice", "polite", or "kind" were used the most to describe it.

3.4. Professional Opinion

3.4.1. Ability to Use the System in an Autonomous Way

Before the experiment, the professional caregivers rated the level of autonomy the users had in their everyday lives while performing any kind of task.

After the usability task, the professional caregivers also rated their clinical judgment about the level of user autonomy using the system, revealing that 46% of the users would be able to autonomously use the system in the future without any kind of support. Only in 14% of the cases did the professional caregivers describe that the users would need frequent support, but they felt that 39% of the sample would always need support.

We conducted a Spearman correlation analysis between the user's general level of autonomy, rated by the professional caregivers and the extent to which they thought the user could use the system autonomously. The correlation was significant and positive ($r_s = 0.45$; $p = 0.016$). This correlation indicates that the professional caregivers thought that users with a high degree of autonomy in their everyday lives could also use the system in a more autonomous way in the future, whereas users with low autonomy in their routines would also have low autonomy in using the system. It seems logical that if the user is not autonomous in his/her daily life, it would be very difficult for him/her to use the system without assistance.

3.4.2. Sessions Needed to Learn to Use the System in an Unassisted Manner

The following analysis evaluates to which extent the professionals believed that the users would be able to use the system on their own with some training. According to the professionals' opinion, 39% of users would always need support to use the system. The also indicated that 36% of users would need more than 10 training sessions to use the system on their own. Finally, they reported that 14% of them would need between 5 and 10 training sessions to use the system autonomously and 11% of them would only need 2 to 4 training sessions (see Figure 6).

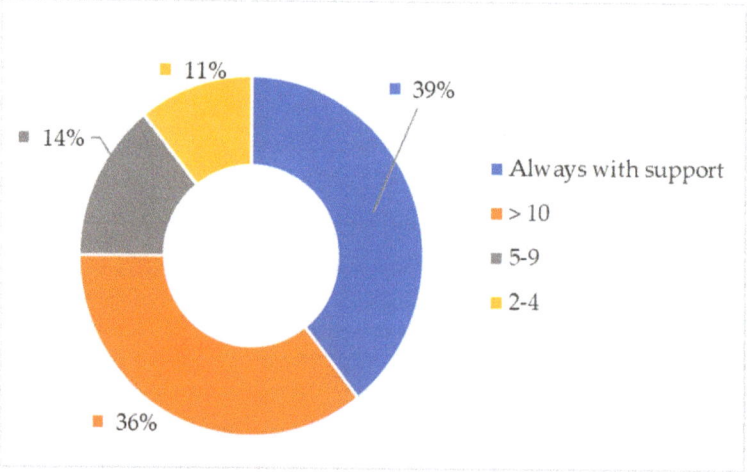

Figure 6. Estimated number of training sessions to use the system in an autonomous way.

3.4.3. Professional Opinion about the Users' Feelings

The professionals also rated how they thought the users felt during the test. We conducted a Spearman correlation analysis between feeling scores given by the user and those given by the professional. The correlation was significant and positive ($r_s = 0.59$; $p = 0.001$), indicating a large agreement between the experienced user feeling and the professional caregiver's impression about the user's feeling.

4. Discussion

The present study aimed to test the usability of a prototype system designed for users with MCI and make adaptations to it based on the results. For this purpose, a functional prototype email system was designed based on the usability design principles of the Butler system (i.e., the design followed the National Institute on Aging checklist [71] and added linear navigation and audio and text help through an avatar) [59]. The system was tested in two nursing homes of the Health Council of the Valencian Community (Spain). The results showed differences between the present study and the findings obtained from previous research with the same web design but a different population (i.e., people without cognitive impairment) [32,46]. The main usability issues revealed in the present study compared with those of users without MCI were the following:

- *Related to spatial abilities and attention.* The results showed a low perception of peripheral elements and the need to place the main interaction elements (e.g., continue the action in the step-by-step navigation) in the center of the screen because less autonomous users showed an attentional focus on this central part of the screen and attentional blindness to the peripheral graphical elements.
- *Related programming interaction.* Given that users expect a real time change in buttons (such as sinking down when pressed), the interaction with the buttons was performed by pressing them for a long time, causing an unexpected interaction result (copying text or activating the secondary browser menu). On the other hand, we observed the user's need to see what they were pressing while touching the buttons. This explains why they clicked outside the buttons.
- *Related audio help.* The standard speed of synthetic speech (3 words per second) was too fast, and most of the users were not able to follow the instructions.

Our findings raise some novel questions about the design of interfaces for MCI users. For example, several studies point out that the use of audio and text support can benefit both novel and experienced older users [72]. However, audio interfaces also could represent a new usability barrier because they force the user to work with memory and mental agility. These new interfaces allow us to avoid the keyboard and present a user interface with less text, but the audio interface adds other difficulties such as having to understand and retain information while making interaction decisions. It is well known that, because speech is linearized, audio instructions as a unimodal strategy impose difficulties in the elderly [73]. In the case of cognitively impaired users, this effort could become another step in the technological barrier stairway. If we take into account that one of the handicaps in MCI is memory loss and a decrease in mental agility, we could encounter a real barrier that goes beyond usability and could become a serious accessibility problem for this kind of user.

Regarding the audio interface to support the interaction, previous studies with elderly users without cognitive impairment suggest that speed adjustment is not necessary [72]. However, our findings showed that it is likely to be necessary to adjust the speed of the speech, as well to add a short time separation between phrases for users with MCI, probably because they need more time to process information. Our study revealed positive results from adjusting the speech speed to 2 words per second and adding 2 s of silence between short sentences, which was done to clearly separate the concepts of the instructions and to give the user time to understand them. At this point, we think it is important to differentiate between input and output audios. Our study only explores this feature as an output of an application, that is, when the user receives information passively (in our case as a complement of the text help). We cannot extrapolate our conclusions to audio inputs, that is, when the user gives audio instructions to the system.

In addition to the findings with the audio interface, our results showed usability difficulties related to the graphic design. A metaphor in this context is how we represent an interaction with the system in an understandable way. For example, a metaphor in a graphic interface could be represented by the buttons and other visual elements like the avatar or the space to write. The commonly used metaphors represented in the technology do not correspond to the previous experience of users with a low technological profile and according literature this can be a barrier [59,74]. This might be the reason why the users in our study made long pulsations while waiting for a change of state in the buttons. These results support the idea that assistive technologies should introduce graphic elements that match the users' previous experience. This opens an avenue for a new dimension that should be considered in the design of this type of technology. Following this need to adapt ICTs to the mental model of the elderly, it could be advisable to represent objects and object behaviours that users could be familiar with. For example, if we represent a button in an application, the feedback when pressing it could be seeing the button sink.

Previous literature highlights the negative effects of age on spatial abilities, memory, attention, and perceptual speed [19,27,75]. Thus, because navigation is one of the greatest difficulties for older users, linear navigation can be useful for improving usability results with elderly users [46,76,77]. Experiencing MCI considerably increases these cognitive and motor difficulties, which adds new challenges in designing webs for this kind of user. Some studies propose linear navigation to avoid spatial disorientation when using websites [75]. However, cognitive impairment influences spatial orientation and, consequently, makes this usability problem even greater. The linear navigation solution cannot fix this because, for users with MCI, spatial orientation might not be limited to navigation among the different parts of the system. The problem could be that, on each screen, the user must make an effort that requires attention and guidance. This idea seems somewhat aligned with the change blindness concept [55] because the users could not find the changes between different screens, and so there was disorientation beyond navigation. A possible solution is to combine different strategies to maintain the attention on interaction effortlessly. For example, one option could be combining the linear navigation with audio and help text and a design in which the main interactions (to continue the task) are placed in the centre of the screen.

Also in relation to cognitive performance, research has evidenced that, when the user is familiar with the learning object, the memory and learning processes are faster [78]. However, cognitive impairments such as memory loss or disorientation could increase the difficulties in recognizing or memorizing objects. Natural interfaces such as speech mode try to replicate a natural and user-friendly interaction. Audio outputs (from the system to the user) can be useful for users who receive help and instructions in real time [72], but audio inputs (from the user to the system) require other mental processes that demand the specific use of memory, such as remembering specific words from the instructions or predicting (or remembering) what step will be next. In this regard, a recent study [39] evidenced significant difficulties in speech recognition in patients with MCI even when embodied conversational agents were successfully implemented. Our study only explored audio outputs, and the results showed that the speech speed could be an important factor in designing audio interfaces.

Another finding was that a positive and significant correlation between the general level of autonomy and the ICT autonomy level was obtained. This result could indicate that the level of autonomy in everyday activities could be a good predictor of the level of user autonomy in the use of assistive technologies, which might have some clinical implications. For example, this could be used as guiding information when having to select the type of interface or amount of support that is provided to users (e.g., those with less daily autonomy should be offered more help or easier interfaces).

From a qualitative point of view, the results of our study showed that users did not perceive the difference between a synthetic voice and a human voice during the testing. These results are important as they suggest that this system can be effectively used in the elderly, which is in line with past literature [72]. This finding supports the idea that the use of mechanical audio interfaces, which are cheaper to develop than audios recorded directly by humans, are suitable for this kind of population. Given that this was perceived like a human voice and did not eliminate emotional qualities, this procedure is promising in this field.

The present study has a number of limitations. First, although the sample size is large enough to obtain usability conclusions, the number of users limits the statistical analysis that can be performed with the data. Additionally, the fact that they all belonged to the same country limits the cultural generalization of the findings. Furthermore, the experimental design limits our conclusions to the specific task of "composing" an email and attaching a picture. Other tasks and interfaces should be used to test our usability recommendations for MCI users. An additional limitation refers to the existence of a single professional rater of the patient's performance. Even though this is the usual practice in clinical settings, the existence of a second evaluator is always preferable for reliability purposes. Finally, this work did not explore in-depth the impact of physical or logical keyboards on performance.

5. Conclusions

In spite of the limitations of this study, the findings resulted in a number of recommendations for the use of ICT in persons with MCI and open the door to exploring new dimensions of spatial orientation on graphic user interfaces. New technologies can help to improve the wellbeing and quality of life of users with MCI or early dementia. However, due to their cognitive impairment, such individuals suffer from a lack of orientation, not only when navigating between screens, but when interacting with a single screen. Simplifying technologies for MCI users should be an important societal goal. The use of linear navigation could be a key element in this direction, but it is not the only one. Designers have a new challenge of "designing interaction in the middle" because the main area of attention for these users was the centre of the screen. Another recommendation is to design the interaction area bigger than the visual button. This should be done because there is a general tendency to press the buttons outside the image in an attempt to see what they are pressing. In addition, the results suggested that natural interfaces, such as audio interfaces, might be useful for these users if the speed is adapted to their cognitive needs. In this sense, text-to-speech technology can be a suitable and cost-effective alternative because users do not distinguish the human voice from a bot. Therefore, based on our findings one recommendable speech speed for similar users and purposes would be 2 words per second and adding 2 s of silence between short sentences. Ultimately, the utility of the results lies in the fact that achieving design interfaces that give MCI users independence could help to prolong the time they live independently at home and might help improve their quality of life. One way of doing this, for instance, would be providing them with a number of alternative care possibilities, such as a cognitive rehabilitation program that they can perform at home autonomously. The main contribution of this study consists of exploring the usability needs of users with MCI on ICT systems and providing some usability recommendations for designing interfaces for this kind of user.

Author Contributions: Conceptualization, D.C., A.G.-P. and C.B.; methodology, D.C. and A.G.-P.; validation, D.C. and I.Z.; formal analysis, D.C. and C.S.-R.; investigation, D.C., C.B., A.G.-P., I.Z. and C.S.-R.; resources, D.C., C.B. and A.G.-P.; data curation, D.C.; writing—original draft preparation, D.C. and I.Z.; writing—review and editing, A.G.-P., C.S.-R. and C.B.; visualization, D.C.; supervision, C.B. and A.G.-P.; project administration, D.C.; funding acquisition, C.B. All authors have read and agreed to the published version of the manuscript.

Funding: This research was funded by European Union's Horizon 2020 research and innovation programme [ehcoBUTLER project, grant agreement No 643566]; Instituto de Salud Carlos III -ISCIII [CIBER of Physiopathology of Obesity and Nutrition, CB06/03/0052].

Acknowledgments: We would like to give special thanks for their interest and professional support to the technical team in charge of ehcoBUTLER programming and development: Rafael Ordóñez, Juan Antonio Grande and Sergio Barrera. Also, we would like to thanks for their involvement and professional support to the staff of the nursing homes that participated in this research: "Residencia de la Tercera Edad y Centro de día "La Vila" (Almussafes, Valencia, Spain) and "Residencia y centro de día de personas mayores dependientes de Chiva" (Chiva, Spain).

Conflicts of Interest: The authors declare no conflict of interest. The funders had no role in the design of the study; in the collection, analyses, or interpretation of data; in the writing of the manuscript, or in the decision to publish the results.

Appendix A

Table A1. Summary of sociodemographic characteristics of the sample.

ID	Number of Iteration	Cognitive Diagnosis	Age	Sex	School-Leaving Age	PC Experience
1	1	MCI	73	M	12	Never
2	1	MCI	83	F	10	Never
3	1	MCI	85	M	Didn't remember	Never
4	1	MCI	71	F	14	Never
5	1	MCI	94	M	14	Never
6	1	MCI	88	M	10	Never
7	1	MCI	95	F	10	Never
8	2	MCI	67	M	14	Never
9	2	MCI	58	M	13	Once
10	2	MCI	89	F	8	Never
11	2	MCI	90	F	14	Never
12	2	MCI	86	F	Didn't go to school	Never
13	2	MCI	89	M	Didn't go to school	Never
14	2	MCI	85	F	Didn't go to school	Never
15	3	MCI	76	F	8	Never
16	3	MCI	70	M	14	Never
17	3	MCI	85	M	7	Never
18	3	MCI	71	F	13	Never
19	3	MCI	69	M	15	Never
20	3	MCI	75	M	Didn't remember	More than 10
21	3	MCI	76	M	14	From 1 to 10
22	4	MCI	81	M	12	Never
23	4	MCI	70	F	16	More than 10
24	4	MCI	88	F	12	Never
25	4	MCI	67	M	20	From 1 to 10
26	4	MCI	81	F	18	Never
27	4	MCI	91	F	11	Never
28	4	MCI	78	F	14	Never

Notes: MCI: Mild Cognitive Impairment. PC experience: number of times that the person used a personal computer before this study. Sex: M = Male, F = Female.

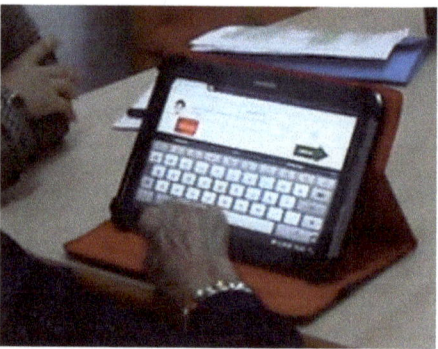

Figure A1. Usability problem on tablets due logic keyboard.

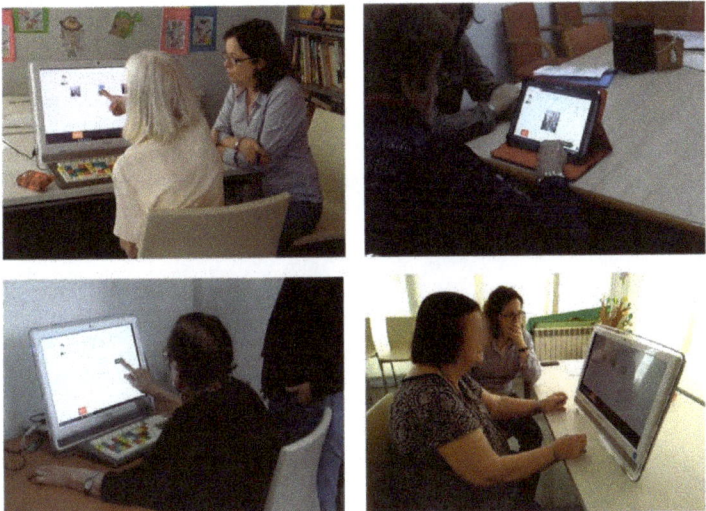

Figure A2. Set-up during usability testing.

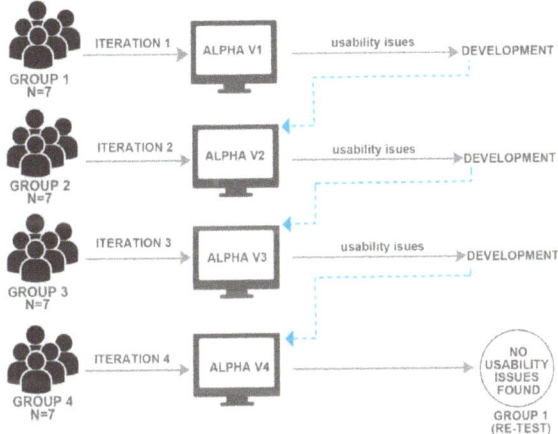

Figure A3. Diagram of iterative cycles performed in the usability test.

References

1. He, W.; Goodkind, D.; Kowal, P. An Aging World: 2015 International Population Reports. In *U.S. Census Bureau, International Population Reports, P95/16-1, An Aging World 2015*; US Government Printing Office: Washington, DC, USA, 2016; p. 204.
2. WHO. Governments Commit to Advancements in Dementia Research and Care. Geneva. Available online: http://www.who.int/mediacentre/news/releases/2015/action-on-dementia/en/ (accessed on 25 November 2017).
3. Fischer, P.; Jungwirth, S.; Zehetmayer, S.; Weissgram, S.; Hoenigschnabl, S.; Gelpi, E.; Tragl, K.H. Conversion from subtypes of mild cognitive impairment to Alzheimer dementia. *Neurology* **2007**, *68*, 288–291. [CrossRef] [PubMed]
4. Martin, M.; Clare, L.; Altgassen, A.M.; Cameron, M.H.; Zehnder, F. Cognition-based interventions for healthy older people and people with mild cognitive impairment. *Cochrane Database Syst. Rev.* **2011**, *19*, CD006220. [CrossRef] [PubMed]

5. Brum, P.S.; Forlenza, O.V.; Yassuda, M.S. Treino cognitivo em idosos com Comprometimento Cognitivo Leve: Impacto no desempenho cognitivo e funcional. *Dement. e Neuropsychol.* **2009**, *3*, 124–131. [CrossRef] [PubMed]
6. Liu, X.Y.; Li, L.; Xiao, J.Q.; He, C.Z.; Lyu, X.L.; Gao, L.; Yang, X.W.; Cui, X.G.; Fan, L.H. Cognitive training in older adults with mild cognitive impairment. *Biomed. Environ. Sci.* **2016**, *29*, 356–364.
7. Zhang, H.; Huntley, J.; Bhome, R.; Holmes, B.; Cahill, J.; Gould, R.L.; Wang, H.; Yu, X.; Howard, R. Effect of computerised cognitive training on cognitive outcomes in mild cognitive impairment: A systematic review and meta-analysis. *BMJ Open* **2019**, *9*, e027062. [CrossRef]
8. Coyle, H.; Traynor, V.; Solowij, N. Computerized and virtual reality cognitive training for individuals at high risk of cognitive decline: Systematic review of the literature. *Am. J. Geriatr.* **2015**, *23*, 335–359. [CrossRef]
9. Franco, M.; Jones, K.; Woods, B.; Gómez, P. Gradior: A personalized computer-based cognitive training programme for early intervention in dementia. In *Early Psychosocial Interventions in Dementia. Evidence-Based Practice*; Moniz-Cook, E., Manthorpe, J., Eds.; Jessica Kingsley Publishers: London, UK, 2009.
10. García-Betances, R.I.; Jiménez-Mixco, V.; Arredondo, M.T.; Cabrera-Umpiérrez, M.F. Using virtual reality for cognitive training of the elderly. *Am. J. Alzheimers Dis. Other Demen.* **2015**, *30*, 49–54. [CrossRef]
11. Palau, F.; Franco, M.; Bamidis, P.; Losada, R.; Parra, E.; Papageorgiou, S.; Vivas, A.B. The effects of a computer-based cognitive and physical training program in a healthy and mildly cognitive impaired aging sample. *Aging Ment. Health* **2014**, *18*, 838–846. [CrossRef]
12. Shuchat, J.; Ouellet, É.; Moffat, N.; Belleville, S. Opportunities for virtual reality in cognitive training with persons with mild cognitive impairment or Alzheimer's disease. *Nonpharmacol. Ther. Dement.* **2012**, *3*, 35.
13. Baecker, R.M.; Marziali, E.; Chatland, S.; Easley, K.; Crete, M.; Yeung, M. Multimedia biographies for individuals with Alzheimer's disease and their families. In Proceedings of the World Congress on Internet in Medicine, Toronto, ON, Canada, 14–19 October 2006.
14. Barban, F.; Annicchiarico, R.; Pantelopoulos, S.; Federici, A.; Perri, R.; Fadda, L.; Carlesimo, G.A.; Ricci, C.; Giuli, S.; Scalici, F.; et al. Protecting cognition from aging and Alzheimer's disease: A computerized cognitive training combined with reminiscence therapy. *Int. J. Geriatr. Psychiatry* **2015**, *31*, 340–348. [CrossRef]
15. Damianakis, T.; Crete-Nishihata, M.; Smith, K.L.; Baecker, R.M.; Marziali, E. The psychosocial impacts of multimedia biographies on persons with cognitive impairments. *Gerontologist* **2010**, *50*, 23–35. [CrossRef]
16. Pino, M.; Boulay, M.; Jouen, F.; Rigaud, A.S. "Are we ready for robots that care for us?" Attitudes and opinions of older adults toward socially assistive robots. *Front. Aging Neurosci.* **2015**, *7*, 1–15. [CrossRef]
17. Cornejo, R.; Tentori, M.; Favela, J. Enriching in-person encounters through social media: A study on family connectedness for the elderly. *Int. J. Hum. Comput. Stud.* **2013**, *71*, 889–899. [CrossRef]
18. Khosravi, P.; Rezvani, A.; Wiewiora, A. The impact of technology on older adults' social isolation. *Comput. Hum. Behav.* **2016**, *63*, 594–603. [CrossRef]
19. Yates, L.A.; Ziser, S.; Spector, A.; Orrell, M. Cognitive leisure activities and future risk of cognitive impairment and dementia: Systematic review and meta-analysis. *Int. Psychogeriatr.* **2016**, *28*, 1791–1806. [CrossRef] [PubMed]
20. Lazar, A.; Thompson, H.; Demiris, G. A systematic review of the use of technology for reminiscence therapy. *Health Educ. Behav.* **2014**, *41*, 51S–61S. [CrossRef] [PubMed]
21. Preschl, B.; Maercker, A.; Wagner, B.; Forstmeier, S.; Baños, R.M.; Alcañiz, M.; Castilla, D.; Botella, C. Life-review therapy with computer supplements for depression in the elderly: A randomized controlled trial. *Aging Ment. Health* **2012**, *16*, 964–974. [CrossRef]
22. Shankar, A.; Hamer, M.; McMunn, A.; Steptoe, A. Social isolation and loneliness: Relationships with cognitive function during 4 years of follow-up in the English Longitudinal Study of Ageing. *Psychosom. Med.* **2013**, *75*, 161–170. [CrossRef]
23. Wang, B.; He, P.; Dong, B. Associations between social networks, social contacts, and cognitive function among Chinese nonagenarians/centenarians. *Arch. Gerontol. Geriatr.* **2015**, *60*, 522–527. [CrossRef]
24. Wilson, R.S.; Boyle, P.A.; James, B.D.; Leurgans, S.E.; Buchman, A.S.; Bennett, D.A. Negative social interactions and risk of mild cognitive impairment in old age. *Neuropsychology* **2015**, *29*, 561–570. [CrossRef]
25. Wilson, R.S.; Krueger, K.R.; Arnold, S.E.; Schneider, J.A.; Kelly, J.F.; Barnes, L.L.; Tang, Y.; Bennett, D.A. Loneliness and Risk of Alzheimer Disease. *Arch. Gen. Psychiatry* **2007**, *64*, 234. [CrossRef] [PubMed]

26. Windsor, T.D.; Gerstorf, D.; Pearson, E.; Ryan, L.H.; Anstey, K.J. Positive and negative social exchanges and cognitive aging in young-old adults: Differential associations across family, friend, and spouse domains. *Psychol. Aging* **2014**, *29*, 28–43. [CrossRef]
27. Boutet, I.; Milgram, N.W.; Freedman, M. Cognitive decline and human (Homo sapiens) aging: An investigation using a comparative neuropsychological approach. *J. Comp. Psychol.* **2007**, *121*, 270–281. [CrossRef] [PubMed]
28. National Collaborating Centre for Mental Health (UK). *Dementia: A NICE-SCIE Guideline on Supporting People with Dementia and Their Carers in Health and Social Care*; British Psychological Society: Leicester, UK, 2007.
29. Sonderegger, A.; Schmutz, S.; Sauer, J. The influence of age in usability testing. *Appl. Ergon.* **2016**, *52*, 291–300. [CrossRef]
30. Wagner, N.; Hassanein, K.; Head, M. The impact of age on website usability. *Comput. Hum. Behav.* **2014**, *37*, 270–282. [CrossRef]
31. Zhou, J.; Rau, P.-L.P.; Salvendy, G. Use and Design of Handheld Computers for Older Adults: A Review and Appraisal. *Int. J. Hum. Comput. Interact.* **2012**, *28*, 799–826. [CrossRef]
32. Castilla, D.; Botella, C.; Miralles, I.; Bretón-lópez, J.; Dragomir-davis, A.; Zaragoza, I.; Garcia-palacios, A. Teaching digital literacy skills to the elderly using a social network with linear navigation: A case study in a rural area. *Int. J. Hum. Comput. Stud.* **2018**, *118*, 24–37. [CrossRef]
33. Dunn, T. Usability for Older Web Users. Available online: https://www.webcredible.com/blog/usability-older-web-users/ (accessed on 25 March 2019).
34. Hogan, M. Age Differences in Technophobia: An Irish Study. In *Information Systems Development*; Springer: Boston, MA, USA, 2009; pp. 117–130.
35. Chua, S.L.; Chen, D.-T.; Wong, A.F.L. Computer anxiety and its correlates: A meta-analysis. *Comput. Hum. Behav.* **1999**, *15*, 609–623. [CrossRef]
36. Wang, C.; Chen, J. Overcoming technophobia in poorly-educated elderly—The HELPS-seniors service learning program. *Int. J. Autom. Smart Technol.* **2015**, *5*, 173–182.
37. Friemel, T.N. The digital divide has grown old: Determinants of a digital divide among seniors. *New Media Soc.* **2016**, *18*, 313–331. [CrossRef]
38. Vroman, K.G.; Arthanat, S.; Lysack, C. "Who over 65 is online?" Older adults' dispositions toward information communication technology. *Comput. Hum. Behav.* **2015**, *43*, 156–166. [CrossRef]
39. Wargnier, P.; Benveniste, S.; Jouvelot, P.; Rigaud, A.S. Usability assessment of interaction management support in LOUISE, an ECA-based user interface for elders with cognitive impairment. *Technol. Disabil.* **2018**, *30*, 105–126. [CrossRef]
40. Campoverde-Molina, M.; Lujan-Mora, S.; Garcia, L.V. Empirical Studies on Web Accessibility of Educational Websites: A Systematic Literature Review. *IEEE Access* **2020**, *8*, 91676–91700. [CrossRef]
41. European Commission Web Accessibility | Shaping Europe's Digital Future. Available online: https://ec.europa.eu/digital-single-market/en/web-accessibility (accessed on 7 July 2020).
42. European Commission. Directive (EU) 2016/2102 of the European Parliament and of the Council of 26 October 2016 on the accessibility of the websites and mobile applications of public. Document 32016L2102 sector bodies. *Off. J. Eur. Union* **2016**, *L327*, 1–15.
43. W3C Web Accessibility Initiative WAI. Web Content Accessibility Guidelines (WCAG) Overview. Available online: https://www.w3.org/WAI/standards-guidelines/wcag/ (accessed on 7 July 2020).
44. W3C Web Accessibility Initiative WAI. Overview of "Web Accessibility for Older Users: A Literature Review". Available online: https://www.w3.org/WAI/older-users/literature/ (accessed on 6 July 2020).
45. W3C Web Accessibility Initiative WAI. Cognitive Accessibility at W3C | Web Accessibility Initiative (WAI) | W3C. Available online: https://www.w3.org/WAI/cognitive/ (accessed on 6 July 2020).
46. Castilla, D.; Garcia-Palacios, A.; Miralles, I.; Breton-Lopez, J.; Parra, E.; Rodriguez-Berges, S.; Botella, C. Effect of Web navigation style in elderly users. *Comput. Hum. Behav.* **2016**, *55*, 909–920. [CrossRef]
47. Arthanat, S. Promoting Information Communication Technology Adoption and Acceptance for Aging-in-Place: A Randomized Controlled Trial. *J. Appl. Gerontol.* **2019**. Available online: https://pubmed.ncbi.nlm.nih.gov/31782347/ (accessed on 6 April 2020).
48. Fernando, S.; Money, A.; Elliman, T.; Lines, L. Developing assistive web-base technologies for adults with age-related cognitive impairments. *Transform. Gov. People Process Policy* **2009**, *3*, 131–143. [CrossRef]
49. Haesner, M.; Steinert, A.; O'Sullivan, J.L.; Steinhagen-Thiessen, E. Evaluating an accessible web interface for older adults—The impact of mild cognitive impairment (MCI). *J. Assist. Technol.* **2015**, *9*, 219–232. [CrossRef]

50. Lauriks, S.; Reinersmann, A.; Van der Roest, H.G.; Meiland, F.J.; Davies, R.J.; Moelaert, F.; Mulvenna, M.D.; Nugent, C.D.; Dröes, R.M. Review of ICT-based services for identified unmet needs in people with dementia. *Ageing Res. Rev.* **2007**, *6*, 223–246. [CrossRef]
51. Jackson, G.R.; Owsley, C. Visual dysfunction, neurodegenerative diseases, and aging. *Neurol. Clin.* **2003**, *21*, 709–728. [CrossRef]
52. Rizzo, M.; Anderson, S.W.; Dawson, J.; Nawrot, M. Vision and cognition in Alzheimer's disease. *Neuropsychologia* **2000**, *38*, 1157–1169. [CrossRef]
53. Rizzo, M.; Sparks, J.; McEvoy, S.; Viamonte, S.; Kellison, I.; Vecera, S.P. Change blindness, aging, and cognition. *J. Clin. Exp. Neuropsychol.* **2009**, *31*, 245–256. [CrossRef]
54. Caird, J.K.; Edwards, C.J.; Creaser, J.I.; Horrey, W.J. Older Driver Failures of Attention at Intersections: Using Change Blindness Methods to Assess Turn Decision Accuracy. *Hum. Factors J. Hum. Factors Ergon. Soc.* **2005**, *47*, 235–249. [CrossRef] [PubMed]
55. Whitenton, K. Change Blindness Causes People to Ignore What Designers Expect Them to See. Available online: https://www.nngroup.com/articles/change-blindness/ (accessed on 25 March 2019).
56. García-Betances, R.I.; Cabrera-Umpiérrez, M.F.; Ottaviano, M.; Pastorino, M.; Arredondo, M.T. Parametric Cognitive Modeling of Information and Computer Technology Usage by People with Aging- and Disability-Derived Functional Impairments. *Sensors* **2016**, *16*, 266. [CrossRef] [PubMed]
57. Contreras-Somoza, L.M.; Irazoki, E.; Castilla, D.; Cristina, B.; Toribio-guzmán, J.M.; Parra-Vidales, E.; Suso-Ribera, C.; Suárez-López, P.; Perea-Bartolomé, M.V.; Franco-Martín, M.Á. Study on the acceptability of an ICT platform for older adults with mild cognitive impairment. *J. Med. Syst.* **2020**, *44*, 120. [CrossRef]
58. European Commission. ehcoBUTLER. A Global Ecosystem for the Independent and Healty Living of Elder People with Mild Cognitive Impairments. | Projects | H2020 | CORDIS | Grant Agreement ID: 643566. 2018. Available online: https://cordis.europa.eu/project/rcn/194077/factsheet/en (accessed on 25 March 2019).
59. Castilla, D.; Garcia-Palacios, A.; Bretón-López, J.; Miralles, I.; Baños, R.M.; Etchemendy, E.; Farfallini, L.; Botella, C. Process of design and usability evaluation of a telepsychology web and virtual reality system for the elderly: Butler. *Int. J. Hum. Comput. Stud.* **2013**, *71*, 350–362. [CrossRef]
60. Nielsen, J. *Usability Engineering*; Academic Press: Boston, MA, USA, 1993.
61. Dumas, J.S.; Redish, J. *A Practical Guide to Usability Testing*; Intellect Books: Exeter, UK, 1999.
62. Mateos, R.; Franco, M.; Sanchez, M. Care for dementia in Spain: The need for a nationwide strategy. *Int. J. Geriatr. Psychiatry* **2010**, *25*, 881–884. [CrossRef]
63. Europe, A. Spain—National Dementia Strategies—Policy in Practice. Available online: https://www.alzheimer-europe.org/Policy-in-Practice2/National-Dementia-Strategies/Spain (accessed on 29 March 2019).
64. Arriola, E.; Carnero, C.; Freire, A.; López-Mogil, R.; López-Trigo, J.A.; Manzano, S.; Olazarán, J. *Deterioro Cognitivo Leve en el Adulto Mayor. Documento de Consenso*; Sociedad Española de Geriatría y Gerontología, Ed.; Sociedad Española de Geriatría y Gerontología: Madrid, Spain, 2017.
65. Botella, C.; Etchemendy, E.; Castilla, D.; Baños, R.M.; García-Palacios, A.; Quero, S.; Alcañiz, M.; Lozano, J.A. An e-health system for the elderly (Butler Project): A pilot study on acceptance and satisfaction. *Cyberpsychol. Behav.* **2009**, *12*, 255–262. [CrossRef] [PubMed]
66. Lorish, C.D.; Maisiak, R. The face scale: A brief, nonverbal method for assessing patient mood. *Arthritis Rheum.* **1986**, *29*, 906–909. [CrossRef]
67. Stern, R.A.; Arruda, J.E.; Hooper, C.R.; Wolfner, G.D.; Morey, C.E. Visual analogue mood scales to measure internal mood state in neurologically impaired patients: Description and initial validity evidence. *Aphasiology* **1997**, *11*, 59–71. [CrossRef]
68. Yang, F.; Dawes, P.; Leroi, I.; Gannon, B. Measurement tools of resource use and quality of life in clinical trials for dementia or cognitive impairment interventions: A systematically conducted narrative review. *Int. J. Geriatr. Psychiatry* **2017**, *33*, 1–11. [CrossRef]
69. Hart, S.; Staveland, L. Development of NASA-TLX (Task Load Index): Results of empirical and theoretical research. In *Human Mental Workload*; Hancock, P., Meshkati, N., Eds.; North Holland Press: Amsterdam, The Netherlands, 1988; pp. 139–183.
70. American Psychological Association. Ethical Principles of Psychologists and Code of Conduct. Available online: https://www.apa.org/ethics/code/ (accessed on 3 February 2020).
71. National Institute on Aging. Making Your Web Site Senior Friendly: A Checklist. Available online: https://www.hsdl.org/?view&did=770661 (accessed on 14 June 2020).

72. Christopher Mayer, C.; Morandell, M.; Gira, M.; Fagel, S. *AAL Joint Programme Ambient Assisted Living User Interfaces AALuis i Project Identification Ambient Assisted Living User Interfaces*; European Commission: Brusels, Belgium, 2011.
73. Freiherr, J.; Lundström, J.N.; Habel, U.; Reetz, K. Multisensory integration mechanisms during aging. *Front. Hum. Neurosci.* **2013**, *7*, 1–6. [CrossRef] [PubMed]
74. Kim, H.; Hirtle, S.C. Spatial metaphors and disorientation in hypertext browsing. *Behav. Inf. Technol.* **1995**, *14*, 239–250. [CrossRef]
75. Techentin, C.; Voyer, D.; Voyer, S.D. Spatial Abilities and Aging: A Meta-Analysis. *Exp. Aging Res.* **2014**, *40*, 395–425. [CrossRef]
76. Barnard, Y.; Bradley, M.D.; Hodgson, F.; Lloyd, A.D. Learning to use new technologies by older adults: Perceived difficulties, experimentation behaviour and usability. *Comput. Hum. Behav.* **2013**, *29*, 1715–1724. [CrossRef]
77. Graf, P.; Mandler, G. Activation makes words more accessible, but not necessarily more retrievable. *J. Verbal Learn. Verbal Behav.* **1984**, *23*, 553–568. [CrossRef]
78. Mandler, G. Recognizing: The judgment of previous occurrence. *Psychol. Rev.* **1980**, *87*, 252–271. [CrossRef]

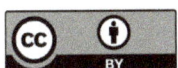

© 2020 by the authors. Licensee MDPI, Basel, Switzerland. This article is an open access article distributed under the terms and conditions of the Creative Commons Attribution (CC BY) license (http://creativecommons.org/licenses/by/4.0/).

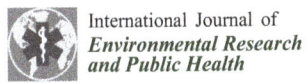

Article

Profiling Dating Apps Users: Sociodemographic and Personality Characteristics

Ángel Castro [1], Juan Ramón Barrada [1,*], Pedro J. Ramos-Villagrasa [2] and Elena Fernández-del-Río [2]

1. Facultad de Ciencias Sociales y Humanas. Universidad de Zaragoza. Calle Atarazanas, 4. 44003 Teruel, Spain; castroa@unizar.es
2. Facultad de Ciencias Sociales y del Trabajo. Universidad de Zaragoza. Calle Violante de Hungría, 23. 50009 Zaragoza, Spain; pjramos@unizar.es (P.J.R.-V.); elenario@unizar.es (E.F.-d.-R.)
* Correspondence: barrada@unizar.es; Tel.: +34-978618101

Received: 8 April 2020; Accepted: 21 May 2020; Published: 22 May 2020

Abstract: The development of new technologies, the expansion of the Internet, and the emergence of dating apps (e.g., Tinder, Grindr) in recent years have changed the way to meet and approach potential romantic and/or sexual partners. The recent phenomenon has led to some gaps in the literature on individual differences (sociodemographic variables and personality traits) between users (previous and current users) and non-users of dating apps. Thus, the aim of this study was to analyze the relationship between using dating apps, sociodemographics (gender, age, sexual orientation, and relationship status), and bright and dark personality traits. Participants were 1705 university students (70% women, 30% men), aged between 18 and 26 ($M = 20.60$, $SD = 2.09$), who completed several online questionnaires. Through multinomial logistic regression analyses, it was found that men, older youth, and members of sexual minorities were more likely to be current and previous dating apps users. Being single and higher scores in open-mindedness were associated with higher probability to be current dating apps user. The dark personality showed no predictive ability. The discussion highlights the usefulness of knowing and considering the sociodemographic background and the characteristics of personality patterns in the design and implementation of preventive and promotion programs of healthy romantic and sexual relationships to improve people's better health and well-being.

Keywords: dating apps; Tinder; Grindr; Big Five; Dark Core; university students

1. Introduction

The development of new technologies has changed people's lives, affecting both their intimacy and how they relate to others. Over the past two decades, the successive popularization of the Internet and smartphone use has changed the way potential couples approach each other for millions of people worldwide. More recently, the use of location-based real-time dating apps has been extended (e.g., Tinder, Grindr), designed to maximize social, romantic, and sexual connections between strangers who are geographically nearby [1–4].

The emergence and development of dating apps have attracted considerable research interest over the past five years. Usage patterns and user profiles have both been studied, as well as the advantages and disadvantages they may have for the mental and relational health of those who use them [5,6]. Among the advantages, their portability, availability, locatability, and multimediality [2] have been highlighted, aspects that facilitate the immediate interaction with possible partners. However, there have also been risks associated with the use of apps, which can affect both mental (e.g., problematic use, related to dark personality patterns) [7] and relational health (e.g., infidelity, performance of risky behaviors, sexual victimization) [5,8].

Previous literature has confirmed that the use of dating apps is associated with different sociodemographic and personality factors. Concerning sex, it has traditionally been considered that men used dating apps more [9]. Currently, it is considered that, although men use them more and more intensely, women use them more selectively and effectively, achieving a greater number of encounters with other users [3,4]. Regarding age, previous studies have mostly evaluated the use of dating apps in college youth aged 18 to 24 [3]. For instance, Shapiro et al. [10] found that 40% of undergraduate students, aged 18–26, used Tinder. However, various investigations suggest that the average age of users could be somewhat older, even up to 31 [1,2,9]. Thus, we expected to find a direct relationship between the age of college students and the use of dating apps.

Sexual orientation also influences the use of these applications. Several studies have found greater use in people of sexual minorities than among heterosexuals [11,12]. Further, it has been emphasized that being able to contact and communicate online can be particularly useful for people of these minorities who have trouble expressing their sexuality and/or finding a partner [13]. Finally, and although there is a stereotype that dating apps are used by singles, several studies have found that a remarkable percentage of users, between 18% and 25%, had a stable partner [4,14]. Nevertheless, it seems that these people use dating apps for different purposes than singles' reasons (e.g., infidelity) [15].

Personality traits play a key role in understanding sexuality and have been essential in the design of sexual health preventive and promotion programs [16]. In the psychosocial area, the personality model that has shown a stronger relationship to a variety of important life outcomes is the five-factor model or the Big Five [17], a taxonomy of five personality traits whose labels can differ according to the authors' denomination (Neuroticism or Negative Emotionality, Extraversion, Openness to Experience or Open-Mindedness, Agreeableness, and Conscientiousness). Thus, for example, the relationship between the Big Five and certain areas of sexuality such as the performance of risky behaviors, sexual functioning, or sexual assault has been studied [16]. However, there is hardly any research to analyze the phenomenon of dating apps in relation to the Big Five traits. The only reference is the study of Timmermans and De Caluwé [18], who found that young single dating apps users scored higher in Extraversion and Open-Mindedness than non-users and obtained lower scores in Conscientiousness.

In recent years, in parallel with the traditional Big Five paradigm, other proposals have emerged focused on the malevolent side of personality, which may be of special interest for the understanding of sexual phenomena [7]. Although some authors defend a multidimensional approach of these socially aversive personality traits (narcissism, Machiavellianism, psychopathy, and sadism), recent evidence about a single common factor, the so-called "Dark Core" [19], based on theoretical and methodological reasons, has gained momentum [19–23]. All of these traits share callousness [24] and the tendency to interpersonal exploitativeness [25]. Previous research found that this dark side of personality was associated with poor quality relationships [26]. Regarding mating behavior, it has been found that people with higher scores in dark personality traits had a less restrictive sociosexuality, more sexual partners, and a greater orientation to short-term mating and casual sexual relationships [27,28]. Concerning the use of dating apps and dark personality, the main conclusions of the few available studies can be summarized in [7,15]: (1) the role of the Dark Core as a single dimension has not been evaluated, but instead, the relationships with the different dark personality traits have been explored; (2) the associations are mediated by the reasons for using the applications, which leads to different relationships depending on the different nature of the personality traits; (3) despite having found partial associations with some patterns (i.e., Machiavellianism), the role of psychopathy has been highlighted, finding higher scores in this personality trait among dating app users than among non-users.

Perhaps due to the recent expansion of the dating apps phenomenon, the existing literature has some gaps. When analyzing the uses and users of dating apps, people who used them at some point and no longer use them have not been included in the same study, nor have they been compared to current users (at the time of study or for a previous short period) [4,8,9,15,18]. To detect possible differences between the two user profiles and to determine their correlates, it would be interesting if research consider both perspectives. In the case of the relationship between the use of dating apps and personality traits, some partial studies either analyze the relationship taking into account only the traits of the Big Five [18] or only the traits of the Dark Tetrad [7]. Only one study has simultaneously contemplated both sides of personality [15]. However, this study is aimed at determining the use of dating apps based on the relational status of the participants and the patterns of infidelity and not so much to explore the differences in individual tendencies between users and non-users.

To fill these gaps, the objective of this study was to analyze the relationship between the previous use and current use (the last three months) of dating apps and the personality traits (Big Five and Dark Core) in a sample of young college students. In this way, we aim to examine the relationships between the use of these applications and personality traits, as well as to know which of those traits can predict the use of dating apps. Further, the predictive role of different sociodemographic variables, such as gender, age, sexual orientation, and relational status, is explored. Knowing the individual tendencies of users of this type of apps can be useful for the design and implementation of preventive and promotion programs for mental health and healthy relationships, both romantic and sexual, in this group.

2. Materials and Methods

2.1. Participants and Procedure

The initial sample comprised 1996 participants. Four inclusion criteria were used: (1) studying a university degree at the time of data collection (76 participants excluded); (2) aged between 18 to 26 years, according to criteria from previous studies with university samples [29–31] (128 participants excluded); (3) labeling themselves as woman or man (13 participants excluded; the small sample size of this group prevented us from incorporating these participants to our analyses); and (4) correctly answering a control question (74 participants excluded; see below).

Considering all these criteria, the final sample included 1705 university students (70% women, 30% men), aged between 18 and 26 ($M = 20.60$, $SD = 2.09$). Of the participants, 70.1% described themselves as heterosexual, 22.5% as bisexual, 5.8% as homosexual, and 1.6% as other orientations. Due to the small sample sizes of non-heterosexual groups, those participants were combined into a sexual minority category (29.9%). Concerning relationship status, 52.9% of the participants had a partner, with an average relationship duration of 26.1 months ($SD = 22.6$), and 47.1% had no partner.

Regarding the procedure, data were collected in December 2019 using a Google Forms survey. To reach participants, a link to the survey was distributed through the e-mail distribution lists of the students of the authors' university. Participants provided informed consent after reading the description of the study, where the anonymity of the responses was clearly stated. The survey remained open for 14 days. This procedure was approved by the Ethics Review Board for Clinical Research of the region (PI18/058).

2.2. Measures

2.2.1. Sociodemographic and Dating App Use Questionnaire

We asked participants about their gender (woman, men, other), age, sexual orientation (heterosexual, homosexual, bisexual, other), and whether they were in a relationship (if they were, for how long). We also asked them whether they had ever used any dating app (Tinder, Grindr or similar) and whether they had used any in the past three months before the study. People who answered "No" to both questions were identified as "nonusers", those who only answered "Yes" to the second one were labeled as "current user", and the rest of the sample were identified as "previous users".

2.2.2. Short Form of the Big Five Inventory–2

This instrument [32] (the short form the original BFI-2) [33] has 30 items that assess the Big Five domains: Negative Emotionality (e.g., "[I am someone who...] is moody, has up and down mood swings"; $\alpha = 0.75$—all reported alpha values correspond to those observed in the current sample); Extraversion (e.g., "is outgoing, sociable"; α = 0.71); Open-Mindedness (e.g., "is curious about many different things"; α = 0.73); Agreeableness (e.g., "is compassionate, has a soft heart"; α = 0.68); and Conscientiousness (e.g., "is systematic, likes to keep things in order"; α = 0.75). These items are rated on a five-point scale, ranging from 1 = *disagree strongly* to 5 = *agree strongly*. The Spanish translation was provided by the first author of the original version of the BFI-2.

2.2.3. Dark Factor of Personality–16

This instrument [20] (a short form of the full 70-item version) has 16 items that assess the dark factor of personality with a single component (e.g., "People who mess with me always regret it"; α = 0.75). These items are rated on a five-point scale, ranging from 1 = *strongly disagree* to 5 = *strongly agree*. Following the original instructions, items were presented in random order for each participant [20]. The translation into Spanish was performed for the present research. In our case, three of the co-authors, all native Spanish speakers, translated the scale from English to Spanish, reviewed the translation together, and agreed on a single version of the scale. Finally, a native professional translator reviewed the correspondence between the English and Spanish versions, which agreed with the translated version. The Spanish version can be seen in Appendix A.

2.2.4. Control Question

Embedded in the questionnaire and to check whether the participants paid enough attention to the wording of the items, we introduced an item asking the participants to respond to it with *strongly disagree*. Those participants responding with an option different from the one requested could be considered distracted.

2.3. Data Analyses

Firstly, we computed descriptives and associations between the different variables. The correlations between dichotomous variables (gender, relationship status, and sexual orientation) with age and the six personality scores were transformed to Cohen's *d* [34]. The effect size measure for the associations between the dating apps use groups (never, previous, current) and age and the six personality scores was the *R* statistic from the ANOVA model of means comparison. The association between the dating apps use groups and dichotomous variables was quantified with Cramer's *V*. We chose the effect measure which we considered to allow a potentially easier interpretation of the results [35].

Secondly, we computed a multinomial logistic regression models, with the dating apps use groups as the criteria—nonusers as the reference group—and gender, relationship status, sexual orientation, age, and personality scores as the predictors. As the metric of the personality scores is not easy to interpret, we standardized them before the regression. By doing so, the odds ratio coefficients of personality variables indicate the change in the odds ratio for increments in units of one standard deviation.

The analyses were performed with R 4.0.0 (R Foundation for Statistical Computing, Vienna, Austria) [36]. No missing data were present in our database. The open database and code files for these analyses are available at the Open Science Framework repository (https://osf.io/wjuh6/).

3. Results

The associations among the different variables, with the descriptives, can be seen in Tables 1 and 2. We will focus our attention on the relationship between dating apps use and sociodemographic characteristics and personality scores.

Table 1. Bivariate relations of the different variables and descriptive statistics.

	1	2	3	4	5	6	7	8	9	10	11
				Pearson r							
1. Negative Emotionality											
2. Extraversion	−0.28										
3. Open-Mindedness	0.01	0.23									
4. Agreeableness	−0.18	0.17	0.17								
5. Conscientiousness	−0.20	0.24	0.02	0.19							
6. Dark Core	0.03	−0.06	−0.15	−0.59	−0.11						
7. Age	−0.05	0.00	0.03	0.02	0.02	−0.02					
				Cohen's d							
8. Men	−0.38	−0.17	−0.01	−0.42	−0.31	0.59	0.02	Pearson r			
9. Single	0.04	−0.08	0.03	−0.20	−0.10	0.13	−0.27	0.15			
10. Sexual minority	0.37	−0.15	0.38	−0.12	−0.24	−0.06	−0.11	−0.03	0.04		
				ANOVA R						Cramer's V	
11. Apps use group	0.07	0.00	0.10	0.08	0.10	0.08	0.24	0.12	0.24	0.25	
Mean	19.02	19.49	22.94	23.16	19.83	27.61	20.60	0.30	0.53	0.30	—
Standard Deviation	4.91	4.54	4.31	3.84	4.75	6.74	2.09	0.46	0.50	0.46	—

Age, measured in years. Men: dummy variable where *women* = 0 and *men* = 1. Single: dummy variable where *in a relationship* = 0 and *single* = 1. Sexual minority: dummy variable where *heterosexual* = 0 and *sexual minority* = 1. ——— = Mean and standard deviation for apps use groups are not reported as this variable was nominal with three levels. Bold values correspond to statistically significant associations ($p < 0.05$).

Table 2. Means and standard deviations (for numerical variables), proportions (for categorical variables), and significance testing according to dating app use.

	Nonusers	Previous Users	Current Users	F	p
	Mean (Standard Deviation)				
Negative Emotionality	18.81 (4.95)	19.52 (4.82)	19.61 (4.71)	4.07	0.017
Extraversion	19.49 (4.49)	19.47 (4.73)	19.48 (4.61)	0.00	0.998
Open-Mindedness	22.74 (4.29)	22.97 (4.52)	24.01 (4.00)	8.04	<0.001
Agreeableness	23.34 (3.80)	22.91 (3.83)	22.49 (3.95)	5.20	0.006
Conscientiousness	20.11 (4.77)	19.25 (4.72)	18.94 (4.56)	7.94	<0.001
Dark Core	27.39 (6.62)	27.59 (6.08)	28.93 (7.94)	4.84	0.008
Age	20.31 (1.98)	21.70 (2.16)	20.86 (2.11)	53.85	<0.001
	Proportion			χ^2	p
Women	0.75	0.15	0.10	23.25	<0.001
Men	0.65	0.17	0.18		
In a relationship	0.79	0.17	0.04	100.51	<0.001
Single	0.65	0.15	0.20		
Heterosexual	0.79	0.13	0.08	108.64	<0.001
Sexual minority	0.55	0.23	0.23		

Nonusers: participants reported having never used dating apps. Previous users: participants reported having used dating apps, but not in the last three months. Current users: Participants reported having used dating apps in the last three months. Age, measured in years. Proportions by row.

Of the participants, 71.5% ($n = 1219$) were nonusers, 15.8% ($n = 270$) were previous dating apps users, and 12.7% ($n = 216$) were current users. All sociodemographic variables were associated with the dating apps users groups. With respect to gender, for women, the distributions by group was $p_{nonuser} = 0.75$, $p_{previous} = 0.15$, and $p_{current} = 0.10$; for men, $p_{nonuser} = 0.65$, $p_{previous} = 0.17$, and $p_{current} = 0.18$; $\chi^2(2) = 23.25$, $p < 0.001$, $V = 0.12$. For those in a relationship, $p_{nonuser} = 0.79$, $p_{previous} = 0.17$, and $p_{current} = 0.04$; for single participants, $p_{nonuser} = 0.65$, $p_{previous} = 0.15$, and $p_{current} = 0.20$; $\chi^2(2) = 100.51$, $p < 0.001$, $V = 0.24$. For heterosexual participants, $p_{nonuser} = 0.79$, $p_{previous} = 0.13$, and $p_{current} = 0.08$; for sexual minority participants, $p_{nonuser} = 0.55$, $p_{previous} = 0.23$, and $p_{current} = 0.23$; $\chi^2(2) = 108.64$, $p < 0.001$, $V = 0.25$. Age was associated with the dating apps users groups, with previous users being the older ones ($M = 21.70$, $SD = 2.16$) and nonusers the youngers ($M = 20.31$, $SD = 1.98$), $F(2, 1702) = 53.85$, $p < 0.001$, $R = 0.24$.

Personality means differed by dating apps users group for all considered variables (all $ps \leq 0.017$), except for Extraversion, $F(2, 1702) = 0.00$, $p = 0.998$. All effect sizes could be considered as rather small ($M_R = 0.07$, range [.00, 0.10]). The higher associations were with respect to Open-Mindedness (higher mean for current users) and Conscientiousness (higher mean for nonusers). We note that Conscientiousness and Dark Core showed a high negative correlation ($r = -0.59$, $p < 0.001$).

Results of the multinomial logistic regression models are shown in Table 3. The explanatory capacity of the model was moderate (Nagelkerke's pseudo-$R^2 = 0.25$, McFadden's pseudo-$R^2 = 0.14$). The explanatory ability was basically provided by the sociodemographic information. Being a member of a sexual minority greatly increased the probability of dating apps use ($OR_{previous} = 3.08$, $p < 0.001$; $OR_{current} = 4.11$, $p < 0.001$). Men had a higher probability of use ($OR_{previous} = 1.44$, $p = 0.029$; $OR_{current} = 1.71$, $p = 0.002$). Increments in age were associated with increments in the probability of use ($OR_{previous} = 1.42$, $p < 0.001$; $OR_{current} = 1.27$, $p < 0.001$). Being single showed a very interesting result, as it had an an important impact on the probability of being a current user ($OR_{current} = 6.48$, $p < 0.001$), but not with being a previous user ($OR_{previous} = 1.22$, $p < 0.177$). To better understand the relevance of these variables, we computed the probability of belonging to each group for an 18-year-old heterosexual woman in a relationship and for a 26-year-old single non-heterosexual man (both with mean scores in all personality variables). For that woman, $p_{nonuser} = 0.95$, $p_{previous} = 0.04$, and $p_{current} = 0.01$; for that man, $p_{nonuser} = 0.12$, $p_{previous} = 0.45$, and $p_{current} = 0.44$. All of the personality scores showed statistically non-significant coefficients (ORs in the range [0.86, 1.19], $ps \geq 0.058$), except for Open-Mindedness with current use ($OR_{previous} = 1.22$, $p = 0.026$).

Table 3. Multinomial logistic regression analyses of use of dating apps.

	Apps Previous Users					Apps Current Users				
	b	SE	OR	95% CI	p	b	SE	OR	95% CI	p
Intercept	−9.44	0.76	0.00	[0.00, 0.00]	<0.001	−8.66	0.88	0.00	[0.00, 0.00]	<0.001
Negative Emotionality	0.15	0.08	1.16	[0.99, 1.36]	0.058	0.13	0.09	1.13	[0.95, 1.35]	0.159
Extraversion	0.15	0.08	1.16	[0.99, 1.35]	0.059	0.15	0.09	1.16	[0.98, 1.38]	0.087
Open-Mindedness	−0.07	0.08	0.93	[0.80, 1.08]	0.340	**0.20**	**0.09**	**1.22**	**[1.02, 1.45]**	**0.026**
Agreeableness	−0.05	0.09	0.95	[0.79, 1.13]	0.555	0.00	0.10	1.00	[0.82, 1.22]	0.989
Conscientiousness	−0.13	0.08	0.88	[0.76, 1.02]	0.085	−0.16	0.09	0.86	[0.72, 1.01]	0.067
Dark Core	−0.02	0.09	0.98	[0.82, 1.17]	0.816	0.17	0.10	1.19	[0.99, 1.44]	0.071
Age	**0.35**	**0.03**	**1.42**	**[1.33, 1.52]**	**<0.001**	**0.24**	**0.04**	**1.27**	**[1.17, 1.37]**	**<0.001**
Men	**0.36**	**0.17**	**1.44**	**[1.04, 1.99]**	**0.029**	**0.53**	**0.18**	**1.71**	**[1.21, 2.41]**	**0.002**
Single	0.20	0.15	1.22	[0.91, 1.62]	0.177	**1.87**	**0.21**	**6.48**	**[4.31, 9.73]**	**<0.001**
Sexual minority	**1.12**	**0.16**	**3.08**	**[2.27, 4.17]**	**<0.001**	**1.41**	**0.17**	**4.11**	**[2.95, 5.75]**	**<0.001**

SE = standard error; OR = odds ratio; CI = odds ratio confidence interval. All personality variables were standarized. Age, measured in years. Men: dummy variable where *women* = 0 and *men* = 1. Single: dummy variable where *in a relationship* = 0 and *single* = 1. Sexual minority: dummy variable where *heterosexual* = 0 and *sexual minority* = 1. Bold values correspond to statistically significant coefficients ($p < 0.05$). Nonusers was the reference group.

Given the relevant correlation between Agreeableness and Dark Core, which could lead to some problems of multicollinearity, we tested a model without dark personality scores. If multicollinearity was a concern, the pattern of results would be changed for this reduced model, but that was not the case. For the full model, the results for Agreeableness were as follows: $OR_{previous} = 0.95$, $p = 0.555$; $OR_{current} = 1.00$, $p = 0.989$; and for the reduced model: $OR_{previous} = 0.96$, $p = 0.589$; $OR_{current} = 0.90$, $p = 0.215$. We did not test a model without Agreeableness as we considered that, theoretically, it made no sense to exclude one of the dimensions of the Big Five.

4. Discussion

The emergence and popularization of dating apps in recent years have changed the way potential romantic and/or sexual partners meet and interact. Due to the recency and relevance of this phenomenon, it is necessary to deepen our knowledge about the profile of dating apps users. Although some studies have pointed out that the use of these applications varies depending on certain sociodemographic variables and personality traits, such studies are still few, and they present partial analyses, significant limitations in sampling, and their results are inconclusive. Therefore, the objective of this study was to analyze the relationship between the use of dating apps—previous and current—and the personality traits (bright and dark), also taking into account the role of sociodemographic variables such as gender, age, sexual orientation, and relational status, in a sample of young university students.

Of the participants, 71.5% were nonusers of dating apps, 15.8% were previous users, and 12.7% were current users (in the last three months). This is a prevalence of medium use, compared with that found in other studies [2,3,18], although it should be noted that, in these studies, sampling was aimed at finding people who used dating apps or it excluded those who had a partner, even with convenience samples. Therefore, although there are different reasons for the lower prevalence of dating app use in this study compared with those in previous works (e.g., participants' age, proportion of people with partners, cultural differences), we consider that our sampling allows us to better estimate the actual percentage of users of these applications.

From the data obtained, a sociodemographic profile of dating app users can be drawn among young Spanish university students. Individuals who are members of sexual minorities, men, and older youths are more likely to use dating apps. Although the results were expected in accordance with the previous literature, it can be stated that these characteristics are consistent for both groups of users (previous and current use) and both in the bivariate and the regression analyses performed.

The past and current likelihood of using dating apps in people from sexual minorities was more than three times greater than that of heterosexual people, in line with existing evidence. As has already been shown, dating apps are a resource widely used by people from sexual minorities, especially those who have more difficulty expressing their sexuality and/or finding a partner [11–13].

Our data support that men use dating apps more than women, as appears in most studies collected in the review of Anzani et al. [1]. As for age, the data revealed that the older the person is, the more likely they are to have used or to use dating apps currently. In the same vein, previous studies found a higher current use in older college students, noting that the phenomenon of dating apps is more prevalent among slightly older youths [1,2,9]. Concerning previous use, it seems logical to think that older youths, due simply to their lifetime, have been more likely to have used a dating app.

Concerning relational status, the results are especially interesting. Being single greatly increased the likelihood of being a current user of dating apps, but not of being a previous user. There exists a stereotype that considers that these apps are used only for casual sex [9] and that dating app users are not interested in long-term relationships. If that was the case, previous users should still be single to a larger extent. These results indicate that dating apps can be used to find long-term relationships or that looking for casual sex is not incompatible with seeking a romantic relationship [37].

We found that 4% of current users were in a relationship. This could be due to the fact that we considered as "current" those who had used in the last three months, so those participants could be single while using the apps, but not when responding to the questionnaires. Other options are people cheating on their partners [15] or in a consensually non-monogamous relationship. Other studies have found that about 20% of dating app users are in a committed relationship [4,38]. Further research is needed to clarify that important difference.

The relationships found between personality traits and the use of dating apps allow us to draw two relevant and surprising conclusions concerning the previous literature, which we will discuss below. First, although all dimensions—but Extraversion—showed statistically significant, although small, associations with dating app use group, those effects disappeared in the regression model. This lack of effect was found for the Big Five domains and for dark personality. The only exception was Open-Mindedness, which emerged as the only personality trait associated with the current use of dating apps, in line with previous studies [18].

Some explanations are plausible to justify why the Open-Mindedness effect was not the same for previous and current use. First, it could be simply interpreted as statistical noise. Second, we cannot discard that some features of Open-Mindedness (i.e., better tolerance of change) have a higher predictive capacity when the criteria refer to more recent behaviors (i.e., use of dating apps in the last three months). To clarify the predictive value of personality traits, future research should examine in greater depth the role of the Big Five in explaining different types of dating apps use (never users vs. experimental users vs. regular users).

The Dark Core of personality was not a significant predictor of previous and current use of dating apps, contrary to previous research [7,15]. This disparity may be due to the conception of dark personality and, consequently, the way of assessing it. Preceding studies addressed the dark personality from a multidimensional approach, using scales that assess four different dark personality traits (i.e., narcissism, Machiavellianism, psychopathy, and sadism). As we mentioned, we conceived the dark personality as a single latent factor called Dark Core, according to the most recent evidence about the theoretical and empirical overlap among the dark traits [19–23]. Further, previous studies [7,15] used the Short Dark Triad-3 (SD-3) [39]. This instrument includes an item that, while measuring psychopathy, clearly overlaps with high sociosexual orientation ("I enjoy having sex with people I hardly know"). Therefore, higher scores for apps users may be indicative of higher dark personality or higher sociosexuality.

We cannot rule out the influence of cultural differences in the relationship between personality and the use of dating apps. Young Spaniards may conceive of intimate relationships through this type of application differently from young people from other contexts where this phenomenon has been studied (Belgium [15]; United Kingdom, United States, and Canada [7]). In the absence of references in a young population similar to the Spanish one, we would need more studies, preferably cross-cultural, to test this hypothesis. Finally, dating app users may not actually differ from non-users in these antagonistic personality traits. If future research corroborated these results, we would have to banish the negative stereotype that is still associated with dating apps and their users [40].

The study has several limitations that need to be taken into account when interpreting the results. The use of dating apps has been evaluated without delving into the variety of uses, from those who used it on a single afternoon as a joke among friends to those who used it for months looking for a romantic relationship. Our estimation of current use is not a punctual prevalence, but with a timeframe of three months. The sample was mostly female, aged between 18 and 26, and coming from a single university. For this reason, it is difficult to generalize the results to the global population of university students and to young people of these ages who do not study at a university. Further, by grouping all the participating members of sexual minorities, we have lost information about the peculiarities of the use of dating apps and the personality patterns of these people depending on whether they are gay/lesbian, bisexual, or of other orientations. As for the instruments used to evaluate the Big Five and the Dark Core, lower levels of reliability were found than those of the original instrument validation studies [20,32]. For Agreeableness, Cronbach's alpha was only 0.68. Reductions in reliability may have led to reductions in the estimated effect sizes and loss of statistical power. For the BFI-2 Short Form, in the German version [41], an even smaller value of Cronbach's alpha was reported for this dimension ($\alpha = 0.65$), so, apparently, these potential problems in reliability cannot be attributed to undetected problems with our sample. Moreover, our study shares with previous studies based on self-selected samples and self-reported measures the limitation due to the response and recall bias. In this sense, it would be interesting to carry out longitudinal studies that would allow evaluating evolution in personality traits, and their influence on the use of dating apps.

Some readers may consider as a problem the inclusion of instruments that have not been validated in Spanish samples, as we did with the BFI-2 or the Dark Factor of Personality–16. We do not share this concern. We cannot take for granted that an instrument that has shown adequate psychometric properties for specific use with a specific sample will show the same results with other samples. For example, if a validation effort is done for the development or adaptation of a Big Five questionnaire with a sample of university students from the north of Spain in 2018, we cannot guarantee that this instrument will be valid for a sample of nurses from the south of Spain in 2020. We have changed occupation, location, and time and we do not know if any of those changes may be relevant.

The essential point is if there are any theoretical or empirical reasons to expect that the validity will be compromised with the intended sample. We consider that this is not the case for our Big Five measure with our sample. As Costa and McCrae have noted, "the [Big Five] factors are found in different age, sex, race, and language groups" [42]. From the same source, "they may be somewhat differently expressed in different cultures". There are strong reasons to not expect this in our case. First, other measures of the Big Five have shown adequate properties in Spanish samples [43,44]. Second, the previous version of the BFI has also shown that "the Spanish BFI may serve as an efficient, reliable, and factorially valid measure of the Big Five for research on Spanish-speaking individuals" [45]. Third, the BFI-2 has shown adequate psychometric properties in different adaptations: German [41] or Russian [46]. In the case of dark personality, other measures of this construct have been previously validated into Spanish without any problem [47]. In any case, all our data are fully available for further research about the psychometric properties of those instruments (https://osf.io/wjuh6/).

Despite the above limitations, the study is considered to make some relevant contributions. First, information on the prevalence of dating apps use among Spanish university students has been provided, and this is one of the first studies to evaluate this phenomenon in Spanish-speaking youth. Second, both previous and current use have been taken into account, a novel aspect with respect to previous research that only evaluated the most recent use. In addition, this has been done in an unbiased sample, in which no attempt was made to overrepresent dating app users, as was the case in previous studies [2,3,18]. Thirdly, a profile of the dating apps user has been developed based on individual differences, with special relevance of sociodemographic variables (gender, age, sexual orientation, and relationship status), as all of them allowed for predicting use. Fourth, the traditional personality traits of the Big Five and dark personality have been simultaneously evaluated. Fifth, it has been found that, among personality dimensions, only Open-Mindedness can help to explain current use, although the contribution is of low magnitude.

5. Conclusions

The findings of this study have allowed us to plot a profile of the dating apps user based on some sociodemographic and personality characteristics. Men, older individuals, without a stable relationship (for current use), and belonging to a sexual minority are more likely to have used and/or to use such applications to relate with others and establish romantic relationships. However, the Big Five personality traits are not associated with past or recent use of dating apps, except for recent use being related to higher Open-Mindedness. Having dark or socially aversive personality traits does not help to explain the use of dating apps. The profile of previous and current users is largely equivalent.

In any case, the results obtained have revealed that the predictive power of personality for past and recent use of dating apps is very small compared to other individual features. In this sense, perhaps it would be appropriate to explore in more detail the influence of cognitive, motivational, and affective elements, more linked to situational and sociocultural influences, and therefore more changeable and adaptable to the characteristics of the environment, rather than focusing on more stable elements (i.e., traits). Although the individual's behavior will depend on the continuous interrelationship of both elements, those who are more easily modifiable will be key aspects of mental and sexual health promotion programs in young people (e.g., negative emotions, low perception of risk of certain behaviors, etc.).

Dating apps, due to their huge use among adolescents and early adults, could be taken into account in the design of mental health protocols, including sexual and reproductive health strategies. For instance, as we found, people from sexual minorities are frequent users of dating apps. Meta-analytic evidence reported elevated risks for different mental health problems for sexual minority individuals [48]. Although dating apps can be useful to express their sexual identity and initiate a romantic relationship, these apps have also some characteristics (e.g., over-exposure) that could increase even more the risk for several mental health problems in vulnerable users (e.g., youth with low self-esteem). However, the popularity of dating apps could be used to promote sexual health among diverse and at-risk populations.

Author Contributions: Conceptualization, Á.C. and J.R.B.; methodology, J.R.B. and P.J.R.-V.; validation, J.R.B.; formal analysis, J.R.B. and P.J.R.-V.; investigation, Á.C. and E.F.-d.-R.; resources, Á.C., J.R.B., P.J.R.-V. and E.F.-d.-R.; data curation, J.R.B.; writing—original draft preparation, Á.C., P.J.R.-V. and E.F.-d.-R.; writing—review and editing, J.R.B., E.F.-d.-R., P.J.R.-V. and Á.C.; project administration, Á.C.; funding acquisition, Á.C. and J.R.B. All authors have read and agreed to the published version of the manuscript.

Funding: This research was funded by: (1) Ministry of Science, Innovation and Universities, Government of Spain (PGC2018-097086-A-I00); and (2) Government of Aragón (Group S31_20D). Department of Innovation, Research and University and FEDER 2014-2020, "Building Europe from Aragón".

Conflicts of Interest: The authors declare no conflict of interest. The funders had no role in the design of the study; in the collection, analyses, or interpretation of data; in the writing of the manuscript, or in the decision to publish the results.

Appendix A

Table A1. Spanish version of the Dark Core Scale [20].

Please read each statement and decide how much you agree or disagree with that statement. Note that there are no "correct" or "incorrect" answers to the statements. Please answer every statement, even if you are not completely sure of your response. If not specified otherwise, the items refer to your behavior (towards others) in general.	Por favor, lee cada oración y decide en qué grado estás de acuerdo o en desacuerdo con la misma. Recuerda que no hay respuestas correctas o incorrectas. Por favor, responde a cada afirmación, aunque no estés completamente seguro/a de tu respuesta. Las preguntas se refieren a tu comportamiento en general con los demás, a menos que se especifique lo contrario.
It is hard for me to see someone suffering.	Me resulta duro ver sufrir a alguien.
Payback needs to be quick and nasty.	La venganza debe ser rápida y cruel.
All in all, it is better to be humble and honest than important and dishonest.	En general, es mejor ser humilde y honesto que ser importante y deshonesto.
My own pleasure is all that matters.	Mi propio placer es lo único que importa.
I cannot imagine how being mean to others could ever be exciting.	NO puedo imaginar cómo ser desagradable con los demás puede ser excitante.
People who get mistreated have usually done something to bring it on themselves.	Las personas que son maltratadas generalmente han hecho algo para provocarlo.
Hurting people would make me very uncomfortable.	Hacer daño a alguien me haría sentir muy incómodo.
It's wise to keep track of information that you can use against people later.	Es inteligente guardar información que puedas utilizar más adelante contra otras personas.
I feel sorry if things I do upset people.	Me siento mal/triste si las cosas que hago molestan a la gente.
People who mess with me always regret it.	La gente que se mete conmigo siempre se arrepiente.
Why should I care about other people, when no one cares about me?	¿Por qué debería preocuparme por otras personas cuando nadie se preocupa por mí?
I would like to make some people suffer, even if it meant that I would go to hell with them.	Me gustaría hacer sufrir a algunas personas, aunque eso significara hundirme con ellas.
Most people deserve respect.	La mayoría de la gente merece respeto.
I make a point of trying not to hurt others in pursuit of my goals.	Procuro NO hacer daño a otras personas mientras persigo mis objetivos.
I would be willing to take a punch if it meant that someone I did not like would receive two punches.	Estaría dispuesto a recibir un puñetazo si eso significara que alguien que NO me gusta recibiera dos puñetazos.
I avoid humiliating others.	Evito humillar a otros.

1 = Totalmente en desacuerdo / 2 = En desacuerdo / 3 = Neutral/Ni de acuerdo ni en desacuerdo / 4 = De acuerdo / 5 = Totalmente de acuerdo.

References

1. Anzani, A.; Di Sarno, M.; Prunas, A. L'utilisation des applis de smartphones pour trouver des partenaires sexuels. *Sexologies* **2018**, *27*, 144–149. [CrossRef]
2. Ranzini, G.; Lutz, C. Love at first swipe? Explaining Tinder self-presentation and motives. *Mob. Media Commun.* **2016**, *5*, 80–101. [CrossRef]
3. Sumter, S.; VandenBosch, L. Dating gone mobile: Demographic and personality-based correlates of using smartphone-based dating applications among emerging adults. *New Media Soc.* **2018**, *21*, 655–673. [CrossRef]
4. Timmermans, E.; Courtois, C. From swiping to casual sex and/or committed relationships: Exploring the experiences of Tinder users. *Inf. Soc.* **2018**, *34*, 59–70. [CrossRef]
5. Albury, K.; Byron, P. Safe on My Phone? Same-Sex Attracted Young People's Negotiations of Intimacy, Visibility, and Risk on Digital Hook-Up Apps. *Soc. Media Soc.* **2016**, *2*, 205630511667288. [CrossRef]
6. Aretz, W.; Gansen-Ammann, D.-N.; Mierke, K.; Musiol, A. Date me if you can: Ein systematischer Überblick über den aktuellen Forschungsstand von Online-Dating. *Z. Sex.* **2017**, *30*, 7–34. [CrossRef]
7. Lyons, M.; Messenger, A.; Perry, R.; Brewer, G. The Dark Tetrad in Tinder: Hook-up app for high psychopathy individuals, and a diverse utilitarian tool for Machiavellians? *Curr. Psychol.* **2020**, 1–8. [CrossRef]
8. Alexopoulos, C.; Timmermans, E.; McNallie, J. Swiping more, committing less: Unraveling the links among dating app use, dating app success, and intention to commit infidelity. *Comput. Hum. Behav.* **2020**, *102*, 172–180. [CrossRef]
9. Lefebvre, L. Swiping me off my feet. *J. Soc. Pers. Relatsh.* **2017**, *35*, 1205–1229. [CrossRef]
10. Shapiro, G.; Tatar, O.; Sutton, A.; Fisher, W.; Naz, A.; Perez, S.; Rosberger, Z. Correlates of Tinder Use and Risky Sexual Behaviors in Young Adults. *Cyberpsychology Behav. Soc. Netw.* **2017**, *20*, 727–734. [CrossRef]
11. Badal, H.J.; Stryker, J.E.; DeLuca, N.; Purcell, D.W. Swipe Right: Dating Website and App Use Among Men Who Have Sex With Men. *AIDS Behav.* **2017**, *22*, 1265–1272. [CrossRef] [PubMed]
12. Ferris, L.; Duguay, S. Tinder's lesbian digital imaginary: Investigating (im)permeable boundaries of sexual identity on a popular dating app. *New Media Soc.* **2019**, *22*, 489–506. [CrossRef]
13. Korchmaros, J.D.; Ybarra, M.L.; Mitchell, K. Adolescent online romantic relationship initiation: Differences by sexual and gender identification. *J. Adolesc.* **2015**, *40*, 54–64. [CrossRef] [PubMed]
14. Orosz, G.; Tóth-Király, I.; Bőthe, B.; Melher, D. Too many swipes for today: The development of the Problematic Tinder Use Scale (PTUS). *J. Behav. Addict.* **2016**, *5*, 518–523. [CrossRef]
15. Timmermans, E.; De Caluwé, E.; Alexopoulos, C. Why are you cheating on tinder? Exploring users' motives and (dark) personality traits. *Comput. Hum. Behav.* **2018**, *89*, 129–139. [CrossRef]
16. Allen, M.S.; Walter, E.E. Linking big five personality traits to sexuality and sexual health: A meta-analytic review. *Psychol. Bull.* **2018**, *144*, 1081–1110. [CrossRef]
17. Ozer, D.; Benet-Martinez, V. Personality and the Prediction of Consequential Outcomes. *Annu. Rev. Psychol.* **2006**, *57*, 401–421. [CrossRef]
18. Timmermans, E.; de Caluwé, E. To Tinder or not to Tinder, that's the question: An individual differences perspective to Tinder use and motives. *Personal. Individ. Differ.* **2017**, *110*, 74–79. [CrossRef]
19. Bertl, B.; Pietschnig, J.; Tran, U.S.; Stieger, S.; Voracek, M. More or less than the sum of its parts? Mapping the Dark Triad of personality onto a single Dark Core. *Personal. Individ. Differ.* **2017**, *114*, 140–144. [CrossRef]
20. Moshagen, M.; Zettler, I.; Hilbig, B.E. Measuring the dark core of personality. *Psychol. Assess.* **2020**, *32*, 182–196. [CrossRef]
21. Muris, P.; Merckelbach, H.; Otgaar, H.; Meijer, E. The Malevolent Side of Human Nature. *Perspect. Psychol. Sci.* **2017**, *12*, 183–204. [CrossRef] [PubMed]
22. O'Boyle, E.H.; Forsyth, D.R.; Banks, G.C.; Story, P.A.; White, C. A Meta-Analytic Test of Redundancy and Relative Importance of the Dark Triad and Five-Factor Model of Personality. *J. Personal.* **2014**, *83*, 644–664. [CrossRef] [PubMed]
23. Volmer, J.; Koch, I.K.; Wolff, C. Illuminating the 'dark core': Mapping global versus specific sources of variance across multiple measures of the dark triad. *Personal. Individ. Differ.* **2019**, *145*, 97–102. [CrossRef]
24. Paulhus, D.L. Toward a Taxonomy of Dark Personalities. *Curr. Dir. Psychol. Sci.* **2014**, *23*, 421–426. [CrossRef]
25. Book, A.; Visser, B.; Blais, J.; Hosker-Field, A.; Methot-Jones, T.; Gauthier, N.Y.; Volk, A.; Holden, R.R.; D'Agata, M.T. Unpacking more "evil": What is at the core of the dark tetrad? *Personal. Individ. Differ.* **2016**, *90*, 269–272. [CrossRef]

26. Ali, F.; Chamorro-Premuzic, T. The dark side of love and life satisfaction: Associations with intimate relationships, psychopathy and Machiavellianism. *Personal. Individ. Differ.* **2010**, *48*, 228–233. [CrossRef]
27. Fernández-Del-Río, E.; Ramos-Villagrasa, P.J.; Castro, Á.; Barrada, J.R. Sociosexuality and Bright and Dark Personality: The Prediction of Behavior, Attitude, and Desire to Engage in Casual Sex. *Int. J. Environ. Res. Public Health* **2019**, *16*, 2731. [CrossRef]
28. Jonason, P.K.; Luevano, V.; Adams, H.M. How the Dark Triad traits predict relationship choices. *Personal. Individ. Differ.* **2012**, *53*, 180–184. [CrossRef]
29. Barthels, F.; Barrada, J.R.; Roncero, M. Orthorexia nervosa and healthy orthorexia as new eating styles. *PLoS ONE* **2019**, *14*, e0219609. [CrossRef]
30. Barrada, J.R.; Castro, Á.; Correa, A.B.; Ruiz-Gómez, P. The Tridimensional Structure of Sociosexuality: Spanish Validation of the Revised Sociosexual Orientation Inventory. *J. Sex Marital. Ther.* **2017**, *44*, 149–158. [CrossRef]
31. Barrada, J.R.; Ruiz-Gómez, P.; Correa, A.B.; Castro, Á. Not all Online Sexual Activities Are the Same. *Front. Psychol.* **2019**, *10*, 339. [CrossRef] [PubMed]
32. Soto, C.J.; John, O.P. Short and extra-short forms of the Big Five Inventory–2: The BFI-2-S and BFI-2-XS. *J. Res. Personal.* **2017**, *68*, 69–81. [CrossRef]
33. Soto, C.J.; John, O.P. The Next Big Five Inventory (BFI-2): Developing and Assessing a Hierarchical Model With 15 Facets to Enhance Bandwidth, Fidelity, and Predictive Power. *J. Personal. Soc. Psychol.* **2017**, *113*, 117–143. [CrossRef] [PubMed]
34. McGrath, R.E.; Meyer, G.J. When effect sizes disagree: The case of r and d. *Psychol. Methods* **2006**, *11*, 386–401. [CrossRef] [PubMed]
35. Wilkinson, L. Statistical methods in psychology journals: Guidelines and explanations. *Am. Psychol.* **1999**, *54*, 594–604. [CrossRef]
36. R Core Team. *R: A Language and Environment for Statistical Computing*; R Foundation for Statistical Computing: Vienna, Austria, 2020.
37. Jackson, J.J.; Kirkpatrick, L.A. The structure and measurement of human mating strategies: Toward a multidimensional model of sociosexuality. *Evol. Hum. Behav.* **2007**, *28*, 382–391. [CrossRef]
38. Orosz, G.; Benyó, M.; Berkes, B.; Nikoletti, E.; Gal, E.; Tóth-Király, I.; Bőthe, B. The personality, motivational, and need-based background of problematic Tinder use. *J. Behav. Addict.* **2018**, *7*, 301–316. [CrossRef]
39. Jones, D.N.; Paulhus, D.L. Introducing the Short Dark Triad (SD3). *Assessment* **2013**, *21*, 28–41. [CrossRef]
40. Choi, E.P.H.; Wong, J.Y.H.; Lo, H.H.M.; Wong, W.; Chio, J.H.M.; Fong, D.-T.; Lo, H.H. Association Between Using Smartphone Dating Applications and Alcohol and Recreational Drug Use in Conjunction With Sexual Activities in College Students. *Subst. Use Misuse* **2016**, *52*, 1–7. [CrossRef]
41. Rammstedt, B.; Danner, D.; Soto, C.J.; John, O.P. Validation of the Short and Extra-Short Forms of the Big Five Inventory-2 (BFI-2) and Their German Adaptations. *Eur. J. Psychol. Assess.* **2020**, *36*, 149–161. [CrossRef]
42. Costa, P.T.; McCrae, R.R. Four ways five factors are basic. *Personal. Individ. Differ.* **1992**, *13*, 653–665. [CrossRef]
43. Ortet, G.; Martínez, T.; Mezquita, L.; Morizot, J.; I Ibáñez, M. Big Five Personality Trait Short Questionnaire: Preliminary Validation with Spanish Adults. *Span. J. Psychol.* **2017**, *20*. [CrossRef] [PubMed]
44. Costa, P.T., Jr.; McCrae, R.R. *Inventario De Personalidad NEO Revisado (NEO PI-R). Inventario NEO Reducido De Cinco Factores (NEO-FFI). Manual 3a Edición [NEO PI-R Revised Neo Personality Inventory and NEO Five-Factor Inventory (NEO-FFI)]*; TEA: Madrid, Spain, 2008.
45. Benet-Martinez, V.; John, O.P. Los Cinco Grandes across cultures and ethnic groups: Multitrait-multimethod analyses of the Big Five in Spanish and English. *J. Personal. Soc. Psychol.* **1998**, *75*, 729–750. [CrossRef]
46. Shchebetenko, S.; Kalugin, A.Y.; Mishkevich, A.M.; Soto, C.J.; John, O.P. Measurement Invariance and Sex and Age Differences of the Big Five Inventory–2: Evidence From the Russian Version. *Assessment* **2019**, *27*, 472–486. [CrossRef] [PubMed]

47. Pineda, D.; Sandín, B.; Muris, P. Psychometrics properties of the Spanish version of two Dark Triad scales: The Dirty Dozen and the Short Dark Triad. *Curr. Psychol.* **2018**, 1–9. [CrossRef]
48. Plöderl, M.; Tremblay, P. Mental health of sexual minorities. A systematic review. *Int. Rev. Psychiatry* **2015**, 27, 367–385. [CrossRef]

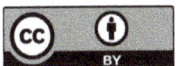

© 2020 by the authors. Licensee MDPI, Basel, Switzerland. This article is an open access article distributed under the terms and conditions of the Creative Commons Attribution (CC BY) license (http://creativecommons.org/licenses/by/4.0/).

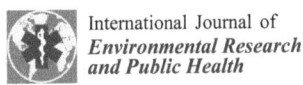

Article

Minding the Gatekeepers: Referral and Recruitment of Postpartum Mothers with Depression into a Randomized Controlled Trial of a Mobile Internet Parenting Intervention to Improve Mood and Optimize Infant Social Communication Outcomes

Kathleen M. Baggett [1,*], Betsy Davis [2], Lisa B. Sheeber [2], Robert T. Ammerman [3], Elizabeth A. Mosley [1], Katy Miller [1] and Edward G. Feil [2]

1. Mark Chaffin Center for Healthy Development, Georgia State University, Atlanta, GA 30303, USA; emosley@gsu.edu (E.A.M.); kspinks@gsu.edu (K.M.)
2. Oregon Research Institute, Eugene, OR 97403, USA; betsy@ori.org (B.D.); lsheeber@ori.org (L.B.S.); edf@ori.org (E.G.F.)
3. Cincinnati Children's Hospital Medical Center, University of Cincinnati College of Medicine, Cincinnati, OH 45229, USA; robert.ammerman@cchmc.org
* Correspondence: Kbaggett@gsu.edu; Tel.: +1-404-413-1571

Received: 16 November 2020; Accepted: 28 November 2020; Published: 2 December 2020

Abstract: Mothers in the United States (U.S.) who are of non-dominant culture and socioeconomically disadvantaged experience depression during postpartum at a rate 3 to 4 times higher than mothers in the general population, but these mothers are least likely to receive services for improving mood. Little research has focused on recruiting these mothers into clinical intervention trials. The purpose of this article is to report on a study that provided a unique context within which to view the differential success of three referral approaches (i.e., community agency staff referral, research staff referral, and maternal self-referral). It also enabled a preliminary examination of whether the different strategies yielded samples that differed with regard to risk factors for adverse maternal and child outcomes. The examination took place within a clinical trial of a mobile intervention for improving maternal mood and increasing parent practices that promote infant social communication development. The sample was recruited within the urban core of a large southern city in the U.S. and was comprised primarily of mothers of non-dominant culture, who were experiencing severe socioeconomic disadvantage. Results showed that mothers self-referred at more than 3.5 times the rate that they were referred by either community agency staff or research staff. Moreover, compared to women referred by research staff, women who self-referred and those who were referred by community gatekeepers were as likely to eventually consent to study participation and initiate the intervention. Results are discussed with regard to implications for optimizing referral into clinical intervention trials.

Keywords: maternal depression; referral; recruitment; mobile intervention; clinical trials

1. Introduction

Ramifications of depressive conditions are quite severe, with depression being a leading cause of disability for women and contributing significantly to the overall burden of disease globally [?]. During the first year after childbirth, women are more likely to develop depression and anxiety than at any other time in their life [?]. Perhaps some of the greatest costs of maternal depression are borne by the children. Perinatal mood and anxiety disorders compromise parenting and adversely affect children's physical and emotional development [? ? ?]. In particular, maternal depression can undermine sensitive and responsive caregiving, parenting behaviors that are key to supporting healthy child development [?]. Hence, it is crucial to provide interventions that both address maternal depression and strengthen skills involved in sensitive and responsive parenting as early as possible in a child's life to promote subsequent maternal and child health and development [?].

Unfortunately, delivering intervention to mothers and children most in need has proven difficult, and few depressed mothers receive treatment [?]. Mothers living in socioeconomic disadvantage and those who are of non-dominant culture are more likely to experience depression compared to higher resourced mothers of the dominant culture [?], but they are far less likely to receive treatment [?]. In the U.S., women of European origin use mental health services at more than twice the rate of Black or Latinx women [?]. This finding is consistent with the more general finding that racial and ethnic minorities are less likely to receive mental health services when compared to non-Latinx White persons after controlling for multiple demographic characteristics and disorder severity [?]. The American Academy of Pediatrics (AAP) and the American College of Obstetricians and Gynecologists (ACOG) [?] have called for women to receive depression screening and referral to intervention during the first year postpartum [?]. Evidence suggests, however, that the majority of women with depressive symptoms do not receive screening and appropriate treatment [?], even within systems reportedly conducting universal screening [?].

According to the Maternal, Infant, and Early Childhood Home Visiting Technical Assistance Coordinating Center [?], mothers who are least likely to enroll and engage in services are those experiencing depression and, because of structural and systemic biases [?], are of non-dominant culture and living within socioeconomic disadvantage. Moreover, in the U.S., redistribution of social safety net resources away from the very poor affect their ability to receive needed mental health and other family services [?]. Issues of diversity and access also come into play in research examining efficacy and effectiveness of interventions [?]. Systemic and structural barriers to recruitment into clinical trials of potential participants from non-dominant cultures exist, including distrust in research as well as costs and logistics that impede participation [?]. Moreover, even when members of non-dominant ethnic and racial groups are included in samples, frequent failure to report ethnic and racial characteristics restricts understanding about service delivery to these populations [?]. In a review of clinical trials for depression spanning a 36-year period [?], researchers reported that over time, participation by persons of low socioeconomic status (SES) and those of minority ethnic and racial backgrounds has increased. Nonetheless, persons of European backgrounds remained the most highly represented group. Moreover, within National Institutes of Health (NIH)-funded clinical trials where racial/ethnic representation in samples is expected and reported [?], researchers often do not examine racial/ethnic status as moderators of treatment effects, such that limited data are available that speak to effectiveness of intervention within these populations [?]. These limitations in the literature leave in question whether access to effective interventions is equitable across populations.

Recruitment of depressed participants, in general, into clinical trials is difficult, spurring conceptual work seeking to understand important gatekeeper-patient factors in recruitment [?] as well as intervention work seeking to modify recruitment behaviors within gatekeeper systems [?]. However, lower resourced individuals are not well-represented within these efforts. One study that directly assessed family general practitioner gatekeeper referrals found substantial disparities in referral and access to mental health services both within and outside of family general practitioner gatekeeper systems [?]. Individuals with greater resource levels were more likely to bypass the gatekeeper system to access directly mental health services, and if these individuals first went to the gatekeeper for referral, they were more likely and more quickly referred to mental health services compared to individuals with lower resource levels [?]. However, this study occurred outside of the U.S. in a country with a profoundly different health service context. In the U.S., large numbers of individuals from non-dominant cultures are under- or uninsured, contributing barriers to health-related service receipt [?] as well as inclusion in clinical trials [?].

Given the ubiquity of digital technologies, mobile health interventions can serve as a way to increase intervention access for those who are traditionally missed [?]. However, there are issues related to what we know about connecting individuals to these interventions. While online recruitment is frequently used in mobile health interventions, very little systematic research exists on this recruitment method [?]. One study comparing recruitment approaches found online paid advertising was more cost effective and timely than provider referral for recruitment to a mobile health early parenting obesity prevention intervention [?]. Another study compared non-paid and paid recruitment approaches to a mobile health smoking cessation intervention and found that online paid advertising and survey panel approaches were best for increasing racial/ethnic diversity in their sample to reach at minimum 25% [?]. Their resultant sample, however, was still primarily White. A recent study describing the recruitment of depressed individuals into a multi-site trial noted that Black participants self-referred into their study at 1.5 times the rate of the local population [?]. However, while self-referral appears an important mechanism for increasing access, the study pertained to a community-based group intervention rather than a mobile health intervention.

At present, existing recruitment studies are extremely limited with regard to implications for referral and recruitment into mobile health intervention trials among non-dominant culture mothers who are depressed and experiencing significant socioeconomic disadvantage. Efforts are needed to identify referral methods that best connect these mothers with intervention and to examine the extent to which various methods are successful at engaging mothers in intervention. We are currently conducting a clinical trial evaluating the efficacy of an integrated internet-based parenting and depression intervention. The intervention is designed to reduce maternal symptomatology and increase sensitive and responsive parenting in mothers of infants. This study, which takes place within the urban core of a large southern city within the U.S., provides a valuable in situ context within which to examine referral and recruitment efforts. Results have the potential to provide information with relevance to improving access to interventions for both depressed women and for women who are socioeconomically disadvantaged, of culturally non-dominant groups, and who continue to have severely unequal access to needed services.

This current study compared three referral approaches to examine their relative success at engaging potential participants in the study. Because researchers may succeed at or fail at engaging women who could benefit from an intervention at multiple points in the recruitment process, we compared the relative success of the referral approaches at several points between initial referral and engagement in the intervention, as described more specifically below. The current study used data from the ongoing clinical trial to examine a year-long period of referral to and recruitment into the intervention trial. The trial provides a unique context within which to compare the success of three referral approaches and examine, in a preliminary way, whether samples referred to the study by different approaches differ on variables associated with adverse maternal and infant outcomes as well as ability to access treatment. The questions we address are:

(1) Are the three referral approaches (i.e., community agency referral, research-team referral, and maternal self-referral) differentially successful as defined by: (a) number of mothers referred; (b) number who complete eligibility screening; (c) number of screenings resulting in eligible participants; (d) number of mothers who consent to participation; and ultimately, (e) number of mothers who initiate intervention?
(2) Do samples referred to the study by different approaches differ on variables associated with maternal or infant outcomes and ability to access treatment, including educational level, relationship status, maternal knowledge of infant development, and severity of maternal symptomatology. Notably, we could not examine income or racial/ethnic differences between groups because of homogeneity in the sample.

2. Materials and Methods

The design of the intervention trial, from which the data presented here were derived, called for recruitment of depressed mothers of infants under one year of age. We focused our recruitment efforts to generate a sample inclusive of mothers from non-dominant cultures who were experiencing socioeconomic disadvantage and elevated maternal depressive symptoms. Inclusion criteria were intended to produce a sample of mother–infant dyads, in which infants were at elevated risk for poor social communication development as a function of maternal depression and adverse mother–infant interactions that exacerbate the detrimental effects of poverty. Prior to initiating human subject activity, all study procedures were approved by the Georgia State University IRB. Potentially eligible women were contacted by research staff who described the project, conducted eligibility screening, and obtained informed consent.

Consented participants were randomized into one of two parallel intervention arms: (1) Mom and Baby Net (MBN) or (2) Depression and Developmental Awareness (DDAS). MBN is a 14-session, coach-facilitated, online intervention that teaches mothers both cognitive-behavioral strategies to reduce depressive symptoms and specific skills for engaging with their infants to promote infant social-communication competencies. DDAS is an informational program designed to improve maternal awareness of depression and understanding of infant developmental milestones. The MBN is a skill-based program designed to promote parental competencies to address affective symptoms and interact positively with their infants. DDAS, on the other hand, is an informational program that provides relevant content but does not shape new skills directly. The two mobile interventions were identical with regard to number of sessions, session length, and delivery mechanisms. For more information about the interventions, see Baggett el al. [?].

In this report, we compared three recruitment strategies for enrolling women into the intervention study. The enrollment period examined herein began one year after initiating outreach to build recruitment capacity and continued for an additional 12 months. Recruitment strategies included the following: (1) community agency referrals; (2) research staff outreach visits to community agencies and community events (i.e., research staff referrals); and (3) maternal self-referral. Outcomes compared across the referral conditions included the following: number referred, number screened, number of eligible screens, number of consented, and number that completed initial session to connect with intervention. We also examined a number of individual characteristics that present risk for maternal depression, adverse mother–infant interactions, and poor infant social communication development. These factors included education level, absence of social support, depression symptom severity, and knowledge about infant social communication development.

2.1. Sample

Participants referred were mothers of infants aged 0–12 months ($N = 203$). Mothers were included in the study sample if they had a score of 3 or more on the Patient Health Questionnaire-2 (PHQ-2) [?] at screening, were a minimum of 18 years old, spoke English, and lived in the local metropolitan area of a large southern city in the U.S. Exclusion criteria included history of psychotic symptoms, residence in homeless or domestic violence shelter, infant receiving intensive medical treatment, and not having permanent legal guardianship of infant. Demographic characteristics for the sample of 86 enrolled mothers are presented in Table ??.

Table 1. Demographic characteristics of the sample recruited into the study.

Variable	Value
Maternal age in years, mean (SD); range	28.12 (5.85); 19.00 to 44.00
Child age in months, mean (SD); range	5.16 (2.82); 2.00 to 12.00
Number of children in the home, mean (SD); range	2.67 (1.45); 1.00 to 6.00
Maternal race (Black) % (n)	95.35% (82)
Maternal ethnicity (Latinx), % (n)	3.49% (3)
Maternal Education (<college degree), % (n)	84.88% (73)
Maternal income, %(n) </=138% Federal Poverty Guideline	85.00% (68)

2.2. Referral

At the onset of study referral, we anticipated enrolling approximately 50 women per year based on referral agreements secured from agencies serving socioeconomically disadvantaged mothers and their infants. However, after one year of community outreach and recruitment capacity building, we had obtained only 5 referrals from community agencies. Moreover, we had received 10 maternal self-referrals, and 19 referrals of women our research team recruited at community events and occasional visits to community agencies to provide support to agency staff making referrals. At this point, we broadened our recruitment strategy to include online maternal self-referral. Referral strategies are described below.

Agency referral: Consistent with the original research plan, the research team encouraged ongoing referral from community agencies serving mothers and infants, such as WIC (Special Supplemental Nutrition Program for Women, Infants, and Children), the regional children's hospital, and medical clinics serving low income women. Partnerships with these agencies were established prior to study initiation for the purpose of participant recruitment. This approach had the potential benefit of reaching women at convenient access points, where they intersected with community agencies designed to promote the health and safety of their children as well as their own well-being. Agencies were provided with information about the project and agreed to screen women with the PHQ-2 and refer potential participants to the project via any of the following mechanisms, as per agency staff preference: (1) use of the project's online screening and referral system; (2) phone; or (3) secure email. However, many agency staff referred mothers without conducting depression screening; in these cases, the research team completed depression screening as part of the overall eligibility assessment and recruitment process.

Research staff outreach and referral: Research staff visited community agencies and attended community events, such as resource fairs, at which service agencies advertise their programs. Staff provided interested women with information about the intervention project, screened for inclusion criteria, and referred mothers to the project coordinator for enrollment.

Online maternal self-referral: The project maintained a self-referral mechanism through its website, which provided the following: (1) access to a brief video describing the intervention programs; (2) information about the project team; (3) depression screening; and (4) a form for providing contact information to research staff. To promote awareness of the online self-referral mechanism, the research team posted information on local community agency websites, social media platforms, and in print material available at local community agencies. We did not use any paid advertising mechanism.

2.3. Measures

To assess maternal progression from referral through successful recruitment into the study intervention, the following variables were documented by date of occurrence or disposition within the project database: referred, screened for eligibility, and eligible after screening. The PHQ-2 was administered online to screen for depression with the established criteria of a score of 3 or higher defined as a positive depression screen. The PHQ-2 is an efficient and well-established measure with strong psychometric characteristics for identifying individuals with depression [?]. At pre-intervention assessment, participants completed a demographic questionnaire to facilitate characterization of the sample with regard to mother's age, ethnicity, race, educational level, income, significant relationship status, and number of children in the home. We also obtained child age in months and child sex.

Additional participant intrapersonal risk characteristics were also assessed at pre-intervention. The Patient Health Question-9 (PHQ-9) was administered to assess depression severity. Endorsement of the PHQ-9 item, "Thoughts that you would be better off dead or of hurting yourself", was viewed as an indicator of self-harm thoughts [?]. The PHQ-9 possesses strong psychometric properties for assessing depression severity; a score at or above 20 is suggestive of severe depression [?]. Participants were also administered the Knowledge of Infant Social communication Development and Competency Promotion, which has demonstrated high internal consistency and sensitivity to intervention change [?].

2.4. Analysis

Using data collected between 21 September 2018 and 20 September 2019 on 203 referred mothers, we viewed the following five progression points into intervention: number of mothers referred from each of the three approaches, the number of mothers screened for eligibility, the number of mothers found to be eligible in screening, the number of mothers who consented to participate in the clinical trial, and the number of mothers who initiated the intervention. For number referred, we do not know the number of mothers within each approach, who could possibly have been referred in order to calculate a relative rate of referral within each approach. We will, therefore, report each approach's contribution of referred mothers to the overall recruited sample and calculate a multiplicative index to reflect any referral number differences between approaches (e.g., one approach contributed 2.7 times the number of referred mothers from other approaches across the same time period). The examination of other successive efficiency progression points is dependent upon the sample sizes resulting from each referral approach. Utilizing G*Power [?] with an overall n of 203, assuming equal numbers of mothers within each referral condition, with $p < 0.05$ two-tailed, we calculated that we would have less than 80% power (i.e., 71%) to detect moderately small effect sizes (d = 0.40), between the three conditions. If sample sizes diverge between the referral approach groups, parametric power would be reduced even further. Hence, to reduce the power burden, we took a conservative approach and limited analysis a priori to a two-group comparison, comparing maternal self-referral and agency referral groups. The a-priori group comparison was based on the fact that the two referral conditions selected are the most salient for referral into intervention research. The Chi Square test was used for the first research question and the Mann–Whitney tests were used for the second research question, given categorical versus ordinal variables, respectively. Working with an equal n two-group design (n = approximately 136), using wmwpow [?] at 80% power, small effect size (d = 0.40), $p < 0.05$ two-tail, and assuming a normal distribution for the two groups, we estimated power = 0.80, an acceptable criterion. If groups sizes differed, however, power was reduced and we focused on reporting effect size estimates, viewing d = 0.30 or higher as potentially meaningful for subsequent examination.

3. Results

With regard to the first research question on referral success, the number of self-referred mothers far surpassed that of mothers referred from traditional agency and research referral gatekeepers, with more than 3.5 times more referrals generated from the self-referral group as compared to referrals from community agency staff or research staff referral groups (see Figure ??).

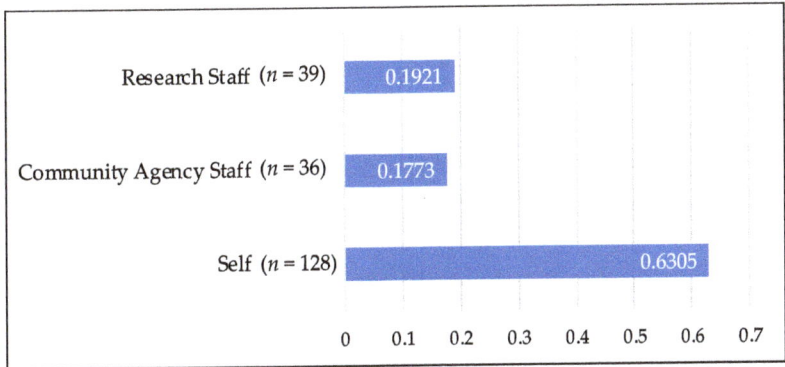

Figure 1. Percentage of each referral group contribution to the total referred sample.

The large difference in the number of cases generated through self-referral, as compared to agency and research staff, had significant impact on the number of cases to be examined at each successive point. Hence, we moved to our most conservative test to reduce burden on power, as described earlier. We conducted four Chi Square tests of between-group examinations and restricted comparisons to the self-referral and agency-referral groups. Table ?? presents the number of mothers within each referral group at each successive point.

Table 2. Number of mothers by referral group meeting each progression point.

Variable	Agency Referral	Research Staff Referral	Mother Self-Referral	Total Referrals
Number referred	36	39	128	203
Number/% screened for eligibility	30 (83.33%)	28 (71.79%)	106 (82.81%)	164 (80.79%)
Number/% eligible based on screening	20 (66.67%)	24 (85.71%)	92 (86.79%)	136 (82.93%)
Number/% who consented	12 (60%)	10 (41.67%)	64 (69.56%)	86 (63.23%)
Number/% who completed initial intervention session	12 (100%)	9 (90%)	62 (96.88%)	83 (96.51%)

Overall, agency-referred and self-referred mothers moved at similar percentage rates through four of the five successive points. The number of women who were eligible to participate based on the screening, however, was significantly higher for the self-referred group as compared to the agency-referred group. This difference reflected a small effect (Chi Square = 6.52, $p = 0.01$, d = 0.45). Figure ?? presents an overall view of the proportion of mothers moving through each point of the recruitment process by referral strategy.

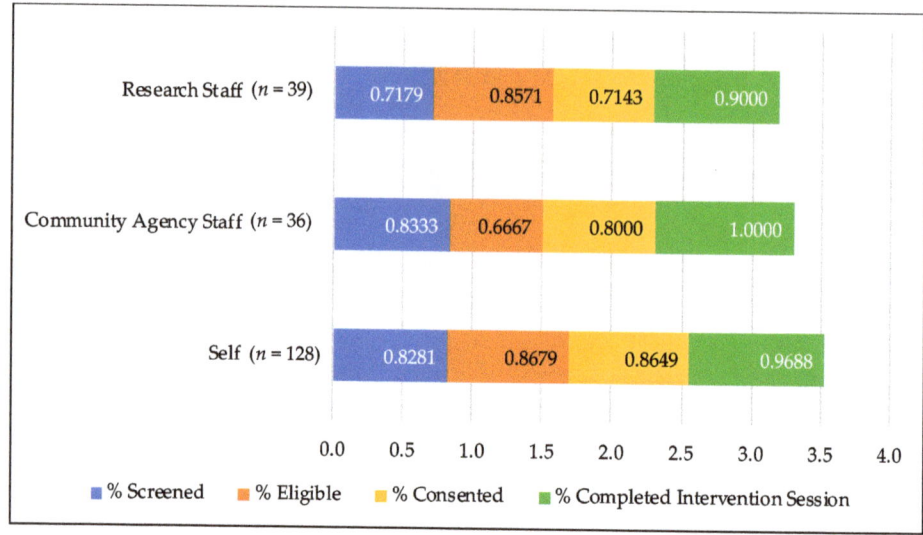

Figure 2. Success of referral to intervention engagement by referral strategy.

Our second question focused on intrapersonal risks experienced by referred mothers. As displayed in the demographics shown in Table **??** above, we achieved our intended sample of mothers, who were primarily of non-dominant culture (Black race) and socioeconomically disadvantaged who, as established in the literature review, experience extreme inequity in accessing depression-focused intervention. We, therefore, created a cumulative intrapersonal risk index to view the level of other risk variables over race and poverty among mothers in our recruited sample (See Table **??**). Each of the five risk variables was dichotomized based on the criterion specified in the table, with 1 representing presence of the characteristic. These variables were summed to produce a risk index range of 0–5.

Table 3. Intrapersonal risk characteristics by referral approach group.

Variable	Agency Referral	Research Staff Referral	Mother Self-Referral
* N/% Less than college degree	12 100%	10 100%	51 79.69%
N/% Severe symptom range	5 41.67%	2 20%	21 32.81%
* N/%Thoughts of self-harm	6 50%	0 0%	11 17.19%
No significant other	9 75%	7 70%	46 71.88%
N/% < 60% Parent knowledge of infant SE development and promotion	11 91.67%	10 100%	53 82.81%

* Significance level <0.05.

Figure ?? presents a plot of the risk index for mothers recruited using each referral strategy. Descriptively, mothers referred by research staff had the lowest and most restricted range of risk. The self-referred mothers had the largest range of risk. Agency-referred mothers demonstrated a slightly higher 75th percentile value (approximately 4.5/5 risks) than those of self-referred mothers (approximately 4/5 risks). For staff-referred, the 75th percentile risk level was approximately the same as the median risk value for agency-referred mothers. We followed the conservative approach to examination and conducted a Mann–Whitney between-group comparison of agency-referred and self-referred mothers. This examination resulted in a small effect size difference (U = 268; p = 0.08, d = 0.39), with agency-referred mothers reporting slightly higher levels of risk.

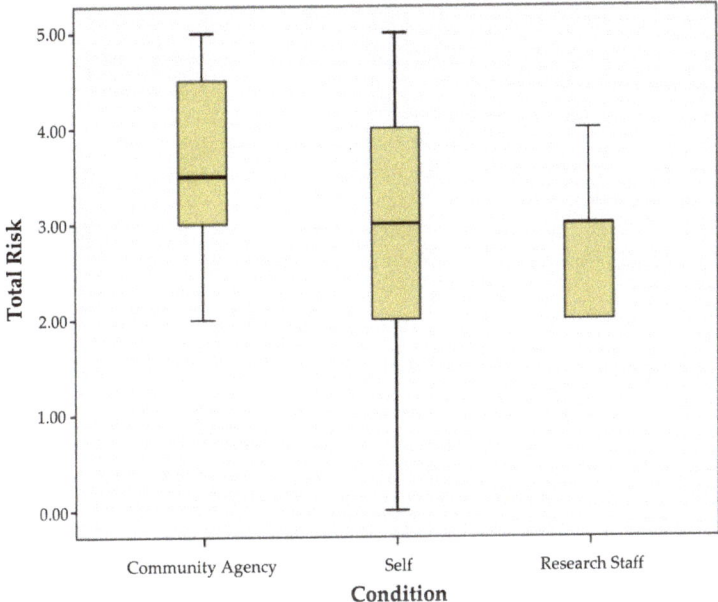

Figure 3. Boxplot of risk for agency, self-referral, and research staff approaches.

4. Discussion

4.1. Summary

The gatekeeper referral systems that relied on agency- and research-staff referrals were less successful compared to mother self-referral. They resulted in substantially fewer initial referrals and experienced losses of potential participants at rates equivalent to or sometimes greater than that of the self-referral system at each stage of the process up through initiation of the intervention. A substantial proportion of mothers across referral groups consented to participation and initiated the intervention. As planned, the final sample across referral groups reflected the population from which they were recruited: non-dominant culture, experiencing severe socioeconomic disadvantage, not having a significant other, and having limited knowledge of infant social-emotional development.

In our preliminary examination of risk factors experienced by mothers, mothers in the self-referred group had the greatest range of risk levels. Though this almost certainly reflects the relatively larger size of the group relative to those referred through other mechanisms, it nonetheless suggests that this approach has potential to result in a somewhat diverse group of participants with regard to these factors. It is important to note that mothers referred by agency staff evidenced a somewhat higher level of risk factors. Though the effect size was small, and the small sample size renders the finding preliminary, it is consistent with prior evidence that individuals with greater resources are more likely to bypass gatekeeper systems to access mental health services directly [?]. We think these findings suggest the potential importance of continuing to try to engage community agency gatekeepers in the referral process. It seems plausible that busy agency staff may be reserving their efforts for women whom they see as most vulnerable. It is also possible that though self-referral is excellent with regard to creating a smooth path to entry for most women (including those who are depressed, of non-dominant culture, and socioeconomically disadvantaged), it is not yet clear the threshold of vulnerability at which entry may require too much initiative for mothers.

4.2. Contributions

Although online recruitment is common in mobile health interventions, there is limited research on recruitment [?]. To our knowledge, this is a first systematic examination of referral processes as they relate to recruitment into intervention for depressed mothers. The existing research on online recruitment into parenting interventions for mothers of newborns has focused nearly exclusively on paid advertising such as through ads on parenting sites and via Facebook [?]. In contrast, our study provides an examination of online recruitment that did not require any paid advertising—a potentially important consideration for cost containment. Although published studies have been reported on the use of non-paid advertising for recruiting into mobile health interventions focused in areas such as smoking cessation [?], they have tended to yield less diverse samples, reflecting primarily dominant culture groups [?]. The present study is unique in that it focuses on a target sample of postpartum women with depression, who are lacking in existing study samples, namely women who identify as non-dominant culture and who are socioeconomically disadvantaged.

4.3. Limitations and Implications for Future Research

The current study has important limitations to note, which reflect that this was a secondary analysis of existing data to address an important research question that was distinct from those of the original parent study. First, relative to race, ethnicity, and income demographics of the sample, our clinical trial is being conducted within an area of concentrated poverty in the urban center of a large southern city, where the population is predominantly Black. Moreover, because we sought to refer and recruit within agencies serving low income individuals within one of the most income disparate cities in the U.S. with a long history of structural and systemic racism [?], the majority of our sample is severely socioeconomically disadvantaged. As such, we cannot adequately examine race and income sample differences by referral group. The current results may not be generalizable to other referral and recruitment efforts taking place within target populations that contain greater diversity in race and income. Of course, it seems unlikely that an approach that worked this successfully in a highly stressed and low resourced population would not be feasible in other samples.

A second limitation is the lack of clinical diagnostic measures. As the aims of the larger study did not necessitate diagnostic interviews, depression is defined here by a well-established questionnaire measure, which, though it has strong concordance with clinically derived diagnoses, is not equivalent and does not provide indices of cooccurring disorders. As such, we do not know how many of the participants met diagnostic criteria for current mood disorders or whether the presence of depressive or comorbid diagnoses influence the success of one or more of the referral processes. Nonetheless, the current results suggest that women experiencing depressive symptoms at levels likely to indicate disorder were enrolled successfully.

Another limitation is the relatively small sample. Clearly, future research on larger samples within more regionally, socioeconomically, and racially diverse target populations is needed to determine generalizability of the current findings and, in particular, to provide stronger data regarding the extent to which diverse recruitment strategies yield equivalent samples. However, based on the current results, we note evidence in support of the possibility that mothers who are Black and socioeconomically disadvantaged can and do self-seek services beyond typical gatekeeper systems to address depression. Studies are needed within community settings, outside of the clinical intervention trial structure, to determine if self-referral into intervention will result in greater racial and ethnic equity in accessing needed community services to reduce depression and strengthen parenting. It is also important to note that our examination of referral progression toward intervention access took place within the framework of a clinical intervention trial. As such, the outcomes may not generalize to processes of community agency and self-referral into community-based clinical intervention services, where there may be less support for moving mothers toward intervention access.

Expanding beyond the current study, other important future research directions to consider include the following: (1) examination of other factors that might influence referral such as insurance status, number of children in the home, or feelings about online interventions; (2) examination of cost effectiveness of various referral approaches; (3) documentation of how self-referring mothers access recruitment websites to self-refer (for example, whether by content searches, service searches, in response to friend suggestions in social communications, or responding to print or electronic links from trusted service providers), and (4) studies that extend beyond the relationship between referral approach and intervention access to include exploration of the relationship between referral approach and study retention, especially with regard to intervention dosage.

5. Conclusions

Results showed that mothers self-referred at more than 3.5 times the rate of referral by community agency staff and research staff. The resultant sample across referral groups reflected mothers of Black race experiencing severe socioeconomic disadvantage. Compared to traditional referral gatekeeper groups, self-referred mothers were equally successful with regard to recruitment into the study intervention.

Author Contributions: Conceptualization, K.M.B., B.D. and L.B.S.; methodology, K.M.B., B.D. and L.B.S.; software, K.M.; formal analysis, K.M.B., B.D., E.A.M. and K.M.; investigation, K.M.B., B.D. and E.G.F.; resources, K.M.B., B.D. and E.G.F.; writing—original draft preparation, K.M.B., B.D., L.B.S., R.T.A. and E.A.M.; writing—review and editing, K.M.B., B.D., L.B.S., R.T.A. and E.A.M.; supervision, K.M.B.; project administration, K.M.B. and B.D.; funding acquisition, K.M.B. All authors have read and agreed to the published version of the manuscript.

Funding: This research was funded by the National Institutes of Health, Eunice Kennedy Shriver National Institute of Child Health and Human Development, grant number R01 HD086894.

Conflicts of Interest: Landry developed the Play and Learning Strategies intervention program. Baggett, Davis, Feil, and Landry are the developers of the InfantNet program, the original intervention platform on which the ePALS Mom and Baby Net program application is based.

References

1. World Health Organization. Depression. World Health Organization: Geneva, Switzerland, January 2020. Available online: https://www.who.int/en/news-room/fact-sheets/detail/depression (accessed on 16 September 2020).
2. Miller, L.J.; LaRusso, E.M. Preventing Postpartum Depression. *Psychiatr. Clin. N. Am.* **2011**, *34*, 53–65. [CrossRef]
3. Mental Health America. Position Statement 49: Perinatal Mental Health. 2018. Available online: https://www.mhanational.org/issues/position-statement-49-perinatal-mental-health (accessed on 30 November 2020).
4. Goodman, S.H.; Simon, H.F.M.; Shamblaw, A.L.; Kim, C.Y. Parenting as a Mediator of Associations between Depression in Mothers and Children's Functioning: A Systematic Review and Meta-Analysis. *Clin. Child Fam. Psychol. Rev.* **2020**, *23*, 427–460. [CrossRef] [PubMed]
5. Rogers, A.; Obst, S.; Teague, S.J.; Rossen, L.; Spry, E.A.; Macdonald, J.A.; Sunderland, M.; Olsson, C.A.; Youssef, G.; Hutchinson, D. Association Between Maternal Perinatal Depression and Anxiety and Child and Adolescent Development: A Meta-analysis. *JAMA Psychiatry* **2020**, *174*, 1082–1092. [CrossRef]
6. Center on the Developing Child at Harvard University, Maternal Depression Can Undermine the Development of Young Children: Working Paper No. 8. 2009. Available online: https://developingchild.harvard.edu/resources/maternal-depression-can-undermine-the-development-of-young-children/ (accessed on 30 November 2020).

7. Goodman, S.H.; Garber, J. Evidence-Based Interventions for Depressed Mothers and Their Young Children. *Child Dev.* **2017**, *88*, 368–377. [CrossRef] [PubMed]
8. Baker, C.E.; Brooks-Gunn, J.; Gouskova, N. Reciprocal Relations between Maternal Depression and Child Behavior Problems in Families Served by Head Start. *Child Dev.* **2020**, *91*, 1563–1576. [CrossRef] [PubMed]
9. National Center for Health Statistics. *Health, United States, 2015: With Special Feature on Racial and Ethnic Health Disparities*; Centers for Disease Control and Prevention: Hyattsville, MD, USA, 2016. Available online: https://www.cdc.gov/nchs/data/hus/hus15.pdf (accessed on 30 November 2020).
10. Grote, N.K.; Zuckoff, A.; Swartz, H.; Bledsoe, S.E.; Geibel, S. Engaging Women Who Are Depressed and Economically Disadvantaged in Mental Health Treatment. *Soc. Work* **2007**, *52*, 295–308. [CrossRef] [PubMed]
11. *Substance Abuse and Mental Health Services Administration, Racial/Ethnic Differences in Mental Health Service Use among Adults*; Substance Abuse and Mental Health Services Administration: Rockville, MD, USA, 2015. Available online: http://www.samhsa.gov/data/ (accessed on 30 November 2020).
12. Ramos, G.; Chavira, D.A. Use of Technology to Provide Mental Health Care for Racial and Ethnic Minorities: Evidence, Promise, and Challenges. *Cogn. Behav. Pract.* **2019**. [CrossRef]
13. Rafferty, J.; Mattson, G.; Earls, M.F.; Yogman, M.W. Incorporating Recognition and Management of Perinatal Depression into Pediatric Practice. *Pediatrics* **2019**, *143*, 31. [CrossRef]
14. American Academy of Pediatrics; American College of Obstetricians and Gynecologists (Eds.) *Guidelines for Perinatal Care*, 8th ed.; American Academy of Pediatrics; The American College of Obstetricians and Gynecologists: Washington, DC, USA, 2017.
15. Allbaugh, L.J.; Marcus, S.M.; Ford, E.C.; Flynn, H.A. Development of a screening and recruitment registry to facilitate perinatal depression research in obstetrics settings in the USA. *Int. J. Gynecol. Obstet.* **2015**, *128*, 260–263. [CrossRef]
16. Byatt, N.; Simas, T.A.M.; Lundquist, R.S.; Johnson, J.V.; Ziedonis, D.M. Strategies for improving perinatal depression treatment in North American outpatient obstetric settings. *J. Psychosom. Obstet. Gynecol.* **2012**, *33*, 143–161. [CrossRef]
17. Maternal, Infant, and Early Childhood Home Visiting Technical Assistance Coordinating Center (MIECHV TACC). *MIECHV Issue Brief on Family Enrollment and Engagement*; Health Resources and Services Administration: Rockville, MD, USA, 2015. Available online: https://mchb.hrsa.gov/sites/default/files/mchb/MaternalChildHealthInitiatives/HomeVisiting/tafiles/enrollmentandengagement.pdf (accessed on 30 November 2020).
18. Bailey, Z.D.; Krieger, N.; Agénor, M.; Graves, J.; Linos, N.; Bassett, M.T. Structural racism and health inequities in the USA: Evidence and interventions. *Lancet* **2017**, *389*, 1453–1463. [CrossRef]
19. Moffitt, R.A. The Deserving Poor, the Family, and the U.S. Welfare System. *Demography* **2015**, *52*, 729–749. [CrossRef]
20. Oh, S.S.; Galanter, J.; Thakur, N.; Pino-Yanes, M.; Barcelo, N.E.; White, M.J.; de Bruin, D.M.; Greenblatt, R.M.; Bibbins-Domingo, K.; Wu, A.H.; et al. Diversity in Clinical and Biomedical Research: A Promise Yet to Be Fulfilled. *PLoS Med.* **2015**, *12*, e1001918. [CrossRef]
21. Durant, R.W.; Wenzel, J.A.; Scarinci, I.C.; Paterniti, D.A.; Fouad, M.N.; Hurd, T.C.; Martin, M.Y. Perspectives on barriers and facilitators to minority recruitment for clinical trials among cancer center leaders, investigators, research staff, and referring clinicians: Enhancing minority participation in clinical trials (EMPaCT): Perspectives on Minority Recruitment. *Cancer* **2014**, *120*, 1097–1105. [CrossRef]
22. Williams, M.; Tellawi, G.; Wetterneck, C.T.; Chapman, L.K. Recruitment of Ethnoracial Minorities for Mental Health Research. *Drugs* **2013**, *67*, 236–244.
23. Polo, A.J.; Makol, B.A.; Castro, A.S.; Colón-Quintana, N.; Wagstaff, A.E.; Guo, S. Diversity in randomized clinical trials of depression: A 36-year review. *Clin. Psychol. Rev.* **2019**, *67*, 22–35. [CrossRef]
24. Kanakamedala, P.; Haga, S.B. Characterization of Clinical Study Populations by Race and Ethnicity in the Biomedical Literature. *Ethn. Dis.* **2013**, *22*, 96.
25. Geller, S.E.; Koch, A.; Pellettieri, B.; Carnes, M. Inclusion, Analysis, and Reporting of Sex and Race/Ethnicity in Clinical Trials: Have We Made Progress? *J. Womens Health* **2011**, *20*, 315–320. [CrossRef]
26. Hughes-Morley, A.; Young, B.; Waheed, W.; Small, N.; Bower, P. Factors affecting recruitment into depression trials: Systematic review, meta-synthesis and conceptual framework. *J. Affect. Disord.* **2015**, *172*, 274–290. [CrossRef]

27. Amorrortu, R.P.; Arevalo, M.; Vernon, S.W.; Mainous, A.G.; Diaz, V.; McKee, M.D.; Ford, M.E.; Tilley, B.C. Recruitment of racial and ethnic minorities to clinical trials conducted within specialty clinics: An intervention mapping approach. *Trials* **2018**, *19*, 115. [CrossRef]
28. Steele, L.; Glazier, R.; Agha, M.; Moineddin, R. The Gatekeeper System and Disparities in Use of Psychiatric Care by Neighbourhood Education Level: Results of a Nine-Year Cohort Study in Toronto. *Healthc. Policy Polit. Santé* **2009**, *4*, e133–e150. [CrossRef]
29. Lillie-Blanton, M.; Hoffman, C. The Role of Health Insurance Coverage in Reducing Racial/Ethnic Disparities in Health Care. *Health Aff. (Millwood)* **2005**, *24*, 398–408. [CrossRef]
30. Cho, H.L.; Danis, M.; Grady, C. The ethics of uninsured participants accessing healthcare in biomedical research: A literature review. *Clin. Trials* **2018**, *15*, 509–521. [CrossRef]
31. Anderson-Lewis, C.; Darville, G.; Mercado, R.E.; Howell, S.; Di Maggio, S. Mobile health Technology Use and Implications in Historically Underserved and Minority Populations in the United States: Systematic Literature Review. *JMIR Mob. Health UHealth* **2018**, *6*, e128. [CrossRef]
32. Lane, T.S.; Armin, J.; Gordon, J.S. Online Recruitment Methods for Web-Based and Mobile Health Studies: A Review of the Literature. *J. Med. Internet Res.* **2015**, *17*, e183. [CrossRef]
33. Laws, R.A.; Litterbach, E.K.V.; Denney-Wilson, E.A.; Russell, C.G.; Taki, S.; Ong, K.L.; Campbell, K.J. A Comparison of Recruitment Methods for an mobile health Intervention Targeting Mothers: Lessons from the Growing Healthy Program. *J. Med. Internet Res.* **2016**, *18*, e248. [CrossRef]
34. Watson, N.L.; Mull, K.E.; Heffner, J.L.; McClure, J.B.; Bricker, J.B. Participant Recruitment and Retention in Remote eHealth Intervention Trials: Methods and Lessons Learned From a Large Randomized Controlled Trial of Two Web-Based Smoking Interventions. *J. Med. Internet Res.* **2018**, *20*, e10351. [CrossRef]
35. Brown, J.S.L.; Murphy, C.; Kelly, J.; Goldsmith, K. How can we successfully recruit depressed people? Lessons learned in recruiting depressed participants to a multi-site trial of a brief depression intervention (the 'CLASSIC' trial). *Trials* **2019**, *20*, 131. [CrossRef]
36. Baggett, K.M.; DiPetrillo, B.; Beacham, C.; Patterson, A.; Miller, K.; Davis, B.; Feil, E.; Sheeber, L. Built Pathways to Resilience: Engaging Mothers with Depression in a Mobile Intervention to Improve Infant Social-Emotional Outcomes. In Proceedings of the Conference on Research Innovations in Early Intervention, San Diego, CA, USA, 27–29 February 2020.
37. Kroenke, K.; Spitzer, R.L.; Williams, J.B.W. The Patient Health Questionnaire-2: Validity of a Two-Item Depression Screener. *Med. Care* **2003**, *41*, 1284–1292. [CrossRef]
38. Wisner, K.L.; Sit, D.K.; McShea, M.C.; Rizzo, D.M.; Zoretich, R.A.; Hughes, C.L.; Eng, H.F.; Luther, J.F.; Wisniewski, S.R.; Costantino, M.L.; et al. Onset Timing, Thoughts of Self-harm, and Diagnoses in Postpartum Women With Screen Positive Depression Findings. *JAMA Psychiatry* **2013**, *70*, 490. [CrossRef]
39. Kroenke, K.; Spitzer, R.L.; Williams, J.B.W. The PHQ-9: Validity of a brief depression severity measure. *J. Gen. Intern. Med.* **2001**, *16*, 606–613. [CrossRef]
40. Feil, E.G.; Baggett, K.; Davis, B.; Landry, S.; Sheeber, L.; Leve, C.; Johnson, U. Randomized control trial of an internet-based parenting intervention for mothers of infants. *Early Child. Res. Q.* **2020**, *50*, 36–44. [CrossRef]
41. Franz, F.; Erdfelder, E.; Lang, A.-G.L.; Buchner, A. G*Power 3: A flexible statistical power analysis program for the social, behavioral and biomedical sciences. *Behav. Res. Methods* **2007**, *39*, 175–191.
42. Mollan, K.R.; Trumble, I.M.; Reifeis, S.A.; Ferrer, O.; Bay, C.P.; Baldoni, P.L.; Hudgens, M.G. Exact Power of the Rank-Sum Test for a Continuous Variable. *arXiv* **2019**, arXiv:1901.04597.
43. Sommeiller, E.; Price, M.; Wazeter, E. *Income Inequality in the U.S. by State, Metropolitan Area, and County*; Economic Policy Institute: Washington, DC, USA, 2016; Available online: https://files.epi.org/pdf/107100.pdf (accessed on 30 November 2020).

Publisher's Note: MDPI stays neutral with regard to jurisdictional claims in published maps and institutional affiliations.

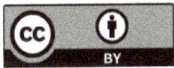

© 2020 by the authors. Licensee MDPI, Basel, Switzerland. This article is an open access article distributed under the terms and conditions of the Creative Commons Attribution (CC BY) license (http://creativecommons.org/licenses/by/4.0/).

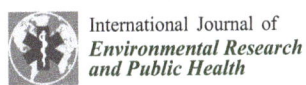

Article

The Use of New Digital Information and Communication Technologies in Psychological Counseling during the COVID-19 Pandemic

Artemisa R. Dores [1,2,*], Andreia Geraldo [2], Irene P. Carvalho [3] and Fernando Barbosa [2]

1. Center for Rehabilitation Research, School of Health, Polytechnic Institute of Porto, 4200-072 Porto, Portugal
2. Laboratory of Neuropsychophysiology, Faculty of Psychology and Education Sciences of University of Porto, 4200-135 Porto, Portugal; g.andreia9@gmail.com (A.G.); fbarbosa@fpce.up.pt (F.B.)
3. CINTESIS and Department of Clinical Neurosciences and Mental Health, School of Medicine, University of Porto (FMUP), 4200-319 Porto, Portugal; irenec@med.up.pt
* Correspondence: artemisa@ess.ipp.pt

Received: 8 September 2020; Accepted: 13 October 2020; Published: 21 October 2020

Abstract: The use of digital information and communication technologies (ICTs) has enabled many professionals to continue to provide their services during the COVID-19 pandemic. However, little is known about the adoption of ICTs by psychologists and the impact of such technologies on their practice. This study aimed to explore psychologists' practices related with the use of ICTs before and during the COVID-19 lockdown, to identify the main changes that the pandemic has brought and the impact that such changes have had on their practice with clients, and also identify the factors that potentially have affected such changes. The Portuguese Psychologists Association announced the study, and 108 psychologists responded to an online survey during the mandatory lockdown. The results showed that these professionals continued to provide their services due to having adopted ICTs. Comparing with face-to-face interventions, psychologists recognized that additional precautions/knowledge were needed to use such technologies. Despite the challenges identified, they described the experience with the use of ICTs as positive, meeting clients' adherence, and yielding positive results. Psychologists with the most years of professional experience maintained their services the most, but those with average experience showed the most favorable attitudes toward the use of technologies and web-based interventions.

Keywords: digital information and communication technologies; psychological counseling; therapy; COVID-19; coronavirus SARS-CoV-2; digital literacy

1. Introduction

The coronavirus disease (COVID-19) pandemic represents an unprecedented global challenge in our era, strongly affecting people's lives, namely, the exercise of various professional activities [1,2]. This unique circumstance, associated with the current availability of several digital tools, has contributed exponentially to the digital revolution that we have witnessed in recent years, with impact on the social, economic, and professional domains of life [3].

In this scenario, e-Health has emerged as one viable solution to allow the continuity of the provision of health services, particularly considering the public health measures that have been taken as a result of the National Emergency State, which has limited people's access to in-person services [4]. E-Health is broadly defined as the provision of services related to health supported by a safe and cost-effective use of information and communications technologies (ICTs) [5].

The path toward the progressive adoption of ICTs in the field of psychology had already begun before the COVID-19 pandemic, albeit in varied degrees across different countries. If documentation guiding and/or regulating professional practice is already available in some countries, a legal or normative void still exists in others. This has implications regarding the availability of the psychological services offered, which are still quite scarce in some countries, as is the case in Portugal. For example, before the COVID-19 pandemic, few Portuguese psychologists adopted guided and unguided psychological internet interventions (1.3% and 1.5%, respectively) [6], despite the already recognized advantages of this type of intervention [7–11].

Many of the guidelines for the online practice of psychology are the result of the work of several national and international associations and bodies (e.g., the American Psychological Association and European Federation of Psychologists' Associations), in an effort to set forth a consensus about the practices that they aim to guide. In Portugal, after a first approval of at-distance interventions by the Ordem dos Psicólogos Portugueses (OPP; transl.: Portuguese Psychologists Association) in 2015, the OPP issued a document with the guidelines for these types of services very recently, precisely at the peak of the COVID-19 pandemic [12,13].

In its first issue, this association claimed that psychological intervention should always be conducted within the same obligations and responsibilities (i.e., ethical principles and deontological and legal norms), regardless of the format of the intervention, as defined in the Code of Ethics. Although the OPP recognized the potential benefits of web-based interventions and use of ITCs, it also launched warnings about the need for a better understanding of the effects of the different modalities of remote intervention (e.g., written, audio or audiovisual support) compared to face-to-face intervention. The OPP additionally warned of the fact that the specificities of cyber space could elude the means of control available to psychologists, which could put privacy and confidentiality at risk [12]. In its second document, entitled "OPP guidelines for professional practice: Provision of psychology services mediated by ICTs" [13], a set of recommendations for the adoption of these technological and digital resources were presented.

In addition to the OPP, other projects have been carried out in Portugal (and elsewhere) with the aim to issue good practices to be adopted for the use of these digital and technological means in the area of health in general, and of psychology in particular. As an example, the European project THERAPY 2.0—Counseling and Therapeutic Interactions with Digital Natives, financed by the ERASMUS + program, sought to issue the appropriate integration of ICTs in counseling and therapy, especially for younger populations and refugees [14,15].

In several countries, an increasing number of studies have also sought to characterize the attitudes of psychologists toward the inclusion of ICTs in their professional practice and to gather evidence about the efficacy and effectiveness of psychological interventions mediated by ICTs (e.g., [7,16–21]). Regarding the psychologists' attitudes, the results of the studies are not consistent (e.g., [6,22]). In Portugal, a recent study assessing psychologists' attitudes revealed a slightly negative/neutral position regarding internet interventions and greater acceptability of blended treatment interventions when compared to standalone internet interventions. However, these attitudes seem to depend on different factors, such as knowledge and training [6]. A study in other countries revealed that, among those who have employed any online means of practicing counseling and therapy, 52.97% had a positive or very positive opinion about the use of these tools. In this study, e-mail was the most widely used online tool, and the computer and smart phone were the most frequently used equipment [14]. Different circumstances and factors seem to contribute to explain the different attitudes and the adoption (or not) of this type of resources [23]. Such factors include the therapist's theoretical model/orientation, geographic area, previous experience with the use of these resources, presence or absence of previous training, perception about the usefulness of these tools, ease with their use, and years of clinical practice [24–31].

Regarding the effectiveness of these online means, in general, studies allow us to conclude that internet interventions may be efficacious and cost-effective [6,16,17,19,20,32–35]. They seemed to be at least as effective as face-to-face interventions in a large group of clients receiving treatment for psychological disorders, namely, for generalized anxiety and other types of anxiety disorders [36–42], depression [43–52], and stress [53,54].

The recognized advantages of using ICTs do not refer merely to their power to compensate for the limitations of traditional interventions (e.g., travelling requirements for customers or therapists), nor to their use as complementary means. There are several advantages associated with implementing internet interventions [8–11,13,14,55]. These include easy accessibility, high adaptability, flexibility and convenience, evolution at the client's pace, easy adherence and treatment monitoring, privacy and possibility of anonymity, cultural adaptability, low cost, and high potential for dissemination [55]. Conversely, the main challenges identified in the use of ICTs include ethical concerns (e.g., security, privacy, confidentiality, and an absence or lack of deontological orientation), clients' ICT illiteracy, and negative attitudes toward internet interventions [6]. Others can be added, such as a lack of access to technological and digital tools by some users, technological problems in their use, and changes to the setting and regarding the therapeutic relationship [8,10,14,26,55–58].

Because different circumstances and factors seem to contribute to explain psychologists' attitudes and the adoption (or not) of this type of resources, it is important to identify potential changes in the use of ICTs during the COVID-19 pandemic. Given the measures of physical distance and isolation that most governments imposed with the state of emergency (e.g., [4]), how have psychologists dealt with the provision of counseling and therapy to their clients? The aims of this work were to (a) analyze how the attitudes of professionals in the field of psychology have changed in relation to the use of ICTs in the context of psychological monitoring during the lockdown; (b) assess whether the practice of psychological counseling and therapy includes greater use of ICTs during the lockdown period; (c) identify the factors that potentially have affected such changes; and (d) study the possible adoption of guidelines for at-distance psychological monitoring by psychologists who are using ICTs during the period of physical distance

2. Materials and Methods

2.1. Participants

The sample in this study comprised 108 psychologists who were registered in the OPP. Most were women (89, or 82.4%). The mean age was 37.20 years old ($SD = 10.05$; $Min = 23$, $Max = 65$), with 55 (50.9%) in the age group between 23 and 35 years, and 53 (49.1%) in the group between 36 and 65 years. The number of years of professional experience ranged between one or less and 33 ($M = 11.52$; $SD = 8.60$). The sample reflects national representation (including continental Portugal and islands), with 19 of the 20 Portuguese districts participating in the study. The most represented districts were Porto ($n = 39$; 36.8%), Lisbon ($n = 21$; 18.9%), Braga ($n = 13$; 12.3%), and Coimbra ($n = 9$; 8.5%). These cities comprehend the national OPP delegations with the most psychologists [59]. Most participants held master's degrees ($n = 69$; 63.9%). Most were specialists in clinical psychology ($n = 60$; 55.6%), and 23 (21.3%) had one or more advanced specialties, including in psychotherapy ($n = 13$; 12.0%), among others.

Participants worked mainly with adults ($n = 81$; 75.0%), followed by adolescents ($n = 52$; 48.1%), children ($n = 46$; 42.6%), and the elderly ($n = 24$; 22.2%), in the areas of anxiety disorders ($n = 91$; 84.3%), mood disorders ($n = 72$; 66.7%), personality disorders ($n = 37$; 34.3%), neurocognitive disorders ($n = 30$; 27.8%), among others. For more information, see Table 1.

Table 1. Socio-demographic characteristics of the participants.

	n/% M/SD
Gender	M: $n = 19$, 17.6% F: $n = 89$, 82.4%
Age	$M = 37.2$; $SD = 10.0$
Education	Graduation: $n = 26$, 24.1% Master: $n = 69$, 63.9% PhD: $n = 13$, 12.0%
Professional Experience	$M = 11.5$; $SD = 8.6$
Clinical and Health Specialty	Y: $n = 60$, 55.6% N: $n = 48$, 44.4%
Advanced Specialties	Neuropsychology: $n = 6$, 5.6% Psychogerontology: $n = 0$ Justice Psychology: $n = 2$, 1.9% Sports Psychology: $n = 0$ Psychotherapy: $n = 13$, 12.0% Sexology: $n = 1$, 0.9% Others: $n = 9$, 8.3%
Population	Children: $n = 46$, 42.6% Adolescents: $n = 52$, 48.1% Adults: $n = 81$, 75.0% Elderly: $n = 24$, 22.2%
Psychological Disorders	Neurodevelopment disorders: $n = 24$, 22.2% Mood disorders: $n = 72$, 66.7% Anxiety disorders: $n = 91$, 84.3% Personality disorders: $n = 37$, 34.3% Substance-related disorders and addictive behaviors: $n = 21$, 19.4% Sleep disorders: $n = 23$, 21.3% Neurocognitive disorders: $n = 30$, 27.8% Others: $n = 10$, 9.3%

2.2. Instruments

A questionnaire was developed for this study and a pilot test was conducted to check its comprehension level and adequacy for the current purposes. The questionnaire included 30 questions divided into three sections: (i) socio-demographic data, with 9 questions; (ii) experience before the COVID-19 pandemic, with 7 questions; and (iii) current experience using ICTs in psychology sessions (namely web-based interventions during the lockdown period), with 14 questions. The questions were designed based on a previous questionnaire developed for the purpose of studying the use of ICTs in the provision of therapy and counseling [14], as well as on the advantages and challenges identified in the literature about the use of these technologies on psychological counseling.

Socio-demographic data included gender, age, education level, number of years of professional experience, district where the respondent was practicing, area of specialization, and targeted population in the respondent's practice (including development stages and most frequent disorders). The remaining two sections of the questionnaire focused on information about the use of ICTs in the respondents' clinical practice. Questions included which tools and devices were used, clients' degree of satisfaction with the use of ICTs, advantages and difficulties identified by the professionals, impact on clients' adherence and on therapeutic results, among others (cf. Appendix A).

2.3. Procedure

This study was approved by the local ethics committee (Approval No.: CE0003A), and the questionnaire was made available at the web-based survey platform LimeSurvey [60]. OPP sent this anonymous online self-report questionnaire to its members via e-mail and published it on its webpage. The questionnaire was also sent to the authors' professional institutions via their mailing lists and was made available via professional social media, such as LinkedIn. This procedure ensured that all psychologists registered at OPP (a mandatory requirement for practicing psychology in Portugal) were invited to take part in this study. The e-mail containing the questionnaire included the study's description and aims, followed by an informed consent form. If the person agreed to participate, a link gave them access to the questionnaire. The data were collected during April and May 2020, precisely at the peak of the Covid-19 pandemic, and during the lockdown period. Data were exported from LimeSurvey [60] into IBM SPSS Statistics 25 Commuter License [61] for analysis.

2.4. Statistical Analysis

Descriptive statistics (e.g., frequency distributions) were conducted for the sample characteristics (e.g., age, gender, educational and professional background)) and for the data pertaining both to the period before and during the COVID-19 pandemic. Data before the COVID-19 pandemic included aspects such as the use of digital tools in professional practice, professional experience with this type of tool, and adherence of clients to therapeutic activities based on digital technologies. During the COVID-19 lockdown, analyses considered the following aspects: maintenance of psychological support services, percentage of clients who have maintained the use of psychological counseling or therapy, frequency and duration of the therapeutic sessions, therapeutic adherence, therapeutic relationship, feedback from the clients, and results of the at-distance sessions.

Additionally, a thematic analysis for the open-type questions was performed on the open-ended questions. Two independent raters (A.G. and I.P.C.) have proceeded to the classification of the categories in each answer. Conflicts were solved by a third rater (A.R.D.).

To explore the correlations between professional experience, age and the selected outcome variables, point-biserial and Spearman correlations were performed.

3. Results

3.1. ICTs in Psychological Counseling and Therapy before the COVID-19 Pandemic

3.1.1. Use of ICTs in Psychological Counseling and Therapy

Regarding the use of digital technologies for providing at-distance psychological counseling and therapy before the COVID-19 pandemic, most ($n = 63$; 58.3%) had rarely or never used digital tools in clinical practice before the COVID-19 pandemic (Table 2).

The reasons pointed out by Portuguese psychologists for never or rarely ($n = 63$) having used digital technologies in psychological counseling and therapy were they considered it very impersonal ($n = 28$; 44.4%), inefficient ($n = 18$; 28.6%), ineffective ($n = 10$; 15.9%), not safe enough ($n = 9$; 14.3%) or ethical ($n = 8$; 12.7%), and for their lack of knowledge on how to apply these technologies in psychological counseling and therapy ($n = 1$; 1.6%). Under "Other", participants additionally shared that they did not feel the need to use these means of providing counseling and therapy before, that these means were not part of their institutions' policies, and that they preferred in-presence interventions.

Table 2. Use of digital information and communication technologies in psychological counseling before and during the COVID-19 pandemic.

		Before the COVID-19	n (%)	During the COVID-19 Confinement Period	n (%)
ICTs use (n = 108)		never	37 (34.3%)	yes (sessions continued)	91 (84.3%)
		rarely	26 (24.1%)	no (sessions discontinued during this period)	15 (15.7%)
		sometimes	26 (24.1%)		
		frequently	14 (13.0%)		
		always	5 (4.6%)		
Tools (n = 71 before) (n = 91 after)		video conferences	50 (70.4%)	video conference	71 (78.0%)
		telephone calls	41 (57.7%)	telephone calls	48 (52.7%)
		e-mails	31 (43.7%)	social networks	35 (38.5%)
		social networks	23 (32.4%)	e-mails	33 (36.3%)
		audio conferences	14 (19.7%)	audio conference	16 (17.6%)
		online intervention platforms	6 (8.5%)	smartphones/tablet apps	7 (7.7%)
		smartphones/tablet apps	6 (8.5%)	online intervention platforms	3 (3.3%)
		online forums	4 (5.6%)	chats	3 (3.3%)
		chats	3 (4.2%)	online forums	1 (1.1%)
		short-message services	2 (1.8%)	virtual rooms	1 (1.1%)
		virtual rooms	1 (0.9%)		
Devices (n = 71 before) (n = 91 after)		computer	62 (87.3%)	computer	80 (87.9%)
		telephone/smartphone	58 (81.7%)	telephone/smartphone	66 (72.5%)
		tablets	9 (12.7%)	tablets	9 (9.9%)
Psychologists' experiences/results (n = 71 before) (n = 91 after)		positive	37 (52.1%)	more or less the same	65 (71.4%)
		neither negative nor positive	21 (29.6%)	better results	4 (4.4%)
		very positive	13 (18.3%)	worse results	22 (24.2%)
		very negative or negative	0 (0%)		
Clients' involvement/adherence (n = 71 before) (n = 91 after)		moderate	28 (39.4%)	more or less the same	52 (57.1%)
		high	18 (25.4%)	decreased	24 (26.4%)
		low involvement	12 (16.9%)	improved	10 (11.0%)
		very low	7 (9.9%)	significantly decreased	5 (5.5%)
		very high	6 (8.5%)	significantly improved	0 (0.0%)

Table 2. Cont.

	Before the COVID-19	n (%)	During the COVID-19 Confinement Period	n (%)
Advantages (n = 108)	geographic flexibility	74 (68.5%)	geographic flexibility	73 (80.2%)
	scheduling flexibility	55 (50.9%)	scheduling flexibility	57 (62.6%)
	reaching new groups	36 (33.3%)	reaching new groups	30 (33.0%)
	easier access to some target-groups	28 (25.9%)	cost-benefit relationship	24 (26.4%)
	cost-benefit relationship	27 (25.0%)	easier access to some target-groups	21 (23.1%)
	new business areas	10 (9.3%)	no advantages	11 (12.1%)
	other	12 (11.1%)	other	2 (2.2%)
Challenges (n = 108)	establishing/maintaining the therapeutic relationship	67 (62.0%)	non-verbal communication	58 (63.7%)
	non-verbal communication	66 (61.1%)	privacy	36 (39.6%)
	therapeutic adherence	52 (48.1%)	establishing/maintaining the therapeutic relationship	34 (37.4%)
	client engagement	50 (46.3%)	session interruptions	31 (34.1%)
	privacy	35 (32.4%)	therapeutic adherence	22 (24.2%)
	session interruption	29 (26.9%)	some problems/topics	19 (20.9%)
	ethical concerns	23 (21.3%)	ethical concerns	19 (20.9%)
	misunderstandings difficulties approach some problems/topics	22 (20.4%)	patient engagement in the sessions	18 (19.8%)
	sessions' frequency	20 (18.5%)	other	
	lack of security	20 (18.5%)		
	establishment of boundaries	19 (17.6%)		
	time management	19 (17.6%)		
	no challenges	12 (11.1%)		
	other	4 (3.7%)		

3.1.2. Tools and Technological Devices Used

Among the Portuguese psychologists who used ICTs to provide at-distance psychological counseling and therapy ($n = 71$), the most often used tools were video conferences ($n = 50$; 70.4%), telephone calls ($n = 41$; 57.7%), e-mails ($n = 31$; 43.7%), and social networks ($n = 23$; 32.4%). Other tools used were audio conferences ($n = 14$; 19.7%), online intervention platforms ($n = 6$; 8.5%), smartphones and tablet apps ($n = 6$; 8.5%), online forums ($n = 4$; 5.6%), chats ($n = 3$; 4.2%), short-message services ($n = 2$; 1.8%), and virtual rooms ($n = 1$; 0.9%). Concerning the technological devices used for providing at-distance psychological counseling and therapy, the most frequently used device was a computer ($n = 62$; 87.3%), followed by a telephone/smartphone ($n = 58$; 81.7%) and by tablets ($n = 9$; 12.7%) (Table 2).

3.1.3. Psychologists' Perceptions about Their Experiences and about Clients' Adherence

Among the psychologists that used digital technologies in psychological counseling and therapy previously to the COVID-19 pandemic ($n = 71$), none considered their experiences with these tools to be negative or very negative. Nevertheless, 21 (of these 71) psychologists (29.6%) considered their experiences to be neither negative nor positive. Most of the respondents considered their experience with digital technologies to be either positive ($n = 37$; 52.1%) or very positive ($n = 13$; 18.3%). Regarding the involvement of their patients in the therapeutic activities that were delivered through digital technologies, most of the psychologists rated it as moderate ($n = 28$; 39.4%), followed by high ($n = 18$; 25.4%) and low involvement ($n = 12$; 16.9%). Only six psychologists (8.5%) considered their patients' involvement in this type of activities very high, and seven psychologists (9.9%) rated their patients' involvement as very low (Table 2).

3.1.4. Advantages and Challenges of ICTs Use

With regard to the advantages that Portuguese psychologists considered might be experienced or already were experienced through the use of ICTs in psychological counseling and therapy, geographic flexibility was the most frequently selected advantage ($n = 74$; 68.5%), followed by scheduling flexibility ($n = 55$; 50.9%), the possibility of them reaching new groups of people in need of psychological counseling and therapy ($n = 36$; 33.3%), and by their easier access to some target-groups, such as persons with disability, refugees, among others ($n = 28$; 25.9%). They added the cost–benefit relationship ($n = 27$; 25.0%) and the possibility of obtaining new business areas ($n = 10$; 9.3%). Twelve (11.1%) of the respondents considered that they have never benefitted, or will never benefit, from any advantage through the use of ICTs in psychological counseling and therapy.

On the contrary, through the analysis of the challenges that psychologists had already faced or were afraid of facing when using new ICTs in psychological counseling and therapy, the most frequently referred challenge was the difficulty in establishing and/or maintaining the therapeutic relationship ($n = 67$; 62.0%), followed by the lack of non-verbal communication ($n = 66$; 61.1%), reduced therapeutic adherence ($n = 52$; 48.1%), reduced client engagement in the sessions ($n = 50$; 46.3%), and reduced privacy ($n = 35$; 32.4%). Other challenges referred by the psychologists were the interruption of the sessions ($n = 29$; 26.9%), ethical concerns ($n = 23$; 21.3%), possible misunderstandings ($n = 22$; 20.4%), difficulties in therapeutically approaching some problems/topics ($n = 20$; 18.5%), the substantial decrease or increase of the sessions' frequency ($n = 20$; 18.5%), lack of security ($n = 19$; 17.6%), establishment of boundaries ($n = 19$; 17.6%), and time management ($n = 12$; 11.1%). Under the category "Other", they also mentioned technical problems. Four (3.7%) respondents considered to never have faced or feared to face challenges in the future related to the use of digital technologies in their professional practice (Table 2).

3.2. ICTs in Psychological Counseling and Therapy during the COVID-19 Pandemic

3.2.1. Use of ICTs in Psychological Counseling and Therapy

During the COVID-19 pandemic, and specifically during the lockdown period, only 17 (15.7%) of the 108 psychologists discontinued the provision of psychological counseling and therapy to their clients (Table 2). These psychologists reported that the main reasons for interrupting their professional activities were the suspension of activities on the part of the institution where they worked, activity suspension on the part of their clients for various reasons (e.g., considering themselves to be info-excluded populations or presenting digital illiteracy, financial difficulties, or sensing that the clinical setting is lacking), psychologists' own personal unavailability during this period (e.g., due to new family responsibilities), and considering that digital means were inadequate for the target population (i.e., children) or clinical condition (e.g., attention deficits) that they were treating. All the other psychologists ($n = 91$, 84.3%) were able to continue the sessions with their cases due to the use of ICTs.

3.2.2. Readiness for the Use of ICTs

Among the 91 psychologists who continued to provide at-distance psychological services, 71 (84.3%) previously read guidelines and other documents that support their at-distance psychological practice. The documents that these psychologists consulted the most were materials made available by the OPP (e.g., written material, videos, and webinars), guidelines from APA and from the International Psychoanalytical Association (IPA), scientific papers, and manuals about online therapeutic interventions (including the Therapy2.0 project).

Regarding additional cautionary procedures implemented by the psychologists for at-distance interventions, respondents referred the careful definition of rules and ethical limits, namely in terms of privacy, confidentiality, security, schedules, forms of contact, session duration and frequency, as well as how to proceed when unforeseen situations occur (e.g., technical failures such as problems with the internet connection, technology problems such as problems with the tools/equipment used, or interruptions). Caution about the type of software and the type of technology used were mentioned, also related with non-exposure of personal life, as well as the conditions of the physical space and the psychologist's personal appearance/presentation, and personal well-being. Psychologists also referred several precautions and procedures associated with the actual therapeutic process, namely regarding verbal and non-verbal communication (e.g., minimizing the occurrence of overlaps, interruptions, and misunderstandings), greater session structuration and directivity (which involved greater previous preparation for some of them), avoidance of emotional themes that require in-person support, which distance prevents, parent follow-up in sessions with children, and assessment of clients' level of comfort with the new format.

3.2.3. Tools and Technological Devices

When focusing on the technological tools used to provide at-distance psychological counseling and therapy, video conference was the most frequently used ($n = 71$; 78.0%), followed by phone calls ($n = 48$; 52.7%), social networks ($n = 35$; 38.5%), e-mail ($n = 33$; 36.3%), audio conference ($n = 16$, 17.6%), smartphones and tablet apps ($n = 7$; 7.7%), online intervention platforms ($n = 3$; 3.3%), chats ($n = 3$; 3.3%), online forums ($n = 1$; 1.1%), and virtual rooms ($n = 1$; 1.1%). Computers were the most frequently used technological device to provide psychological services during the COVID-19 pandemic ($n = 80$; 87.9%), followed by telephones/smartphones ($n = 66$; 72.5%) and tablets ($n = 9$; 9.9%) (Table 2).

3.2.4. Impact of the COVID-19 on the Psychologists' Practice

Most of the respondents ($n = 53$; 58.2%) have continued to provide their services to most of their clients, i.e., twenty-seven (29.7%) of the psychologists continued to provide counseling and therapy to between 51% and 75% of their clients, and 26 psychologists (28.6%) to between 76% and 100% of their clients. However, for 23 psychologists (25.3%), the number of clients decreased to a range of between 0% and 25%, and for another 15 psychologists (16.5%) that number diminished to a range of between 26% and 50%. These psychologists referred, as main reasons for these reductions, low client adherence, lack of client's necessary privacy, confidentiality and non-interruption conditions at home, the fact that clients preferred in-presence contacts (considering such forms of intervention to be more effective than, or feeling uncomfortable with, the new format), had financial difficulties, had difficulties managing the new routines (including caring for the children at home), and lacked the technological means for at-distance sessions. In some cases, the client's condition was stable, and the therapeutic process had come to an end, or it was requiring no immediate sessions.

Considering the frequency of the counseling and therapy sessions among the clients who continued to use this service, a small majority of the psychologists ($n = 48$; 52.7%) referred that their clients have maintained the previous frequency, but 29 psychologists (31.9%) reported a decrease in the number of sessions, and six (6.6%) reported a significant decrease in that number. Despite that, seven psychologists (7.7%) reported an increase in the number of sessions during the COVID-19 pandemic, and one (1.1%) reported a significant increase. The same pattern was found for the duration of the counseling and therapy sessions, with 55 (60.4%) psychologists reporting a maintenance of the duration of each session, 20 (22.0%) reporting a decrease, and 4 (4.4%) reporting a significant decrease in the duration of the sessions. Nevertheless, 12 psychologists (13.2%) stated that the duration of the counseling and therapy sessions increased during the COVID-19 pandemic.

3.2.5. Psychologists' Perception about Their Experiences and about Clients' Adherence

Regarding the results of the current therapeutic sessions, when compared to former in-presence sessions, most psychologists ($n = 65$; 71.6%) considered the results to be more of less the same, four (4.4%) reported obtaining better results with at-distance sessions, and 22 (24.2%) considered that at-distance sessions have yielded worse results than in-presence sessions. Similarly, from the points of views that clients shared with their psychologists, at-distance and in-person sessions were more or less the same ($n = 71$; 78.0%). Six (6.6%) of the respondents reported receiving better feedback (i.e., the clients preferred the online sessions), and one (1.1%) received much better feedback. Even so, 13 (14.3%) psychologists received worse feedback from their clients about this type of intervention.

In what concerns therapeutic adherence to the ICT sessions, the majority of psychologists considered it to be more or less the same during the COVID-19 pandemic, comparing to the pre-COVID sessions ($n = 52$; 57.1%), and 10 psychologists (11.0%) reported an improvement. Nevertheless, other psychologists reported a decrease ($n = 24$; 26.4%) or a significant decrease ($n = 5$; 5.5%) in the therapeutic adherence of their clients (Table 2). The vast majority of respondents considered that the therapeutic relationship between the psychologists and their clients was maintained ($n = 77$; 84.6%), with only three (3.3%) psychologists reporting an improvement in those relationships. However, 11 (12.1%) psychologists considered that those relationships have worsened during this period.

3.2.6. Advantages and Challenges of the ICTs Use

Regarding the advantages that Portuguese psychologists viewed as associated with their current use of new ICTs in psychological counseling and therapy, geographic flexibility was the most frequently selected ($n = 73$; 80.2%), followed by scheduling flexibility ($n = 57$; 62.6%) and the possibility of reaching new groups of persons in need of psychological counseling and therapy ($n = 30$; 33.0%). Other advantages that they mentioned were the cost–benefit relationship ($n = 24$; 26.4%), the easier access of psychologists to some target groups, such as persons with disability and refugees, among others ($n = 21$; 23.1%), and the possibility of obtaining new business areas ($n = 11$; 12.1%). Under the category "Other", they further mentioned the possibility of providing secure interventions in the current COVID-19 pandemic context, which ensured the possibility of maintaining the interventions. Only two (2.2%) respondents considered that at-distance psychological counseling and therapy does not offer any advantages.

Through the analysis of the challenges that psychologists currently face when they provide at-distance psychological counseling and therapy sessions, the most frequently referred difficulty was lack of non-verbal communication ($n = 58$; 63.7%), followed by reduced privacy ($n = 36$; 39.6%), the difficulty in establishing and/or maintaining the therapeutic relationship ($n = 34$; 37.4%), session interruptions ($n = 31$; 34.1%), reduced therapeutic adherence ($n = 22$; 24.2%), difficulties in approaching some problems/topics therapeutically ($n = 19$; 20.9%), ethical concerns ($n = 19$; 20.9%), and a reduction in patient engagement in the sessions ($n = 18$; 19.8%) (Table 2). Other challenges that counsellors referred to (under the category "Other") were the establishment of boundaries ($n = 17$; 18.7%), the significant decrease or increase in session frequency ($n = 16$; 14.8%), the time management of the sessions ($n = 15$; 16.5%), possible misunderstandings ($n = 14$; 15.4%), and lack of security ($n = 10$; 11.0%). Under this category, they additionally mentioned technology problems (e.g., equipment adjustments) and technical failures (e.g., internet connection). Five respondents (5.5%) did not report any difficulty or challenge in providing at-distance psychological counseling and therapy.

In Table 2, the psychologists' practices are presented pre- and post-COVID-19 for easy comparison of the main results described previously.

3.3. Variables Associated with Psychologist' Attitudes and Practices

Significant point-biserial correlation coefficient were positive between the aspect "continue to provide psychological counseling to customers regularly" and years of professional experience, $r_{pb} = 0.296$, $p = 0.002$. Significant correlations were negative between "frequency of psychological counseling sessions" and both years of professional experience, $r_s = -0.341$, $p < 0.001$, and age, $r_s = -0.229$, $p = 0.017$. The aspect, "duration of psychological counseling sessions" also displayed a significant negative correlation with age, $r_s = -0.209$, $p = 0.030$. Thus, regarding respondents' professional experience, psychologists with more years of experience maintained their professional services during the COVID-19 pandemic more than professionals with less years of experience. Nevertheless, the frequency of the sessions decreased for the professionals who had more years of professional experience. Regarding age, older psychologists reported a decrease in session frequency and duration. No significant results were found in any of the other variables analyzed.

4. Discussion

This study aimed to explore psychologists' attitudes and practices related with the use of ICTs before and during the COVID-19 pandemic lockdown period, for identification of the main changes that have occurred in the provision of counseling and therapy. The impact of age and years of professional experience on the use of ICTs was also inspected.

In this study, psychologists' use of ICTs in their professional activity before the COVID-19 pandemic is in accordance with the literature, namely in terms of previous experience of their use, tools, devices, professionals' satisfaction with their use, advantages, and perceived challenges. These results reproduce those by Mendes-Santos (2020), in which only 29.6% of the inquired Portuguese psychologists admitted to having used digital technologies in their professional practice. The results of the present study also showed that most Portuguese psychologists had never or rarely used digital technologies as a means of delivering psychological counseling and therapy before the COVID-19 pandemic [6]. There is also a high degree of similarity between the tools most frequently used in our study and the tools used, the resources that psychologists most recommend to their clients (e.g., telephone calls, e-mails, video conferences, social networks, and apps) [6], and the most used devices (e.g., computers and smart phones) reported in other research (e.g., [14]). Additionally, according to previous studies, accessibility/geographic flexibility, convenience/(scheduling) flexibility, and cost-effectiveness/low cost are amongst the most recognized advantages of using ICTs (e.g., [6,55]). Regarding the disadvantages, the major challenges in this study, pertaining to ethical concerns and to the difficulty in establishing and/or maintaining the therapeutic relationship due to different reasons, were also identified in the literature [6,8,10,14,26,55–58].

The analysis of the reasons given for not using ICTs before the COVID-19 pandemic revealed that lack of knowledge and training about the correct use of ICTs was particularly relevant, which might explain professionals' concerns about efficiency, effectiveness, and ethical issues. These same factors were associated with more negative attitudes toward the use of technologies in a previous study [6]. Training thus seems to be a necessary step in order to increase the use of ICTs. However, before the COVID-19 pandemic, available training was scarce, perhaps also because the professionals themselves perceived the use of ICTs as unnecessary, as they indicated in this study.

The emergence of the COVID-19 pandemic brought about relevant changes in the use of ICTs. Barriers to their use by both professionals and clients have been reduced, as the availability of information about their use in various formats has increased. The percentage of psychologists who have adopted ICTs in their practice during the lockdown period was very high in this study, and the vast majority of respondents were able to maintain their professional activity due to the inclusion of these means in their practice. This shows an enormous capacity of adaptation and flexibility, both on the psychologists' and clients' parts. This phenomenon was observed not only in Portugal but in other countries too, such as the United States, where the provision of at-distance psychological services has been raised from 7.07% to 85.53% [62]. Additionally, other health services are also adopting the online modalities, namely in medicine [63,64], with the professionals reporting positive perceptions regarding the telehealth services. However, the implementation of ICTs in such a short period of time leads to questions about the conditions under which they were implemented.

Our results showed that more than half of the psychologists have read about the use of ICTs, and some had already used these tools, even if not exclusively, in their professional practice before, which is consistent with a previous study [6]. They additionally identified a number of materials that were informative of at-distance psychological practice. These materials also contained information on additional care that needs to be adopted in at-distance psychological monitoring sessions and that is different from the procedures that these professionals might have adopted in the use of digital technologies in the context of their social relationships.

Their concerns about web-based session pertained to a diversity of aspects considered to be critical in the e-Health literature (e.g., the clear definition of rules and ethical limits) that can be different from face-to-face services [13]. However, it is noteworthy that most professionals have not offered any input on any additional measures that they might have adopted (e.g., use end-to-end encrypted technology), nor has it been possible, within the scope of this work, to identify how psychologists were capable of responding effectively to the new requirements and specificities that they reported they have adopted. Despite the great availability of webinars and the training and specialty documents made available during this period (e.g., [13]) by accredited entities, often free of charge, little is known about how such information transfer to the professional contexts.

This study provides important information in that regard by confirming the pertinence and usefulness of such materials among the psychologists. In general, the tools and devices used before the lockdown period were the same that were used during the COVID-19 pandemic, although there was an increase in the use of several of them during the COVID-19 pandemic (e.g., video conferences, computers, and telephones/smartphones). The primary use of computers and smartphones in this study is in line with the findings from previous research, although psychologists in our study used mostly video conference and telephone calls, whereas e-mail was the most widely used tool in a previous study [14].

Psychologists who do use ICTs in their practice tended to report a positive or very positive experience regarding the use of these online technologies in counseling and therapy. Similarly, a study focused on the attitudes of psychotherapists towards online therapy during the COVID-19 pandemic have also found a positive attitude of the professionals with regard to this therapy modality [65]. Research has recognized several advantages associated with using ICTs in such contexts, and participants in our sample identified equivalent advantages [8–11,13,14,55]. Their reported advantages were the same before and during the lockdown period, although they added a new advantage during the lockdown period, i.e., the possibility to conduct secure interventions. The number of professionals who did not see any advantage in the use of ICTs after the pandemic decreased to a practically residual value. However, the implementation of these modalities was not without difficulties. Both before and during the pandemic, psychologists identified a set of challenges in the adoption of DICTS in professional practice. Some decreased during the pandemic, possibly due to the professionals' increased experience (e.g., establishing/maintaining the therapeutic adherence). However, others were particularly worsened during the period of mandatory lockdown (e.g., loss of privacy and risk of interruption).

Although generally positive, the results regarding psychologists' experiences/results and clients' adherence to therapeutic activities based on digital technologies were variable, as reported in previous studies (e.g., [36–54] and [6,55] respectively). It is important in the future to understand which ingredients explain this variability, both in relation to individual and to disorder aspects, and to work with the group of clients who have failed to adhere to the new format. From the limitations identified in this study, some clients might benefit from better advertisement of this type of services and of the scientific evidence of its effects, together with the possibility of receiving a reduction in the price of the services provided. Increasing clients' digital literacy will also contribute to their adherence to web-based interventions. This is already happening among the new generations, whose members are already known as digital natives [14,15], but it is still difficult when working with specific populations, such as the elderly and people that live in rural areas, or when performing some psychological acts, such as psychological assessment and rehabilitation practices [62]. Additionally, other challenges might be more difficult to overcome, such as the sense that an adequate therapeutic setting is lacking. This aspect has been particularly exacerbated by the situation of mandatory lockdown that has brought together all who live in the same physical space, namely risking privacy.

Regarding the correlations between the professionals' characteristics (i.e., age and years of professional experience) and the use of ICTs in professional practice, the results showed that were the professionals with more professional experience who presented greater maintenance of psychological support services, but less frequently. However, because it was also the professionals with more professional experience who presented greater maintenance of psychological support services, the decrease in the frequency of the sessions reported by them might have been an intentional procedure to help their own and their clients' adaptation to the new format.

The results failed to show a correlation between age and the use of ICTs, except for frequency and duration of the therapeutic sessions, which was significantly shorter for the oldest than for the youngest psychologists. The decrease in these aspects in the group of older psychologists from the pre- to the during-lockdown period could be possibly explained by the greater discomfort that these professionals experienced with the use of ICTs. The influence of the personal characteristics of the professionals in their attitude towards online psychological counseling was also reported in another study [65], with the psychotherapists who had previous experience with online psychotherapy, who thought that the patients they attend to had positive experiences in this modality, that adopted cognitive behavioral therapy in their practices (in comparison to psychodynamic therapists), and that lives in North America (in comparison to Europe) exhibiting a more positive attitude towards online psychotherapy.

This work has some limitations, namely the sample size and the use of a questionnaire that has not been previously validated to study the attitudes of psychologists toward ICTs (namely toward web-based interventions). However, the data collection took place during the period of absolutely unique and exceptional sanitary measures to prevent the pandemic dispersion of the coronavirus SARS-CoV-2, which causes COVID-19. To understand the impact of these circumstances on professionals' practice is of the utmost relevance, despite the fact that these same circumstances have limited the time to conduct the data collection and the availability of participants in the study. Still, the collaboration of the OPP in this scenario, advertising the study and making the questionnaire available to all its members, contributed to ensure national representation of the participants. The process of adapting an existing instrument, namely obtaining the respective authorizations, would require an extended period of time that would risk missing this window of opportunity. Instead, the questionnaire was adapted from an instrument that was previously used by the authors and that was tested in a pilot-study. Future studies could focus on exploring the reasons that seem to be interfering either negatively or positively with clients' adherence to, and satisfaction with, ICT sessions, so that personalized healthcare services can be provided and tailored to the specificities of each case.

5. Conclusions

It is widely known that the COVID-19 pandemic and associated restrictive measures of physical contact have significantly changed many professional activities. The current work has contributed to our understanding of that impact in the practice of psychology and psychotherapy, in close relation with the use of ICTs. Awareness of these changes can guide future professional practice by allowing the replication of the best practices and experiences shared by the psychologists during the period of maximum lockdown. It can also help to overcome the main difficulties and limitations experienced, for example, by guiding future training in this area, stimulating the creation of guidelines for ICT-based professional practice in different countries, and of measures to promote knowledge of and adherence to these guidelines that are becoming increasingly available.

Author Contributions: Conceptualization, A.R.D. and F.B.; methodology, A.R.D. and A.G.; formal analysis, A.G.; investigation, A.R.D. and A.G.; resources, A.R.D.; data curation, A.R.D.; writing—original draft preparation, A.R.D. and A.G.; writing—review and editing, I.P.C.; visualization, A.R.D. and A.G.; supervision, F.B.; project administration, A.R.D. and F.B.; funding acquisition, A.R.D. All authors have read and agreed to the published version of the manuscript.

Funding: This research was supported by Fundação para a Ciência e Tecnologia (FCT) through R&D Units funding (UIDB/05210/2020), and through a doctoral grant (SFRH/BD/138723/2018) awarded to Andreia Geraldo.

Acknowledgments: The authors wish to thank Ordem dos Psicólogos Portugueses (T.N: the Portuguese Psychologists Association) for advertising the present study to its members.

Conflicts of Interest: The authors declare no conflict of interest.

Appendix A

The Use of New Digital Information and Communication Technologies in Psychological Counseling during the COVID-19 Pandemic

This project is conducted by researchers at the Center for Rehabilitation Research of the School of Health, Polytechnic Institute of Porto, and at the Laboratory of Neuropsychophysiology of the Faculty of Psychology and Education Sciences, University of Porto. Its main goal is to study the use of digital technologies in psychological counseling during the COVID-19 pandemic (SARS-CoV-2) in Portugal. To attain this goal, a questionnaire has been developed, targeting psychologists who are effective members of the Portuguese Psychologists Association.

Although the completion of the questionnaire is anonymous, some socio-demographic and professional data will be requested, as well as answers to closed- and open-ended questions. These questions focus on the use of digital technologies in psychological counseling. Please read each question carefully. It is important that your answers are sincere.

If you accept to participate in this study, please click on "Next" to proceed to the informed consent.

Informed Consent

All data will be collected and processed in an anonymous and confidential way, so you will never be asked for your name, professional number, or other personal data that could identify you. The data will be used for research purposes and will never be analysed at the individual level. Your participation is completely voluntary, and your contribution is very important for us, to better understand the role of digital technologies in confinement situations like the one we are going through now. Although you can quit answering the survey at any time without any consequences, we really appreciate your collaboration.

If you want to clarify any question or if you need more information, please contact: Andreia Geraldo (andreiageraldo.psic@gmail.com).

We appreciate your cooperation.

Andreia Geraldo, researcher

Artemisa R Dores, responsible for the project

If you intend to participate in this study, select the option below to proceed to the survey.

I declare that I have read the information above, have become aware of the research aims, and agree to participate in this study.

Socio-demographic and professional data

1. Gender:

    Man
    Woman
    Other

2. Age (years):
3. Education:

    Graduation
    Master's
    PhD

4. Year of completion of the course [please consider the first degree that have allowed you to practice Psychology in Portugal (e.g., Pre-Bologna graduation; Post-Bologna Master's Degree)]:
5. Number of years of professional experience [please count from the moment you started the practice of Psychology services]:
6. Distrit(s) in which you practice Psychology:

    Aveiro
    Beja
    Braga
    Bragança
    Castelo Branco
    Coimbra
    Évora
    Faro
    Guarda
    Leiria
    Lisboa
    Portalegre
    Porto
    Santarém
    Setúbal
    Viana do Castelo
    Vila Real
    Viseu

7. Are you a specialist in Clinical and Health Psychology accredited by the Portuguese Psychologists Association?

   Yes
   No (Note: In case the answer above is Yes, the next question appears)
   Do you have an advanced specialty recognized by the Portuguese Psychologists Association?
   Yes
   No
   If yes, which one(s) of them? (you can choose several)
   Neuropsychology
   Psychogerontology
   Justice Psychology
   Sports Psychology
   Psychotherapy
   Sexology
   Other

8. Select the age group(s) of the population your work with most often (you can choose several):

   Children
   Adolescents
   Adults
   Elderly

9. Indicate which psychological disorders you assess and intervene most often (you can choose several):

   Neurodevelopment disorders
   Mood disorders
   Anxiety disorders
   Personality disorders
   Substance-related disorders and addictive behaviours
   Sleep disorders
   Neurocognitive disorders
   Other(s): (please specify)

   Use of Digital Technologies in Psychological Counselling We ask you to consider your entire professional career as a psychologist, prior to the confinement measures imposed by the declaration of the State of Emergency in Portugal, to answer the following questions.

10. Have you used digital tools to conduct at-distance psychological counselling?

    Never
    Rarely
    Sometimes
    Often
    Always

    (Note: If the previous answer was Never or Rarely, the next question appears. If the answer is no, after responding to 10.1, the participants go directly to question no. 15)

10.1. Which are the main reasons for you having never or rarely used this kind of tools?

    I don't know how to apply them in my work
    I don't consider them efficient (i.e., the adequate use of the necessary resources for the intervention/treatment)
    I don't consider them effective (i.e., the ability of a given program to produce benefit when applied under ideal conditions)
    I find them very impersonal
    I don't consider them safe enough
    I don't consider them ethical enough
    I find them very expensive
    Other(s): (please specify)

11. Which tool(s) have you already used in at-distance psychological counselling?

E-mail
Audio-conference (e.g., Skype, Facetime, Zoom)
Videoconference (e.g., Skype, Facetime, Zoom)
Online platforms
Online forum
Chat
Social networks (e.g., Facebook, Twitter, WhatsApp, Instagram, LinkedIn)
Smartphone and tablet apps
Virtual rooms (e.g., Second Life)
Telephone calls
Other(s): (please specify)

12. Which device(s) have you already used to maintain at-distance psychological counselling?

Computer
Tablet
Telephone/smartphone
Other(s): (please specify)

13. How do you rate your experience using this type of tools for conducting at-distance psychological counselling before the imposition of confinement measures by the declaration of the national state of emergency?

Very negative
Negative
Neither negative nor positive
Positive
Very positive

14. How do you rate your clients' involvement in therapeutic activities that use this kind of tools before the imposition of confinement measures by the declaration of the national state of emergency?

Very low
Low
Moderate
High
Very high

15. What are the advantages that you have already benefited from, or that you consider you could have benefited from, by using this type of tools in psychological counselling, before the imposition of confinement measures by the declaration of the national state of emergency? Geographic flexibility, both for professionals and clients (i.e., they can interact from any location)

    Time flexibility
    Cost-benefit ratio
    To be able to reach new groups of people in need of psychological counselling
    Easy access to some target groups (e.g., people with anxiety, people with disabilities, refugees)
    New business areas
    None
    Other(s): (please specify)

16. Which are the challenges that you have faced or feared to face with the use of this kind of tools in psychological counselling processes before the imposition of the confinement measures by the declaration of the national state of emergency?

    Reduced therapeutic adherence
    Difficulty in establishing or maintaining the therapeutic relationship
    Significant decrease or increase in the frequency of the sessions
    Temporal management of the sessions
    Setting boundaries
    Interruption of the sessions
    Less client involvement in and commitment to the session
    Lack of non-verbal communication
    (Possible) misunderstandings
    Difficulty in therapeutically approaching a problem/topic
    Lack of security
    Reduced privacy
    Ethical concerns
    None
    Other(s): (please specify)

    Considering the challenges imposed to all psychologists by the COVID-19 pandemic situation (SARS-CoV-2), we ask you to answer the following questions according to your current professional practices.

17. Have you continued to provide psychological counselling to your clients regularly?

    Yes
    No

    (Note: If the answer to the previous question is no, the next question appears, and the participant has finished his/her questionnaire)

    17.1. Which are the reasons that have led you to suspend your professional activity?

18. Have you consulted any supporting documents or guidelines for at-distance psychological counselling or psychological counselling in crisis and catastrophe situations?

    Yes
    No

    (Note: If the answer to the previous question is yes, the next question appears)

18.1. Please insert the name and/or link of the document(s) you consulted.

19. Currently, which percentage of your clients do you continue to monitor regularly when compared to the period before the declaration of the state of emergency in Portugal?

    Between 0% and 25%
    Between 26% and 50%
    Between 51% and 75%
    Between 76% and 100%

20. If there was a significant reduction in the percentage of clients that you regularly monitor, which are the main reasons that you identify for this to have happened?

21. The frequency of the psychological counselling sessions with each client that you continue to monitor

    Diminished a lot
    Diminished
    Remained the same
    Increased
    Increased a lot

22. The duration of the psychological counselling with each client that you continue to monitor

    Diminished a lot
    Diminished
    Remained the same
    Increased
    Increased a lot

23. Which tool(s) do you use to provide regular at-distance psychological counselling to your clients?

    E-mail
    Audio-conference (e.g., Skype, Facetime, Zoom)
    Video-conference (e.g., Skype, Facetime, Zoom)
    Online platforms
    Online forum
    Chat
    Social networks (e.g., Facebook, Twitter, WhatsApp, Instagram, LinkedIn)
    Smartphone and tablet apps
    Virtual rooms (e.g., Second Life)
    Telephone calls
    Other(s): (please specify)

24. Which device(s) have you already used to maintain at-distance psychological counselling?

    Computer
    Tablet
    Telephone/smartphone
    Other(s): (please specify)

25. How do you rate the therapeutic adherence of your clients currently, when compared to in-presence sessions?

    Much smaller

Smaller
More or less the same
Greater
Much greater

26. How do you rate the therapeutic relationship with your clients currently, when compared to in-presence sessions?

Much worse
Worse
More or less the same
Better
Much better

27. How do you rate the results of each therapeutic session currently, when compared to in-presence sessions?

Much worse
Worse
More or less the same
Better
Much better

28. How do you rate the feedback of your clients, when compared to in-presence sessions?

Much worse
Worse
More or less the same
Better
Much better

29. In case you consider that you have adopted some additional precautions in at-distance psychological counselling, when compared to those you adopt in relation to the use of digital technologies in the context of your social relationships, please indicate them.

30. What are the advantages that you identify in at-distance psychological counselling? Geographic flexibility, both for professionals and clients (i.e., they can interact from any location)

Time flexibility
Cost-benefit ratio
To be able to reach new groups of people in need of psychological counselling
Easy access to some target groups (e.g., people with anxiety, people with disabilities, refugees)
New business areas
Other(s): (please specify)

31. Which are the difficulties that you face in promoting at-distance psychological counselling sessions?

Reduced therapeutic adherence
Difficulty in establishing or maintaining the therapeutic relationship
Significant changes in the frequency of the sessions
Temporal management of the sessions
Setting boundaries
Interruption of the sessions

Less client involvement in and commitment to the session
Lack of non-verbal communication
(Possible) misunderstandings
Difficulty in therapeutically approaching a problem/topic
Lack of security
Reduced privacy
Ethical concerns
Other(s): (please specify)

32. What are the difficulties that are reported by your clients in relation to maintaining at-distance psychological counselling?

Thank you for your collaboration.

References

1. An Early View of the Economic Impact of the Pandemic in 5 Charts. International Monetary Fund IMFBlog. Available online: https://blogs.imf.org/2020/04/06/an-early-view-of-the-economic-impact-of-the-pandemic-in-5-charts/ (accessed on 2 May 2020).
2. How the Economy Will Look after the Coronavirus Pandemic: The Pandemic Will Change the Economic and Financial Order Forever. Available online: https://foreignpolicy.com/2020/04/15/how-the-economy-will-look-after-the-coronavirus-pandemic/ (accessed on 2 May 2020).
3. Mühleisen, M. The long and short of the digital revolution. *Financ Dev.* **2018**, *55*, 5–8.
4. Diário da República Eletrónico. (DRE; 18 March 2020). Decreto do Presidente da República n.º 14-A/2020. Available online: https://dre.pt/web/guest/home/-/dre/130399862/details/maximized (accessed on 12 June 2020).
5. WHO. *Fifty-Eighth World Health Assembly: Resolutions and Decisions Annex*; WHO: Geneva, Switzerland, 2005; pp. 108–109.
6. Mendes-Santos, C.; Weiderpass, E.; Santana, R.; Andersson, G. Portuguese Psychologists' attitudes towards internet interventions: An exploratory cross-sectional study. *JMIR Ment. Health* **2020**, *7*, e16817. [CrossRef] [PubMed]
7. Andersson, G. Internet-delivered psychological treatments. *Annu. Rev. Clin. Psychol.* **2016**, *12*, 157–179. [CrossRef] [PubMed]
8. Andersson, G.; Titov, N. Advantages and limitations of Internet-based interventions for common mental disorders. *World Psychiatry* **2014**, *13*, 4–11. [CrossRef] [PubMed]
9. Carlbring, P.; Andersson, G. Internet and psychological treatment. How well can they be combined? *Comput. Hum. Behav.* **2006**, *22*, 545–553. [CrossRef]
10. Schröder, J.; Berger, T.; Westermann, S.; Klein, J.P.; Moritz, S. Internet interventions for depression: New developments. *Dialogues Clin. Neurosci.* **2016**, *18*, 203–212.
11. Wolvers, M.; Bruggeman-Everts, F.Z.; Van der Lee, M.L.; Van de Schoot, R.; Vollenbroek-Hutten, M.M. Effectiveness, mediators, and effect predictors of internet interventions for chronic cancer-related fatigue: The design and an analysis plan of a 3-armed randomized controlled trial. *JMIR Res. Protoc.* **2015**, *4*, e77. [CrossRef]
12. OPP. Parecer 21/CEOPP/2015 da Ordem dos Psicólogos Portugueses (OPP). [Document 21/CEOPP/2015 of the OPP]. Available online: https://www.ordemdospsicologos.pt/ficheiros/documentos/p_21_intervena_aao_aa_disntaancia.pdf (accessed on 3 May 2020).
13. OPP. Linhas de Orientação para a Prática Profissional OPP: Prestação de Serviços de Psicologia Mediados por Tecnologias da Informação e da Comunicação (TIC). [Guidelines for Professional Practice OPP: Provision of Psychology Services Mediated by Information and Communication Technologies (ICT)]. Available online: https://www.ordemdospsicologos.pt/ficheiros/documentos/linhasorientacao_prestacaoservicos_opp_1.pdf (accessed on 15 May 2020).
14. Dores, A.R.; Barbosa, F.; Silva, R. Chegar mais perto dos que estão longe: Therapy 2.0 [Getting Closer to Those Who Are Far: Therapy 2.0]. *Rev. Estud. Investig. Psicol. Educ.* **2017**. [CrossRef]

15. Drda-Kühn, K.; Dores, A.R.; Schlenk, E. Online interventions: Counteracting the exclusion of young people in counselling and therapy. In *Digital Diversity Bildung und Lernen im Kontext Gesellschaftlicher Transformationen*; Angenent, A., Heidkamp, B., Kergel, D., Eds.; Springer: Wiesbaden, Germany, 2019; pp. 321–330. [CrossRef]
16. Andersson, G.; Cuijpers, P. Internet-based and other computerized psychological treatments for adult depression: A meta-analysis. *Cogn. Behav. Ther.* **2009**, *38*. [CrossRef]
17. Barak, A.; Hen, L.; Boniel-Nissim, M.; Shapira, N.A. A comprehensive review and a meta-analysis of the effectiveness of internet-based psychotherapeutic interventions. *J. Technol. Hum. Serv.* **2008**, *26*, 109–160. [CrossRef]
18. Dowling, M.; Rickwood, D. Online counseling and therapy formental health problems: A systematic review of individual synchronous interventions using chat. *J. Technol. Hum. Serv.* **2013**, *31*, 1–21. [CrossRef]
19. Olthuis, J.V.; Watt, M.C.; Bailey, K.; Hayden, J.A.; Stewart, S.H. Therapist-supported internet cognitive behavioural therapy for anxiety disorders in adults. *Cochrane Database Syst. Rev.* **2016**, *3*. [CrossRef] [PubMed]
20. Richards, D.; Richardson, T. Computer-based psychological treatments for depression: A systematic review and meta-analysis. *Clin. Psychol. Rev.* **2012**, *32*, 329–342. [CrossRef]
21. Richards, D.; Viganó, N. Online counseling: A narrative and critical review of the. Literature. *J. Clin. Psychol.* **2013**, *69*, 994–1011. [CrossRef] [PubMed]
22. Topooco, N.; Riper, H.; Araya, R.; Berking, M.; Brunn, M.; Chevreul, K.; Kleiboer, A. Attitudes towards digital treatment for depression: A European stakeholder survey. *Internet Interven.* **2017**, *8*, 1–9. [CrossRef] [PubMed]
23. Schuster, R.; Pokorny, R.; Berger, T.; Topooco, N.; Laireiter, A.R. The advantages and disadvantages of online and blended therapy: Survey study amongst licensed psychotherapists in Austria. *J. Med. Internet Res.* **2018**, *20*, e11007. [CrossRef]
24. Mora, L.; Jeffrey, N.; Chaplin, W. Psychologist treatment recommendations for Internetbased therapeutic interventions. *Comput. Hum. Behav.* **2008**, *24*, 3052–3062. [CrossRef]
25. Wangberg, S.C.; Gammon, D.; Spitznogle, K. In the eyes of the beholder: Exploring psychologists' attitudes towards and use of e-therapy in Norway. *Cyberpsychol. Behav.* **2007**, *10*, 418–423. [CrossRef] [PubMed]
26. Perle, J.G.; Langsam, L.C.; Randel, A.; Lutchman, S.; Levine, A.B.; Odland, A.P.; Marker, C.D. Attitudes toward psychological telehealth: Current and future clinical psychologists' opinions of internet-based interventions. *J. Clin. Psychol.* **2013**, *69*, 100–113. [CrossRef]
27. Vigerland, S.; Ljótsson, B.; Gustafsson, F.B.; Hagert, S.; Thulin, U.; Andersson, G.; Serlachius, E. Attitudes towards the use of computerized cognitive behavior therapy (cCBT) with children and adolescents: A survey among Swedish mental health professionals. *Internet Interv.* **2014**, *1*, 111–117. [CrossRef]
28. Schröder, J.; Berger, T.; Meyer, B.; Lutz, W.; Hautzinger, M.; Späth, C.; Moritz, S. Attitudes towards internet interventions among psychotherapists and individuals with mild to moderate depression symptoms. *Cognit. Ther. Res.* **2017**, *41*, 745–756. [CrossRef]
29. Lamela, D.; Neves, F.R.P. O Efeito da Prática Profissional Baseada na Evidência Nas Atitudes dos Psicólogos Face à Intervenção Psicológica Eletrónica. Master's Thesis, Universidade Lusófona, Porto, Portugal, 2017.
30. Simms, D.; Gibson, K.; O'Donnell, S. To Use or Not to Use: Clinicians' Perceptions of Telemental Health. *Can. Psychol. Psychol. Can.* **2011**, *52*, 41–51. [CrossRef]
31. Bruno, R.; Abbott, J.-A.M. Australian health professionals' attitudes toward and frequency of use of internet supported psychological interventions. *Int. J. Ment. Health* **2015**, *44*, 107–123. [CrossRef]
32. Hadjiconstantinou, M.; Byrne, J.; Bodicoat, D.H.; Robertson, N.; Eborall, H.; Khunti, K.; Davies, M.J. Do web-based interventions improve well-being in type 2 diabetes? A systematic review and meta-analysis. *J. Med. Internet Res.* **2016**, *18*, e270. [CrossRef]
33. Agboola, S.O.; Ju, W.; Elfiky, A.; Kvedar, J.C.; Jethwani, K. The Effect of technology-based interventions on pain, depression, and quality of life in patients with cancer: A systematic review of randomized controlled trials. *J. Med. Internet Res.* **2015**, *17*, e65. [CrossRef] [PubMed]
34. Kuijpers, W.; Groen, W.G.; Aaronson, N.K.; van Harten, W.H. A systematic review of web-based interventions for patient empowerment and physical activity in chronic diseases: Relevance for cancer survivors. *J. Med. Internet Res.* **2013**, *15*, e37. [CrossRef] [PubMed]

35. Loucas, C.E.; Fairburn, C.G.; Whittington, C.; Pennant, M.E.; Stockton, S.; Kendall, T. E-therapy in the treatment and prevention of eating disorders: A systematic review and meta-analysis. *Behav. Res. Ther.* **2014**, *63*, 122–131. [CrossRef] [PubMed]
36. Andersson, G.; Paxling, B.; Roch-Norlund, P.; Östman, G.; Norgren, A.; Almlöv, J.; Carlbring, P. Internet-based psychodynamic versus cognitive behavioral guided self-help for generalized anxiety disorder: A randomized controlled trial. *Psychother. Psychosom.* **2012**, *81*, 344–355. [CrossRef]
37. Hedman, E.; Ljótsson, B.; Rück, C.; Bergström, J.; Andersson, G.; Kaldo, V.; El Alaoui, S. Effectiveness of Internet-based cognitive behaviour therapy for panic disorder in routine psychiatric care. *Acta Psychiatr. Scand.* **2013**, *128*, 457–467. [CrossRef]
38. Mansson, K.N.T.; Frick, A.; Boraxbekk, C.J.; Marquand, A.F.; Williams, S.C.R.; Carlbring, P.; Furmark, T. Predicting long-term outcome of internet-delivered cognitive behavior therapy for social anxiety disorder using fMRI and support vector machine learning. *Transl. Psychiatry* **2015**, *5*, e530. [CrossRef]
39. Carlbring, P.; Gunnarsdóttir, M.; Hedensjö, L.; Andersson, G.; Ekselius, L.; Furmark, T. Treatment of social phobia: Randomised trial of internet-delivered cognitive-behavioural therapy with telephone support. *Br. J. Psychiatry* **2007**, *190*, 120–138. [CrossRef] [PubMed]
40. Paxling, B.; Almlov, J.; Dahlin, M.; Carlbring, P.; Breitholtz, E.; Eriksson, T.; Andersson, G. Guided internet-delivered cognitive behavior therapy for generalized anxiety disorder: A randomized controlled trial. *Cogn. Behav. Ther.* **2011**, *40*, 159–173. [CrossRef] [PubMed]
41. Carlbring, P.; Maurin, L.; Törngren, C.; Linna, E.; Eriksson, T.; Sparthan, E.; Andersson, G. Individually-tailored, Internet-based treatment for anxiety disorders: A randomized controlled trial. *Behav. Res. Ther.* **2011**, *49*, 18–24. [CrossRef] [PubMed]
42. Spence, J.; Titov, N.; Dear, B.F.; Johnston, L.; Solley, K.; Lorian, C.; Schwenke, G. Randomized controlled trial of Internet-delivered cognitive behavioral therapy for posttraumatic stress disorder. *Depress. Anxiety* **2011**, *28*, 541–550. [CrossRef]
43. Andersson, G.; Hesser, H.; Veilord, A.; Svedling, L.; Andersson, F.; Sleman, O.; Lamminen, M. Randomised controlled non-inferiority trial with 3-year follow-up of internet-delivered versus face-to-face group cognitive behavioural therapy for depression. *J. Affect. Disord.* **2013**, *151*, 986–994. [CrossRef]
44. Berger, T.; Hämmerli, K.; Gubser, N.; Andersson, G.; Caspar, F. Internet-based treatment of depression: A randomized controlled trial comparing guided with unguided self-help. *Cogn. Behav. Ther.* **2011**, *40*, 251–266. [CrossRef]
45. Carlbring, P.; Hägglund, M.; Luthström, A.; Dahlin, M.; Kadowaki, Å.; Vernmark, K.; Andersson, G. Internet-based behavioral activation and acceptance-based treatment for depression: A randomized controlled trial. *J. Affect. Disord.* **2013**, *148*, 331–337. [CrossRef]
46. Ly, K.H.; Carlbring, P.; Andersson, G. Behavioral activation-based guided self-help treatment administered through a smartphone application: Study protocol for a randomized controlled trial. *Trials* **2012**, *13*. [CrossRef]
47. Mohr, D.C.; Duffecy, J.; Ho, J.; Kwasny, M.; Cai, X., Burns, M.N.; Begale, M. A randomized controlled trial evaluating a manualized TeleCoaching protocol for improving adherence to a web-based intervention for the treatment of depression. *PLoS ONE* **2013**, *8*, e70086. [CrossRef]
48. O'Mahen, H.A.; Richards, D.A.; Woodford, J.; Wilkinson, E.; McGinley, J.; Taylor, R.S.; Warren, F.C. Netmums: A phase II randomized controlled trial of a guided Internet behavioural activation treatment for postpartum depression. *Psychol. Med.* **2014**, *44*, 1675–1689. [CrossRef]
49. Perini, S.; Titov, N.; Andrews, G. Clinician-assisted Internet-based treatment is effective for depression: Randomized controlled trial. *Aust. N. Z. J. Psychiatry* **2009**, *43*, 571–578. [CrossRef] [PubMed]
50. Ruwaard, J.; Schrieken, B.; Schrijver, M.; Broeksteeg, J.; Dekker, J.; Vermeulen, H.; Lange, A. Standardized web-based cognitive behavioural therapy of mild to moderate depression: A randomized controlled trial with a long-term follow-up. *Cogn. Behav. Ther.* **2009**, *38*, 206–221. [CrossRef] [PubMed]
51. Vernmark, K.; Lenndin, J.; Bjarehed, J.; Carlsson, M.; Karlsson, J.; Öberg, J.; Andersson, G. Internet administered guided self-help versus individualized e-mail therapy: A randomized trial of two versions of CBT for major depression. *Behav. Res. Ther.* **2010**, *48*, 368–376. [CrossRef] [PubMed]
52. Wagner, B.; Horn, A.B.; Maercker, A. Internet-based versus face-to-face cognitive-behavioral intervention for depression: A randomized controlled non-inferiority trial. *J. Affect. Disord.* **2014**, *152–154*, 113–121. [CrossRef]

53. Ly, K.H.; Asplund, K.; Andersson, G. Stress management for middle managers via an acceptance and com¬mitment-based smartphone application: A randomized controlled trial. *Internet Interv.* **2014**, *1*, 95–101. [CrossRef]
54. Zetterqvist, K.; Maanmies, J.; Strom, L.; Andersson, G. Randomized controlled trial of internet-based stress management. *Cogn. Behav. Ther.* **2003**, *32*, 151–160. [CrossRef]
55. Feijt, M.A.; de Kort, Y.A.; Bongers, I.M.; IJsselsteijn, W.A. Perceived Drivers and Barriers to the Adoption of eMental Health by Psychologists: The Construction of the Levels of Adoption of eMental Health Model. *J. Med. Internet Res.* **2018**, *20*, e153. [CrossRef]
56. Glueckauf, R.L.; Maheu, M.M.; Drude, K.P.; Wells, B.A.; Wang, Y.; Gustafson, D.J.; Nelson, E.L. Survey of psychologists' telebehavioral health practices: Technology use, ethical issues, and training needs. *Prof. Psychol. Res. Pract.* **2018**, *49*, 205–219. [CrossRef]
57. Evans, D.J. South African psychologists' use of the Internet in their practices. *S. Afr. J. Psychol.* **2014**, *44*, 162–169. [CrossRef]
58. Cipolletta, S.; Mocellin, D. Online counseling: An exploratory survey of Italian psychologists' attitudes towards new ways of interaction. *Psychother. Res.* **2018**, *28*, 909–924. [CrossRef]
59. OPP. Os Números da Associação. Censo dos Membros Efectivos da OPP [Association Numbers. Census of Effective Members of the OPP]. Available online: https://issuu.com/ordemdospsicologos/docs/dossier-censo-web (accessed on 14 June 2020).
60. LimesurveyGmbH. *LimeSurvey: An Open Source Survey Tool*; LimeSurvey GmbH: Hamburg, Germany, 2019.
61. IBMCorp. *IBM SPSS Statistics for Windows 25*; IBM Corp: Armonk, NY, USA, 2017.
62. Pierce, B.S.; Perrin, P.B.; Tyler, C.M.; McKee, G.B.; Watson, J.D. The COVID-19 telepsychology revolution: A national study of pandemic-based changes in U.S. mental health delivery. *Am. Psychol.* **2020**. [CrossRef] [PubMed]
63. Helou, S.; Helou, E.E.; Abou-Khalil, V.; Wakim, J.; Helou, J.E.; Daher, A.; Hachem, C.E. The effect of the COVID-19 pandemic on physicians' use and perception of telehealth: The case of Lebanon. *Int. J. Environ. Res. Public Health* **2020**, *17*, 4866. [CrossRef] [PubMed]
64. Uscher-Pines, L.; Sousa, J.L.; Raja, P.; Mehrotra, A.; Barnett, M.L.; Huskamp, H.A. Suddenly becoming a "virtual doctor": Experiences of psychiatrists transitioning to telemedicine during the COVID-19 pandemic. *Psychiat. Serv.* **2020**. [CrossRef]
65. Békés, V.; Doorn, K.A. Psychotherapists' attitudes toward online therapy during the COVID-19 pandemic. *J. Psychother. Integr.* **2020**, *30*, 238–247. [CrossRef]

Publisher's Note: MDPI stays neutral with regard to jurisdictional claims in published maps and institutional affiliations.

© 2020 by the authors. Licensee MDPI, Basel, Switzerland. This article is an open access article distributed under the terms and conditions of the Creative Commons Attribution (CC BY) license (http://creativecommons.org/licenses/by/4.0/).

MDPI
St. Alban-Anlage 66
4052 Basel
Switzerland
Tel. +41 61 683 77 34
Fax +41 61 302 89 18
www.mdpi.com

International Journal of Environmental Research and Public Health Editorial Office
E-mail: ijerph@mdpi.com
www.mdpi.com/journal/ijerph